Adrenal Cortical Neoplasia

Editor

ALICE C. LEVINE

ENDOCRINOLOGY AND METABOLISM CLINICS OF NORTH AMERICA

www.endo.theclinics.com

Consulting Editor
DEREK LEROITH

June 2015 • Volume 44 • Number 2

ELSEVIER

1600 John F. Kennedy Boulevard • Suite 1800 • Philadelphia, Pennsylvania, 19103-2899

http://www.theclinics.com

ENDOCRINOLOGY AND METABOLISM CLINICS OF NORTH AMERICA Volume 44, Number 2
June 2015 ISSN 0889-8529, ISBN 13: 978-0-323-38884-9

Editor: Jessica McCool
Developmental Editor: Meredith Clinton

Endocrinology and Metabolism Clinics of North America (ISSN 0889-8529) is published quarterly by Elsevier Inc., 360 Park Avenue South, New York, NY 10010-1710. Months of issue are March, June, September, and December. Periodicals postage paid at New York, NY and additional mailing offices. Subscription prices are USD 330.00 per year for US individuals, USD 581.00 per year for US institutions, USD 165.00 per year for US students and residents, USD 415.00 per year for Canadian individuals, USD 718.00 per year for Canadian institutions, USD 480.00 per year for international individuals, USD 718.00 per year for international institutions, and USD 245.00 per year for international and Canadian and foreign students/residents. To receive student/resident rate, orders must be accompanied by name of affiliated institution, date of term, and the signature of program/residency coordinator on institution letterhead. Orders will be billed at individual rate until proof of status is received. Foreign air speed delivery is included in all *Clinics* subscription prices. All prices are subject to change without notice. **POSTMASTER:** Send address changes to *Endocrinology and Metabolism Clinics of North America*, Elsevier Health Sciences Division, Subscription Customer Service, 3251 Riverport Lane, Maryland Heights, MO 63043. **Customer Service: Telephone: 1-800-654-2452** (U.S. and Canada); **1-314-447-8871** (outside U.S. and Canada). **Fax: 1-314-447-8029. E-mail: journalscustomerservice-usa@elsevier.com (for print support); journalsonlinesupport-usa@elsevier.com (for online support).**

Reprints. For copies of 100 or more, of articles in this publication, please contact the Commercial Rights Department, Elsevier Inc., 360 Park Avenue South, New York, NY 10010-1710; phone: +1-212-633-3874; fax: +1-212-633-3820; E-mail: reprints@elsevier.com.

Endocrinology and Metabolism Clinics of North America is covered in *MEDLINE/PubMed (Index Medicus), EMBASE/Excerpta Medica, Current Contents/Clinical Medicine, Current Contents/Life Sciences, Science Citation Index, ISI/BIOMED, BIOSIS,* and *Chemical Abstracts.*

Contributors

CONSULTING EDITOR

DEREK LEROITH, MD, PhD
Director of Research, Division of Endocrinology, Diabetes and Bone Diseases, Icahn School of Medicine at Mount Sinai, New York, New York

EDITOR

ALICE C. LEVINE, MD
Professor of Medicine; Co-Director of the Adrenal Center, The Hilda and J. Lester Gabrilove Division of Endocrinology, Diabetes and Bone Diseases, Department of Internal Medicine, Icahn School of Medicine at Mount Sinai, New York, New York

AUTHORS

ABIR AL GHUZLAN, MD
Department of Pathology, Gustave Roussy, Université Paris Sud, Paris, France

YOICHI ARAI, MD, PhD
Professor, Department of Urology, Tohoku University Graduate School of Medicine, Sendai, Japan

RICHARD J. AUCHUS, MD, PhD
Professor, Division of Metabolism, Endocrinology, and Diabetes, Department of Internal Medicine; Department of Pharmacology, University of Michigan, Ann Arbor, Michigan

ERIC BAUDIN, MD, PhD
Department of Endocrine Oncology and Nuclear Medicine, Gustave Roussy; Faculté de Médecine, INSERM UMR 1185, Université Paris Sud, Paris, France

AMANDINE BERDELOU, MD
Department of Endocrine Oncology and Nuclear Medicine, Gustave Roussy, Université Paris Sud; Faculté de Médecine, Paris, France

JÉRÔME BERTHERAT, MD, PhD
Cochin Institut, INSERM U1016; Cochin Institut, CNRS UMR8104; Paris Descartes University; Endocrinology Department, Center for Rare Adrenal Diseases, Hôpital Cochin, Assistance Publique Hôpitaux de Paris, Paris, France

ISABELLE BORGET, PharmD
Department of Statistics, Gustave Roussy, Université Paris Sud, Paris, France

CAROLINE CARAMELLA, MD
Department of Imaging, Gustave Roussy, Université Paris Sud, Paris, France

DESIRÉE DEANDREIS, MD
Department of Endocrine Oncology and Nuclear Medicine, Gustave Roussy, Université Paris Sud, Paris, France

FREDERIC DESCHAMPS, MD
Department of Interventional Radiology, Gustave Roussy, Université Paris Sud, Paris, France

ERIC DEUTSCH, MD, PhD
Department of Radiotherapy, Gustave Roussy, Université Paris Sud, Paris, France

FREDERIC DUMONT, MD
Department of Surgery, Gustave Roussy, Université Paris Sud, Paris, France

DEIRDRE COCKS ESCHLER, MD
Assistant Professor of Medicine, Endocrinology Division, Department of Medicine, Stony Brook University School of Medicine, Stony Brook, New York

STÉPHANIE ESPIARD, MD
Cochin Institut, INSERM U1016; Cochin Institut CNRS UMR8104; Paris Descartes University, Paris, France

SAULO J. FELIZOLA, MD, PhD
Department of Pathology, Tohoku University Graduate School of Medicine, Sendai, Japan

GUSTAVO G. FERNANDEZ RANVIER, MD
Division of Metabolic, Endocrine and Minimally Invasive Surgery, Department of Surgery, Mount Sinai Hospital, Icahn School of Medicine at Mount Sinai, New York, New York

SARA GALAC, DVM, PhD
Assistant Professor, Department of Clinical Sciences of Companion Animals, Faculty of Veterinary Medicine, Utrecht University, Utrecht, The Netherlands

SANDI-JO GALATI, MD
Endocrine and Diabetes Specialists of CT, Trumbull, Connecticut

GILLIAN M. GODDARD, MD
The Hilda and J. Lester Gabrilove Division of Endocrinology, Diabetes and Bone Diseases, Department of Internal Medicine, Icahn School of Medicine at Mount Sinai; Attending Physician, Lennox Hill Hospital, North Shore-LIJ Health System, New York, New York

GARY D. HAMMER, MD, PhD
Director, Endocrine Oncology Program; Director, Center for Organogenesis, Millie Schembechler Professor of Adrenal Cancer, University of Michigan, Ann Arbor, Michigan

AMIR H. HAMRAHIAN, MD, FACE
Chief, Endocrinology; Professor of Medicine, Cleveland Clinic Abu Dhabi, Abu Dhabi, United Arab Emirates

SEGOLENE HESCOT, MD
Department of Endocrine Oncology and Nuclear Medicine, Gustave Roussy, Université Paris Sud; Faculté de Médecine, INSERM UMR 1185, Université Paris Sud, Paris, France

WILLIAM B. INABNET III, MD, FACS
Eugene W Friedman Professor of Surgery, Chairman, Department of Surgery, Mount Sinai
Beth Israel, Icahn School of Medicine at Mount Sinai, New York, New York

ADRIANA G. IOACHIMESCU, MD, PhD, FACE
Associate Professor of Medicine and Neurosurgery, Emory University School of Medicine,
Atlanta, Georgia

KAZUE ISE
Department of Pathology, Tohoku University Graduate School of Medicine, Sendai,
Japan

NINA KOGEKAR, BA
Department of Medicine, Icahn School of Medicine at Mount Sinai, New York, New York

SOPHIE LEBOULLEUX, MD, PhD
Endocrine Oncology and Nuclear Medicine, Gustave Roussy, Université Paris Sud, Paris,
France

ANTONIO M. LERARIO, MD, PhD
Visiting Scholar, Internal Medicine, Medical School, University of Michigan, Ann Arbor,
Michigan

ALICE C. LEVINE, MD
Professor of Medicine; Co-Director of the Adrenal Center, The Hilda and J. Lester
Gabrilove Division of Endocrinology, Diabetes and Bone Diseases, Department of
Internal Medicine, Icahn School of Medicine at Mount Sinai, New York, New York

ROSSELLA LIBE, MD
Coordinator of the French Network of Adrenal Tumors (Inca-COMETE), Cochin, Paris
University; Gustave Roussy, Université Paris Sud, Villejuif, France

MARC LOMBES, MD, PhD
Faculté de Médecine, INSERM UMR 1185, Université Paris Sud, Paris, France

RYO MORIMOTO, MD, PhD
Division of Nephrology, Endocrinology, and Vascular Medicine, Department of Medicine,
Tohoku University Graduate School of Medicine, Sendai, Japan

YASUHIRO NAKAMURA, MD, PhD
Department of Pathology, Tohoku University Graduate School of Medicine, Sendai,
Japan

ANGELO PACI, PharmD
Department of Pharmacology, Gustave Roussy, Université Paris Sud, Paris,
France

RACHEL PESSAH-POLLACK, MD, FACE
Endocrinology Division, Department of Medicine, Icahn School of Medicine at Mount
Sinai, New York, New York; Department of Endocrinology, ProHealth Care Associates,
Lake Success, New York

WILLIAM RAINEY, PhD
Departments of Molecular & Integrative Physiology and Internal Medicine, University of
Michigan, Ann Arbor, Michigan

AARTI RAVIKUMAR, MD
The Hilda and J. Lester Gabrilove Division of Endocrinology, Diabetes and Bone Diseases, Department of Internal Medicine, Icahn School of Medicine at Mount Sinai, New York, New York

ERICK M. REMER, MD, FACR
Professor of Radiology, Imaging Institute, Cleveland Clinic, Cleveland, Ohio

HIRONOBU SASANO, MD, PhD
Professor, Department of Pathology, Tohoku University Graduate School of Medicine, Sendai, Japan

FUMITOSHI SATOH, MD, PhD
Division of Nephrology, Endocrinology, and Vascular Medicine, Department of Medicine, Tohoku University Graduate School of Medicine, Sendai, Japan

MARTIN SCHLUMBERGER, MD, PhD
Endocrine Oncology and Nuclear Medicine, Gustave Roussy, Université Paris Sud, Paris, France

JEAN-YVES SCOAZEC, MD, PhD
Department of Pathology, Gustave Roussy, Université Paris Sud, Paris, France

ADINA F. TURCU, MD
Clinical Instructor, Division of Metabolism, Endocrinology, and Diabetes, Department of Internal Medicine, University of Michigan, Ann Arbor, Michigan

DAVID B. WILSON, MD, PhD
Associate Professor, Departments of Pediatrics and Developmental Biology, St. Louis Children's Hospital, Washington University, St Louis, Missouri

YEWEI XING, PhD
Research Fellow, Internal Medicine, Medical School, University of Michigan, Ann Arbor, Michigan

YUTO YAMAZAKI, MD
Department of Pathology, Tohoku University Graduate School of Medicine, Sendai, Japan

JACQUES YOUNG, MD, PhD
Faculté de Médecine, INSERM UMR 1185, Université Paris Sud; Department of Endocrinology, Faculté de Médecine, Université Paris Sud, Paris, France

Contents

The human adult adrenal cortex is composed of the zona glomerulosa (zG), zona fasciculata (zF), and zona reticularis (zR), which are responsible for production of mineralocorticoids, glucocorticoids, and adrenal androgens, respectively. The final completion of cortical zonation in humans does not occur until puberty with the establishment of the zR and its production of adrenal androgens; a process called adrenarche. The maintenance of the adrenal cortex involves the centripetal displacement and differentiation of peripheral Sonic hedgehog–positive progenitors cells into zG cells that later transition to zF cells and subsequently zR cells.

Adrenal steroidogenesis is a dynamic process, reliant on de novo synthesis from cholesterol, under the stimulation of ACTH and other regulators. The syntheses of mineralocorticoids, glucocorticoids, and adrenal androgens occur in separate adrenal cortical zones, each expressing specific enzymes. Congenital adrenal hyperplasia (CAH) encompasses a group of autosomal-recessive enzymatic defects in cortisol biosynthesis. 21-Hydroxylase (21OHD) deficiency accounts for more than 90% of CAH cases and, when milder or nonclassic forms are included, 21OHD is one of the most common genetic diseases. This review discusses in detail the epidemiology, genetics, diagnostic, clinical aspects and management of 21OHD.

This comparative review highlights animal models of adrenocortical neoplasia useful either for mechanistic studies or translational research. Three model species—mouse, ferret, and dog—are detailed. The relevance of each of these models to spontaneous and inherited adrenocortical tumors in humans is discussed.

Advances in genomics accelerated greatly progress in the study of the genetics adrenocortical tumors. Bilateral nodular hyperplasias causing

uncommon in pregnancy; a high degree of clinical suspicion must exist. Physiologic changes to the hypothalamus-pituitary-adrenal axis in a normal pregnancy result in increased cortisol, renin, and aldosterone levels, making the diagnosis of CS and PA in pregnancy challenging. However, catecholamines are not altered in pregnancy and allow a laboratory diagnosis of pheochromocytoma that is similar to that of the nonpregnant state. Although adrenal tumors in pregnancy result in significant maternal and fetal morbidity, and sometimes mortality, early diagnosis and appropriate treatment often improve outcomes.

Adrenocortical carcinoma (ACC) is a malignant neoplasm often associated with an aggressive biological behavior. The histologic differentiation between ACC and adrenocortical adenoma (ACA) is largely determined by employing the Weiss criteria, although this classification may not apply to all the cases. Additionally, various genomic features of ACC could be an auxiliary mode to establish the diagnosis of ACC. Most ACC cases are hormonally functional, and immunohistochemical analysis of steroidogenic enzymes has provided pivotal information as to the analysis of intratumoral production of steroids. This article summarizes the current status of the histopathological diagnosis, molecular pathogenesis, and hormonal features of ACC.

Recent developments in the treatment of adrenocortical carcinoma (ACC) include diagnostic and prognostic risk stratification algorithms, increasing evidence of the impact of historical therapies on overall survival, and emerging targets from integrated epigenomic and genomic analyses. Advances include proper clinical and molecular characterization of all patients with ACC, standardization of proliferative index analyses, referral of these patients to large cancer referral centers at the time of first surgery, and development of new trials in patients with well-characterized ACC. Networking and progress in the molecular characterization of ACC constitute the basis for significant future therapeutic breakthroughs.

Adrenocortical carcinoma (ACC) is rare but one of the most malignant endocrine tumors. This article reviews and summarizes the current knowledge about the treatment of ACC. The epidemiology and molecular events involved in the pathogenesis of ACC are briefly outlined. The different diagnostic tools to distinguish benign from malignant adrenocortical tumors, including biochemical analysis and imaging, are discussed. The surgical treatment of ACC has evolved in the last 2 decades. The different surgical alternatives for the treatment of ACC in the context of primary, recurrent, or metastatic disease are reviewed, and the remaining challenges and controversies are discussed.

ENDOCRINOLOGY AND METABOLISM CLINICS OF NORTH AMERICA

FORTHCOMING ISSUES

September 2015
Postmenopausal Endocrinology
Nanette Santoro and
Lubna Pal, *Editors*

December 2015
Reproductive Endocrinology
Peter Lee and
Christopher P. Houk, *Editors*

RECENT ISSUES

March 2015
Pituitary Disorders
Anat Ben-Shlomo and Maria Fleseriu,
Editors

December 2014
Lipids
Donald A. Smith, *Editor*

RELATED INTEREST

Surgical Pathology Clinics, Volume 7, Issue 4 (December 2014)
Endocrine Pathology
Peter M. Sadow, *Editor*
Available at: http://www.surgpath.theclinics.com/

VISIT THE CLINICS ONLINE!
Access your subscription at:
www.theclinics.com

Foreword

Adrenal Cortical Neoplasia

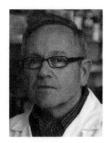

Derek LeRoith, MD, PhD
Consulting Editor

This issue on adrenal cortical tumors, expertly edited by Dr Alice C. Levine, brings together a number of important topics for the basic scientist and the practicing clinician, both endocrinologists and endocrine surgeons. We believe that the readers will appreciate the updates on the topics and find them of practical importance.

In their opening article on adrenal cortical development, Drs Xing, Lerario, Rainey, and Hammer focus on adrenal cortical zonal development. During the late fetal period, the zona glomerulosa and fasciculata develop; the former produces mineralocorticoids and the latter produces glucocorticoids. The zona reticularis only develops near puberty and is responsible for androgen production. This important differentiation into these zones is maintained by progenitor cells, identified as hedgehog positive, that are distributed by centripetal forces. As described in the article, there are numerous transcription factors, pituitary, and other hormones involved in both differentiation and production of these essential adrenal hormones. Furthermore, the various syndromes of adrenal insufficiency or excess hormone production apparently arise from mutations in stem progenitor cells.

Drs Turcu and Auchus continue the concept of steroidogenesis in a zone-specific manner and describe in more detail the enzymatic pathways in each zone that leads from cholesterol to aldosterone, cortisol, and dehydroepiandrosterone, respectively. The article also discusses congenital adrenal hyperplasia, the most common form being 21-hydroxylase deficiency. They describe the genetics, the clinical presentations, diagnosis, and management of the disorder, including prenatal treatment with dexamethasone.

Animal models of human disease may be extremely useful in understanding the pathophysiology of the disease, as discussed by Drs Galac and Wilson. Mouse models, in particular, are readily manipulated by transgenic and gene-deletion technology as well as surgical and medical means. Xenografic models are used to introduce human adrenal cortical cancer (ACC) cells in immunodeficient mice. Drugs have then been used to inhibit the growth of the tumors, including IGF-1 receptor blockers,

Endocrinol Metab Clin N Am 44 (2015) xiii–xv
http://dx.doi.org/10.1016/j.ecl.2015.03.003
0889-8529/15/$ – see front matter © 2015 Published by Elsevier Inc.

thiazolidinediones, and mTOR inhibitors. Transgenic models include, for example, SV40 large T-Ag under the control of the inhibin promoter or a transgenic with multiple copies of the steroidogenic factor-1, while others involve mutations in the cAMP signaling pathways. Finally, they also describe ACCs in other animal species as potentially useful for studies.

Drs Espaird and Bertherat, in their article, pursue the description of the genetic basis to adrenocortical tumors. Benign adrenal adenomas may be discovered as incidentalomas in 1% to 7% of the population, whereas ACCs are extremely rare. Bilateral adenomas associated with Cushing syndrome often have mutations in the cAMP/PKA signaling pathway, whereas primary macronodular adrenal hyperplasia often demonstrates an inactivating mutation of the tumor suppressor gene ARMC5. There are other mutations seen in adenomas of the cortex, both benign and malignant. It is hoped that as more of the genetics are discovered that there may be an improvement in diagnostic acumen and this may relate to therapeutic advantages and improved outcomes.

Adrenal incidentalomas are quite commonly found on adrenal imaging, reaching almost 4% of the population, especially in middle age. Drs Ioachimescu, Remer, and Hamrahian discuss that incidentalomas may also harbor a significant number of hormonal secretory adenomas and thus there is need for further clinical, biochemical, and radiological evaluation to exclude subclinical Cushing or pheochromocytoma. In addition, evaluation of the lipid content of the adrenal is important when consideration is given for the possibility of malignancy. Surgical management is dependent on hormonal status or if a suspicion of malignancy exists. Medical management is discussed in later articles in detail.

Although primary aldosteronism was previously thought to be a rare cause of hypertension, clinical studies conducted over the past 20 years indicate that perhaps 10% of patients with hypertension may have primary aldosteronism, according to Dr Galati. Bilateral adrenal hyperplasia accounts for almost two-thirds of cases and, interestingly, most cases do not present with the classic feature of hypokalemia. The majority of the remaining cases are due to aldosterone-producing adenomas, with malignancies being extremely rare. Hereditary cases have been described but are also rare. The standard screening used is the aldosterone-to-renin ratio (ARR), and if the ARR raises suspicion, then the adrenal venous sampling (AVS) may be valuable in distinguishing unilateral from bilateral disease if surgical resection is under consideration. Surgical cure is often the first choice for AVS-confirmed aldosteronomas, although medical therapies are also an option, including spironolactone or eplerenone and, of course, antihypertensive agents.

Drs Goddard, Ravikumar, and Levine describe a rather controversial aspect of adrenal adenomas and mild hypercorticolism. The importance of this topic is in regard to both its description as "subclinical Cushing syndrome" as well as recent reports demonstrating deleterious long-term effects of even mild chronic elevations in cortisol on the cardiovascular system. Treatment options include surgical resection of the affected adrenal gland or medical therapies that block either cortisol production or action at the receptor level.

Adrenal tumors in pregnancy present a specific problem diagnostically as well as therapeutically. As discussed by Drs Cocks Eschler, Kogekar, and Pessah-Pollack, the hypothalamic-adrenal axis is affected resulting in elevated levels of cortisol, aldosterone, and renin, making the diagnosis a challenge. Since adrenal adenomas, ACC, pheochromocytoma, and other adrenal pathologies are rare in pregnancy, a high level of suspicion is warranted. Many of the pathologies are harmful to mother and infant and require intervention either surgically or medically.

Molecular pathogenesis of ACC is described in the article by Drs Nakamura, Yamazaki, Felizola, Ise, Morimoto, Satoh, Arai, and Sasano. As discussed elsewhere, ACC is a rare but extremely malignant tumor. Immunohistochemical analysis of steroid hormones in adrenal cortical tumors may provide insight into cell of origin, prognosis, and possible new treatment options and may serve as an adjunct to the Weiss criteria in distinguishing benign from malignant lesions.

Drs Baudin and colleagues discuss issues related to ACC diagnosis and management. Since the tumors are so rare, making clinical trials difficult, they suggest a concerted effort by various groups to collaborate. Studies have demonstrated that several key pathways, including the p53, Wnt/β-catenin, and IGFII pathways, are involved, whereas genes such as *CDKN2A*, *RB1*, *TERT*, and *MENIN* are involved and hypermethylation of CIMP in up to 50% of ACC has also been described.

While a very rare condition, ACC is extremely malignant, as discussed by Drs Fernandez Ranvier and Inabnet. The 5-year survival rate is between 32% and 50% for patients with resectable tumors, and less than 1 year for patients who present with metastatic disease. Once biochemical and imaging studies have identified ACC, surgical resection remains the primary form of therapy, with open resection preferred over laparoscopic resection. Staging of the disease also determines postoperative medical therapy.

We greatly appreciate the hard work and contributions by the issue editor and the authors for this most timely and appropriate issue on adrenal cortical tumors.

Derek LeRoith, MD, PhD
Division of Endocrinology, Diabetes
and Bone Diseases
Icahn School of Medicine at Mount Sinai
1 Gustave Levy Place (1055)
Atran B4-35
New York, NY 10029, USA

E-mail address:
derek.leroith@mssm.edu

Preface

Genetics and the Clinical Approach to Adrenal Cortical Neoplasia: Connecting the Dots

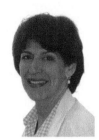

Alice C. Levine, MD
Editor

Although Eustacius first described the anatomy of the adrenal glands over 450 years ago, it was not until the mid-nineteenth century that their functional role was elucidated. In 1856, Brown-Sequard first demonstrated that the adrenal cortex is essential for life. In the nineteenth century and early twentieth century, scientific reports of the ravages of too little (Addison) or too much (Cushing) glucocorticoid production established that there is a delicate balance of these compounds. In 1936, Seyle demonstrated that this system is elegantly regulated during periods of stress via positive and negative feedback involving the brain, pituitary, and the adrenal cortex. In the mid-twentieth century, ACTH (Li et al) and adrenal steroids were isolated and demonstrated to have anti-inflammatory effects (Hench, Kendall, and Reichstein), and the adverse effect of aldosterone on blood pressure was described (Conn). From 1980 to the present, the molecular era of scientific research resulted in the cloning and functional characterization of steroid receptors, steroidogenic enzymes, and essential nuclear transcription factors that modulate the production and actions of the adrenal cortex.

This issue of *Endocrinology and Metabolism Clinics of North America* brings us up-to-date on this, arguably, most important endocrine gland. Recent basic science research that utilizes the tools of molecular genetics has uncovered heritable mutations underlying many adrenal cortical neoplasias that also align with somatic mutations discovered in those same tumors. Recent clinical research studies challenge the long-held assumption that mild elevations in adrenal cortical steroids are rare and of minimal clinical significance. Indeed, with the increase in the reported incidence of both adrenal incidentalomas and the metabolic syndrome worldwide, a connection

Endocrinol Metab Clin N Am 44 (2015) xvii–xviii
http://dx.doi.org/10.1016/j.ecl.2015.03.002
0889-8529/15/$ – see front matter © 2015 Published by Elsevier Inc.

endo.theclinics.com

between these two disorders may lead to a more targeted and effective approach to prevent cardiovascular morbidity and mortality.

In this issue, a panel of expert authors from around the globe has collaborated to give an up-to-date, translational view of adrenal cortical neoplasia in the twenty-first century. I am grateful for their contributions that include insights into the development, pathology, molecular genetics, clinical presentations, and treatments for adrenal cortical tumors. This volume demonstrates the tremendous strides that have been made but it also points to where knowledge gaps still exist. The clinical applicability of molecular genetics and the consequences of mild adrenal cortical steroid overproduction need to be further investigated so that guidelines for screening and timing and type of intervention are established. We still need to connect the dots.

Alice C. Levine, MD
Professor of Medicine
Co-Director of the Adrenal Center
The Hilda and J. Lester Gabrilove
Division of Endocrinology, Diabetes
and Bone Diseases
Department of Internal Medicine
Icahn School of Medicine
at Mount Sinai
One Gustave L. Levy Place
Box 1055
New York, NY 10029-6574, USA

E-mail address:
alice.levine@mountsinai.org

Development of Adrenal Cortex Zonation

Yewei Xing, PhD[a], Antonio M. Lerario, MD, PhD[a], William Rainey, PhD[a,b], Gary D. Hammer, MD, PhD[c],*

KEYWORDS

- Adrenal cortex • Zonation • Development • Steroidogenesis

KEY POINTS

- The human adult adrenal cortex is composed of 3 different zones: zona glomerulosa (zG), zona fasciculata (zF), and zona reticularis (zR). These zones are responsible for production of mineralocorticoids, glucocorticoids, and adrenal androgens, respectively.
- The establishment of the adrenal zG and zF occurs late in fetal development with a transition from the fetal to adult cortex; however, the final completion of cortical zonation in humans does not occur until puberty with the establishment of the zR and its production of adrenal androgens; a process called adrenarche.
- The maintenance of the adrenal cortex involves the centripetal displacement and differentiation of peripheral Sonic hedgehog–positive progenitors cells into zG cells that later transition to zF cells and subsequently zR cells.

FETAL AND EARLY ADULT DEVELOPMENT OF THE ADRENAL CORTEX
Formation of the Adrenal Cortex

Origin of the adrenogonadal primordium

The adrenal glands develop from 2 separate embryologic tissues: the medulla is derived from neural crest cells originating in proximity to the dorsal aorta, whereas the cortex develops from the intermediate mesoderm.[1] The appearance of the adrenal gland in the form of the adrenogonadal primordium (AGP) at 28 to 30 days postconception (dpc) in humans (embryonic day [E] 9.0 in mice) is marked by the expression of steroidogenic factor 1 (SF1; NR5A1), a nuclear receptor essential for adrenal development and steroidogenesis.[2,3] The bilateral AGP first appears as a thickening of the coelomic epithelium between the urogenital ridge and the dorsal mesentery. Each

Disclosures: The authors have nothing to disclose.
Funding sources: A.M. Lerario is supported by CAPES, grant number BEX 8726/13-2.
[a] Internal Medicine, Medical School, University of Michigan, 109 Zina Pitcher Place, 1860 BSRB, Ann Arbor, MI 48109, USA; [b] Department of Molecular & Integrative Physiology, University of Michigan, 2560D MSRB II, 1150 W. Medical Center Dr., Ann Arbor, MI 48109-5622, USA; [c] Endocrine Oncology Program, Center for Organogenesis, University of Michigan, 109 Zina Pitcher Place, 1528 BSRB, Ann Arbor, MI 48109-2200, USA
* Corresponding author.
E-mail address: ghammer@umich.edu

Endocrinol Metab Clin N Am 44 (2015) 243–274
http://dx.doi.org/10.1016/j.ecl.2015.02.001
0889-8529/15/$ – see front matter
endo.theclinics.com

AGP contains a mixed population of adrenocortical and somatic gonadal progenitor cells. SF1-positive AGP cells then delaminate from the epithelium and invade the underlying mesenchyme of the intermediate mesoderm.[4]

Separation of adrenogonadal primordium (formation of the adrenal gland)

Following delamination, most AGP cells migrate dorsolaterally to form the gonadal anlagen (gonadal primordial [GP]). A subset of AGP cells that express higher levels of SF1 migrate dorsomedially to form the adrenal anlagen (adrenal primordial [AP] or adrenal fetal zone [FZ]), ultimately settling ventrolateral to the dorsal aorta.[3] At about 48 dpc in humans (E11.5–E13.5 in mice), neural crest cells migrate from the dorsal midline just lateral to the neural tube to the area where the AP is developing.[5] These cells persist as discrete islands scattered throughout the embryonic adrenal until birth and ultimately coalesce and differentiate into the catecholamine-producing chromaffin cells of the adrenal medulla.[6,7] Meanwhile, the adrenal gland starts to separate from surrounding mesenchyme and becomes encapsulated with the formation of a fibrous layer overlying the developing cortical cells, a process largely complete by 52 dpc in humans (E14.5 in mice).[8]

Adrenocortical and chromaffin cells have an intimate relationship during embryonic development and postnatal homeostasis. Adrenal glucocorticoids play an essential role in chromaffin cell hormone production by regulating the expression of phenylethanolamine N-methyltransferase, which results in epinephrine (as opposed to norepinephrine) being the dominant catecholamine produced in the postnatal adrenal medulla.[9,10] However, mutant mice lacking the glucocorticoid receptor show normal embryonic neural crest cell migration to the adrenal and normal early fetal chromaffin cell development.[11] Similarly, even in the setting of a hypoplastic (*Sf1* heterozygous [*Sf1*$^{+/-}$] mice) or aplastic (*Sf1* null [*Sf1*$^{-/-}$] mice) adrenal cortex, a rudimentary adrenal medulla develops,[12] albeit in an ectopic location in the hypoplastic gland.[12,13] Further studies are needed to yield insights into the molecular mechanisms that dictate the interplay between the steroidogenic adrenocortical cells and the catecholamine-producing chromaffin cells of the adrenal gland.[14,15]

Fetal Development of the Adrenal Cortex

Fetal zone formation and function

After encapsulation, the embryonic adrenal cortex expands rapidly. In humans, the enlargement of the fetal cortex (FZ) accounts for most of the prenatal growth, especially during the last 6 weeks of gestation. The human fetal adrenal is one of the largest organs at term (0.2% of total body weight and nearly the size of the kidney), with 80% of the gland composed of FZ cells.[16] These large steroidogenic cells (20–50 mm) show a high cytoplasmic/nuclear ratio and robustly express cytochrome P450 17 alpha (CYP17), a bifunctional enzyme with both 17 hydroxylase and 17,20 lyase activities that convert pregnenolone to dehydroepiandrosterone (DHEA). Because of the high activity of CYP17 at this stage, the human fetal adrenal cortex produces large amounts of DHEA and DHEA-sulfate (S), which is then converted by the placenta to estrogens for the maintenance of normal pregnancy. Although large amounts of other sulfated Δ5 steroids, including pregnenolone sulfate and 17α-hydroxypregnenolone sulfate are also produced by FZ cells, it is unclear whether such steroids play a functional role in human biology.

Emergence of the definitive zone

By the eighth week of gestation, new adrenocortical cells emerge between the capsule and FZ, forming the definitive zone (DZ), which later develops into the adult cortex. The DZ is composed of SF1-positive, densely packed basophilic cells arranged in a narrow band of cellular clusters.[17,18] Small in size (10–20 mm), DZ cells are lipid poor during midgestation and show structural characteristics typical of cells in a proliferative state. However, as gestation advances, inner cells of the DZ form arched cords with fingerlike columns of cells reaching the outer rim of the FZ. During the third trimester, the cells of these cords continue to expand and begin producing cortisol under the regulation of adrenocorticotropin hormone (ACTH), defining the emergence of the zF of the adult adrenal cortex.

Factors involved in fetal adrenal development (regulatory mechanism)

Steroidogenic factor 1 The nuclear receptor SF1 (also known as NR5A1) has emerged as a pivotal factor for the initiation and fetal maturation of the adrenal cortex. In the absence of SF1 expression, the adrenal gland does not form (adrenal aplasia in *Sf1*-knockout mice[3] and most human patients[19,20]). Moreover, Sf1 haploinsufficiency (*Sf1*[+/-]) results in delayed and incomplete development of the adrenal gland in mice,[21] whereas overexpression of Sf1 results in aberrant proliferation, gonadal differentiation, and ultimately neoplasia in the mouse adrenal.[22]

The regulation of *Sf1* gene expression is complex, with different enhancer elements controlling the spatial and temporal expression in the developing adrenal. Current data indicate that although Wilms tumor 1 (WT1) regulates *Sf1* expression in the AGP, Cbp/ P300-interacting transactivator with Glu/Asp-Rich carboxy-terminal domain 2 (CITED2) expression in the AGP is necessary for proper differentiation of the AP or FZ.[23,24] Zubair and colleagues[25] identified the mouse fetal adrenal-specific enhancer (FAdE) in the *Sf1* gene as the critical mediator of *Sf1* gene expression in the AP. The transcription complex containing the homeobox protein PKNOX1 (Prep1), homeobox gene 9b (Hox9b), and pre–B-cell leukemia transcription factor 1 (Pbx1) initiates FAdE-mediated *Sf1* expression in the AGP.[25] Sf1 subsequently regulates itself by maintaining FAdE-mediated *Sf1* expression in the AP. After E14.5 in mice, FAdE is no longer used.[26] In the emerging DZ, *Sf1* regulation is shifted to a different definitive enhancer that has not yet been characterized. In humans, no similar FAdE or DZ enhancers have yet been confirmed.[25]

Dax1 An Sf1 target gene, *Dax1* (dosage-sensitive sex reversal, adrenal hypoplasia critical region, on chromosome X, gene 1, Nr0b1), is an orphan nuclear receptor. *DAX1* was first cloned as the gene responsible for X-linked cytomegalic adrenal hypoplasia congenita.[27,28] In the adrenal, Dax1 primarily serves as a corepressor of Sf1-mediated transcription of steroidogenic genes.[4,19,29] Consistent with this role and the enriched expression of Dax1 in the outer cortex, knockdown of *Dax1* results in premature differentiation of mouse adrenocortical progenitor cells. However, this occurs at the expense of depleting this essential cell population, ultimately resulting in adrenal failure.[30] As such, Dax1 plays an essential role in the maintenance of stem/progenitor cell pluripotency. Moreover, Dax1 may serve as the repressor for FAdE activity in the mouse adrenal gland during the FZ to DZ transition.[26] The relationships between Dax1, Sf1, ACTH, and Wnts are summarized in **Fig. 1**.

Regulation of *Dax1* expression is therefore predicted to be a dynamic process, balancing progenitor renewal and adrenocortical differentiation/steroidogenesis. Sf1 activates *Dax1* transcription in cooperation with paracrine Wnt signaling and glucocorticoids that are synthesized in the differentiated adult cortex.[31] In contrast, ACTH, the well-established glucocorticoid stimulator, has been shown to effect release of Sf1 complexes from the *Dax1* promoter, thus leading to effective inhibition of *Dax1* transcription. This process is predicted to promote the response of Sf1-positive progenitor cells to ACTH and subsequently initiate steroidogenesis. In an analogous fashion,

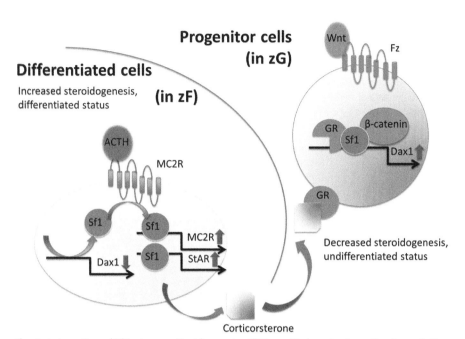

Fig. 1. Interaction of Sf1, glucocorticoid receptor (GR), and beta-catenin on Dax1 regulation.

Dax1 plays a similar role in mouse embryonic stem (ES) cells. It is transcriptionally activated by the other member of the NR5A family, liver receptor homolog 1 (LRH1), and the homeobox transcription factor Nanog.[32] Moreover, knockdown of *Dax1* leads to premature spontaneous differentiation of ES cells into cells of all 3 germ layers, establishing Dax1 as a critical mediator of stem/progenitor cell pluripotency.[33]

Adrenocorticotropic hormone and other hormonal factors ACTH is a 39-amino-acid peptide secreted from the anterior pituitary gland under control of corticotropin-releasing hormone (CRF or CRH).[34] As a major component in the hypothalamic-pituitary-adrenal (HPA) axis, ACTH binds to the transmembrane receptor melanocortin receptor 2 (MC2R) specifically in adrenocortical cells and exerts its effect through downstream cAMP and Ras/MEK/ERK signaling pathways.[35] Although adrenocortical growth and differentiation are independent of ACTH during the first trimester of human pregnancy, ACTH begins to play an essential role in the morphologic and functional development of the adrenal gland after 15 weeks of gestation.[36] The growth-promoting effects of ACTH are mediated in part through the stimulation of locally produced growth factors such as insulinlike growth factor (IGF) 2 and fibroblast growth factor (FGF) beta.[37,38] During development, as the outer DZ emerges, ACTH participates in the regulation of steroidogenesis, cell differentiation, and cell growth.[39–41]

As mentioned earlier, CRH, a 41-amino-acid peptide, is commonly considered to regulate adrenal function indirectly through the central nervous system (CNS) via the HPA axis.[42] Secreted by the parvocellular neurons of the paraventricular nucleus in the hypothalamus in response to central and peripheral stimuli, CRH stimulates corticotroph cells in the anterior pituitary to produce Pro-opiomelanocortin (POMC), which is subsequently cleaved to ACTH.[43]

CRH, CRH-homologous peptides (Urocortin [UCN]1-3), and their receptors (CRF1 and CRF2 receptor) are all found locally in the both adult and fetal adrenal gland with different distribution patterns.[44,45] In adults, although CRH is expressed throughout the gland, UCN1 mainly presents in chromaffin cells in the medulla.[43,46] In contrast, UCN2 is observed in all 3 zones of the human cortex but is only weakly expressed in adrenal medulla, and UCN3 also seems to be expressed in human adrenals.[44,46] The expression patterns of CRF and UCNs in fetal adrenals parallel the developmental changes in humans, in which UCN1, UCN3, and the CRF1 and CRF2 receptors all seem to be expressed in both the FZ and DZ of the adrenal cortex.[45,47]

The presence of all CRH peptides and their receptors in the adrenal suggests that the CRH system can function locally within human and rodent adrenals. Another important source of CRH is the human placenta, which releases CRH into the fetal circulation. As gestation advances CRH concentration increases: the remarkable increase in placental CRH production at the end of gestation has been suggested to contribute to the parturition process by forming a feed-forward loop that leads to increased productions of cortisol and DHEA/DHEA-S in human fetal adrenals. Studies have shown that CRH stimulates cortisol production in primary cultures of fetal adrenocortical cells by increasing the messenger RNA (mRNA) levels of steroidogenic acute regulatory protein and other steroidogenic enzymes, including hydroxy-delta-5-steroid dehydrogenase (*HSD3B2*), *CYP21*, and *CYP11B1*.[48] In addition, CRH enhances the adrenal response to ACTH, further driving the production of cortisol and DHEA/DHEA-S.[48,49] A further study has shown that the stimulatory effect of CRH on cortisol production may require the presence of chromaffin cells,[50] consistent with the potential paracrine relationship between cortex and medulla.

Insulinlike growth factor 2 Both IGF1 and IGF2 are mitogens expressed in the adrenal gland. IGFs bind dimeric/heterodimeric cell surface receptors (insulin receptor [IR] or IGF receptor 1 [IGF1R]) and induce autophosphorylation of the intracellular portion of the receptor, leading to activation of Ras/MEK/ERK and PI3K/AKT.[51,52] Although both IGF1 and IGF2 are present during human adrenal development, IGF2 is more highly expressed in early fetal development, in which it likely plays a major role.[53–55] In contrast, IGF1 is dominant in the adult adrenal gland, functioning as a regulator of postnatal growth maintenance. Although at lower levels compared with fetal adrenal cortex, IGF2 is expressed in the adult adrenal gland with expression restricted to the peripheral cortex and capsule of the adult adrenal, coinciding with the stem/progenitor cell niche.[52] However, in the mouse, the expression pattern is a little different: in the fertilized mouse embryo, mRNA transcripts encoding *Igf2* are present in low amounts almost as soon as the embryonic genome is activated, at the 2-cell to 4-cell stage, whereas the *Igf1* mRNA appears later, around the time of implantation at 8 to 9 days of gestation. Besides their mitogenic effects, IGFs and FGF have been shown to be essential factors for maintenance of the stem cell niche in multiple other organ systems,[55,56] supporting a potential role for IGF2 in adrenal stem/progenitor cell maintenance. A more recent study found the IGF pathway essential in adrenogonadal development and primary sex determination, because knocking down the receptors causes adrenal agenesis, possibly by decreased expression of Sf1 in AGP and subsequent failure of adrenal primordia specification. Growth retardation, male/female sex reversal, and delayed ovarian development are additionally observed in these mice.[57]

Transition of fetal zone to definitive zone /adult cortex
Studies by Zubair and colleagues[25,26,58,59] provided significant insights into the relationship between the FZ and the DZ/adult cortex. Using the FAdE-Cre mouse model, these investigators observed proliferating cells in a scattered pattern throughout the adrenal gland until E13.5.[13,59] At later time points, proliferating cells assembled in the periphery of the adrenal gland.[60] Similar to the developing human adrenal cortex,

the mouse FZ is first encapsulated by surrounding cells of the intermediate mesoderm. Following encapsulation a second group of cells emerge as the densely packed DZ or definitive (adult) cortex. As previously noted, *Sf1* is activated by FAdE only in the FZ before E14.5 but this enhancer does not activate *Sf1* expression in the DZ. By breeding a Rosa26 mouse with a transgenic mouse harboring the Cre-recombinase gene driven by a basal *Sf1* promoter and the FAdE enhancer, Zubair and colleagues[59] traced the fate of FZ cells during development. Their results showed that all DZ cells are derived from FAdE-expressing cells of the fetal adrenal. To complement these experiments, Zubair and colleagues also used a tamoxifen-inducible FAdE-Cre mouse model. DZ staining was only observed when tamoxifen was administrated early in embryogenesis (E11.5–E12.5). No LacZ-positive cells were found when tamoxifen was administered after E14.5. These results are consistent with the absence of FAdE activity during later developmental stages and support the conclusion that the FZ gives rise to the DZ.

In contrast, studies focused on a downstream activator of the hedgehog pathway, glioma-associated oncogene homolog 1 (zinc finger protein) (Gli1) provide evidence that the adrenal capsular cells also give rise to the DZ.[61,62] Gli1-expressing cells are specifically located in the adrenal capsule and do not express Sf1. As shown by King and colleagues,[62] this subpopulation of cells is capable of giving rise to Sf1-expressing, differentiated adrenocortical cells during embryonic development. However, these data are in conflict with the lineage tracing experiments mentioned earlier using FAdE-LacZ reporter mouse that revealed that all DZ cells arise from FZ cells. Although these apparently conflicting observations may reflect 2 temporally distinct lineages of the definitive cortex, in which both the Sf1-positive FZ and the Sf1-negative capsule cells can give rise to Sf1-positive DZ adrenocortical cells, recent studies support a single developmental and homeostatic mechanism of adrenal growth. Wood and colleagues[63] showed that FZ cells that once expressed *Sf1* under control of the FAdE enhancer gave rise to a subset of capsular cells. These FZ cell descendants within the adrenal capsule express Gli1, suggesting that some FZ cells can transition into Sf1-negative capsular cells that in turn can give rise to the underlying DZ/adult cortex (**Fig. 2**).

Postnatal Adrenal Development

The human adrenal gland continues to undergo significant remodeling during neonatal and pubertal periods. Immediately after birth, cells within the FZ undergo apoptosis, resulting in involution of the remaining FZ.[64] In contrast, under the influence of the trophic hormones angiotensin II (AngII) and ACTH, the adult zona glomerulosa (zG) and zona fasciculata (zF) mature. Later, at 6 to 8 years of age in girls and 7 to 9 years of age in boys, the adrenal zona reticularis (zR) begins to form between the zF and the medulla. This process, known as adrenarche,[65] is characterized by increased proliferation and production of adrenal androgens. Because of zR hormonal influence, secondary sexual characteristics appear, particularly development of pubic hair and altered sweat composition, which produces adult body odor. In addition, increased oiliness of the skin and hair and mild acne may occur.[66] In most boys, these changes are indistinguishable from early testicular testosterone effects occurring at the beginning of gonadal puberty. In girls, adrenal androgens from adrenarche drive most of the early androgenic changes of puberty. Adrenarche occurs prematurely in many children who are overweight and/or born small for gestational age, suggesting links between placental hormones, intrauterine growth retardation, metabolic disease, and zG function.[67–70] However, the exact mechanisms for zR growth and the control factors for adrenarche remain elusive.

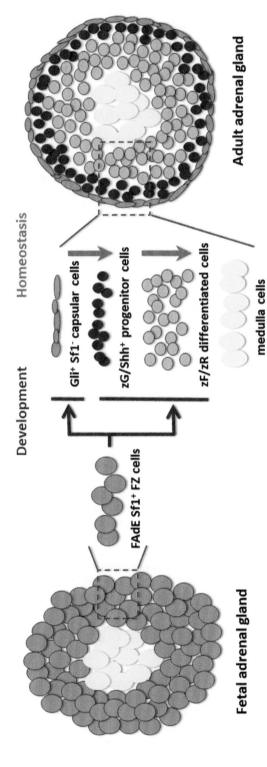

Fig. 2. Stem cell theory of adrenal development and homeostasis.

In rodents, the remaining remnants of the FZ (classically called the x-zone in mice) ultimately regress at the onset of puberty in boys and during the first pregnancy in women.[71,72] However, because FAdE activity is lost by E14.5, a definitive enhancer likely begins functioning before birth. Current efforts aim to identify and characterize a definitive/adult *Sf1* enhancer in rodents. **Fig. 3** summarizes the major stages of human and mouse adrenal gland development.

STRUCTURE AND FUNCTION OF THE ADULT ADRENAL CORTEX
Adrenal Cortical Zonation

Anatomy
In conjunction with FZ regression, the DZ forms discrete functional compartments within the adrenal cortex, termed the zG and the zF. The zG, composed of ovoid cells, is the most outer layer. Although in children with low-salt diets, zG is normally presented as a full zone, because of the high salt levels in the Western diet, zG cells in adults are scattered in clusters with a width of 200 to 1300 μm and a depth of 100 to 500 μm beneath the capsule.[73–75] These aldosterone-producing cell clusters express the CYP11B2 enzyme and are responsible for aldosterone production.[73] The zF constitutes most of the adrenal cortex, positioned directly under the zG. zF cells are large cells organized into bundles, which led to the name fascicles. In addition, zR constitutes the innermost layer of the adrenal cortex, between the zF and the adrenal medulla. Here, zR cells are arranged as cords that project in different directions, resulting in the netlike appearance that gives the zone its name (reticulum means net).

Extracellular matrix Extracellular matrix (ECM), which is composed of glycoproteins and associated integrin receptors, has been shown to play an important role in both the fetal and adult adrenal.[76] Using second-trimester human fetal adrenal glands, in situ studies have shown that collagen type IV is the major ECM glycoprotein present in the fetal adrenal and that it is evenly distributed throughout the gland. In contrast, other ECM glycoproteins, including laminin and fibronection, show more restricted expression patterns. Specifically, laminin is mainly expressed in the early expanding DZ, whereas fibronectin has a gradient that is highest in the FZ and decreases in the outer layers. The receptors for ECM components (integrin subunits) are also distributed in different zones of the human fetal adrenal. Integrin alpha-1 chain is found primarily in the DZ, whereas alpha-2 subunits are found abundantly at the interface of the FZ/DZ. The alpha-3 chain (a low-affinity ligand for fibronectin), is observed in the DZ/FZ and FZ. Consistent with this pattern, in vitro studies using primary human fetal adrenal cells cultured on matrix-coated dishes found that the ECM not only contributes to maintenance of cell morphology of primary cultures but also influences cellular behavior. For example, increased proliferation rates are observed on laminin-coated or collagen-coated dishes, whereas fibronectin supports higher levels of apoptosis.[77] In addition, collagen IV strongly enhances ACTH-stimulated DHEA/DHEA-S as well as cortisol secretion[77,78]; fibronectin increases DHEA and DHEA/DHEA-S secretion through increased P450C17 gene expression.[78] These studies show that the unique ECM environment within each region of the fetal adrenal gland supports zone-specific cellular behavior.

Similar to its effects in the fetal gland, the ECM is also thought to influence behavior and function within the adult adrenal gland. Studies in adult rat adrenal glands have shown varying expression gradients for all 4 major glycoproteins. In adult rat adrenal glands, collagen I is the major glycoprotein in the outer capsule, with moderate levels of collagen IV, fibronectin, and laminin also present. Collagen IV, fibronectin, and laminin surround each glomerulosa cell in the zG. In the zG, collagen IV is present as thick

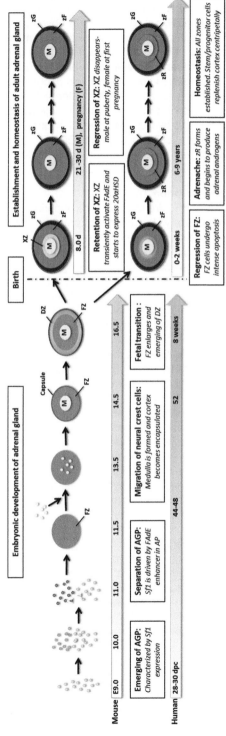

Fig. 3. Development and zonation of the adrenal gland. DZ, definitive zone; FZ, fetal zone; XZ, remnant of fetal zone (x-zone); zF, zona fasciculata; zG, zona glomerulosa; zR, zona reticularis.

fibrils, whereas fibronectin and laminin transition to discontinuous and short fibrils, respectively. The expression of each of these glycoproteins progressively decreases in the inner cortex regions. In the zR, only collagen IV is observed. In addition to varying expression patterns, ECM components also have distinct effects on adult adrenal function in vitro.[79] Specifically, fibronectin, collagen I, and collagen IV increase 3β-HSD expression and subsequent aldosterone production in zG cells as well as corticosterone secretion in zF cells. In contrast, laminin decreased protein synthesis, 3β-HSD expression, and corticosteroid release.[79] Morphologic changes are also detected on cells growing on different ECMs, indicating potential changes in function as well. Similarly, induction of 11β-hydroxylase and 21-hydroxylase enzyme expression is observed in bovine adrenal cells cultured with ECMs.[80] These results suggest that complex interactions between different matrix gradients likely contribute to the precise control of cellular behaviors within each zone.

Adrenal blood supply and innervation

Three critical arteries supply each adrenal gland: the superior suprarenal artery provided by the inferior phrenic artery, the middle suprarenal artery provided by the abdominal aorta, and the inferior suprarenal artery provided by the renal artery. Perhaps because of the energy-intensive nature of steroidogenesis, the adrenal glands have one of the greatest blood supplies per gram of tissue of any organ, with up to 60 arterioles entering each adrenal gland, which may account for the high prevalence of cancer metastases found in the adrenal gland.[81–83] Arterial blood first reaches the outer surface of adrenal cortex where the cortical arteries branch to form the subcapsular capillary plexus.[84] Most of the subcapsular plexus become fenestrated capillaries that follow the cordlike structures of the ZF down into the ZR before dumping into the medullary veins, which then form the suprarenal veins. Some of the arterioles continue through the cortex and provide blood directly to parts of the medulla. The right suprarenal vein drains into the inferior vena cava and the left suprarenal vein drains into the left renal vein or the left inferior phrenic vein.[85–88] This unique anatomy of blood supply in the adrenal cortex provides an interesting spatial gradient of adrenal steroids in different zones and may be a contributing regulatory mechanism for the distinct characters of cells in each zone.

The adrenal gland is also richly innervated, with most of the nerve plexuses located in the capsular region. Their fibers mainly originate from the greater splanchnic nerve and associated abdominal plexuses of the sympathetic autonomic nervous system, together with some parasympathetic contributions from the phrenic and vagal nerves. The nerve bundles penetrate the cortex, mostly in association with blood vessels.[89] Similar to the vasculature structure, most of these postganglionic nerves terminate in the medulla. Although controversial, it has been hypothesized that the innervation of the superficial blood vessels regulates blood flow in the cortical capillary bed. Moreover, in vitro studies have reported the regulation of cortical blood flow by neuropeptides released in response to splanchnic nerve stimulation. Specifically, vasoactive intestinal polypeptide and Met-enkephalin levels increase, whereas neuropeptide Y levels decrease, cortical flow rate.[90] In addition, although of unclear pathophysiologic relevance, these same neuropeptides are present at lower levels in associated nerve fibers in hyperplastic cortical tissue.[91]

Function of Adrenal Cortical Zones

The main function of the adrenal cortex is to produce a variety of steroids hormones. Although each zone uses cholesterol as the precursor molecule, distinct steroids result from differential enzyme expression.

Mineralocorticoids

Angiotensinogen (synthesized in the liver) is converted by renin (from the juxtaglomerular cells of the kidney) to angiotensin I, which is later converted to AngII by angiotensin-converting enzyme in the lung. Aldosterone is the primary mineralocorticoid produced by zG cells under the control of AngII and extracellular potassium.[92–95] Aldosterone functions as the ligand for the nuclear receptor MR (mineralocorticoid receptor) in target tissues that include the colon, salivary gland, and the renal distal convoluted tubule and collecting ducts, where it causes increased reabsorption of sodium and increased excretion of both potassium (by principal cells) and hydrogen ions (by intercalated cells of the collecting duct).

Glucocorticoids

Glucocorticoids are produced by zF cells at a basal level, but can be stimulated by ACTH secreted from the anterior pituitary under stress.[96–98] In humans, cortisol is the main glucocorticoid produced by the adrenal cortex under normal conditions and its actions include mobilization of fats, proteins, and carbohydrates.[99–101] In mice and rats, because of the lack of *Cyp17* gene expression, corticosterone is the major glucocorticoid produced and used.[102–104] Once produced and released into the bloodstream, glucocorticoids facilitate the release of energy stores for use during stress. Integral to the feedback control of the activated HPA axis, glucocorticoids inhibit production and secretion of ACTH from the HPA axis.[105,106]

Adrenal androgens

In primates, cells in the zona reticularis produce precursor androgens, including DHEA and androstenedione.[107–109] DHEA is further converted to DHEA-sulfate by the action of dehydroepiandrosterone sulfotransferase (SULT2A1). These precursors are weak androgens and get released into the bloodstream and are taken up in peripheral tissues, including hair follicles, genital skin, and prostate, for production of more potent androgens, including testosterone.[110–112] Recent work using human adrenal vein sampling has detected testosterone and other downstream androgen metabolites from the adrenal cortex, suggesting the presence of a wider variety of adrenal androgens than previously appreciated.[113] The regulatory mechanism of adrenal androgen production has not been fully elucidated. However, luteinizing hormone (LH)/human chorionic gonadotropin (hCG) receptors have been shown to be present in zR[114] and hCG can stimulate DHEA-sulfate synthesis in cultured human fetal adrenals.[115,116] This finding suggested that LH/hCG might regulate androgen synthesis in an ACTH-independent manner. Moreover, the illicit action of LH has been implicated in excess cortisol production in patients with primary macronodular adrenal hyperplasia (PMAH).[117]

Homeostasis of Adult Cortex

Homeostatic maintenance of the definitive zone/adult cortex

After the functional adult adrenocortical zones are established, they are maintained by stem or progenitor cells. Since the 1930s, numerous studies have suggested that cells from the outer region of the adrenal cortex proliferate and migrate to repopulate the adrenal cortex.[118–120] Several studies show that most proliferating cells are located in the outer layer of the mature adrenal gland, whereas most cell death occurs near the boundary of cortex and medulla. These historical data are consistent with the presence of a stem/progenitor cell population in or directly under the capsule of the cortex.[121–124]

Shh pathway In 2009, 3 laboratories independently used lineage tracing to provide evidence that the Shh signaling pathway was essential for mouse adrenal gland development and maintenance.[62,125,126] In these studies, Shh was found in the adrenal gland at E11.5, primarily in the subcapsular zG where stem/progenitor cells reside. In adult adrenal glands, Shh colocalizes with Sf1 in nonsteroidogenic cortical cells of the zG region but not in differentiated zG or zF cells, which express both Sf1 and markers of fully differentiated steroidogenic cells (Cyp11b2 and Cyp11b1, respectively). However, descendants of Shh-expressing cells express adrenocortical differentiation markers, suggesting that Shh-positive cells serve as progenitor cells for the adrenal cortex.[62] Mice in which *Shh* is ablated specifically in *Sf1*-expressing cells reveal marked adrenal hypoplasia, decreased proliferation, and a thin capsule.[125] However, despite a decrease in size, the adrenal glands in these mice maintain proper zonation, suggesting that Shh does not have a role in the initiation of differentiation. Together, these data implicate the Shh pathway in actively promoting maintenance of the adrenal cortex.

Wnt pathway The Wnt/beta-catenin signaling pathway is also critical for adrenocortical homeostasis. Studies performed in the mouse adrenal revealed that beta-catenin expression and activity is present early in the fetal cortex. By E18.5, with the emergence of the DZ, beta-catenin is restricted to the subcapsular zG.[127] Using a cre-lox technology to ablate beta-catenin specifically in Sf1-expressing cells of the adrenal cortex, Kim and colleagues[128] observed adrenal aplasia at birth in mice expressing a highly penetrant *Sf1*-cre transgene. Careful examination of these mice showed normal adrenal development until E12.5, after which adrenal failure became evident precisely as DZ cells emerged between the coalescing capsule and the FZ. In mice that bear a weakly penetrant *Sf1*-cre transgene (express beta-catenin in about half of the adrenocortical cells), adrenal development progresses normally. However, as the mice age (ie, 30 weeks) a progressive cortical thinning and a decreased steroidogenic capacity is observed. This progressive failure of the cortex is hypothesized to be a result of the loss of adrenocortical progenitor cells.

Additional support for a role of Wnt/beta-catenin signaling pathway in the maintenance of adrenocortical stem/progenitor cells comes from studies in which the pathway has been genetically overactivated in the mouse adrenal cortex. In these studies, both an expansion of undifferentiated progenitorlike cells and ultimate tumor formation are observed. In one model of increased Wnt signaling, hyperaldosteronism caused by zG-specific expansion is characterized.[128,129] Moreover, activation of the Wnt pathway is frequently observed in adrenocortical neoplasms.[130–132] Although the exact function of Wnt/beta-catenin signaling in the adrenal cortex remains unknown, beta-catenin and Sf1 can directly activate *Dax1*, which suggests that Dax1 may be a critical mediator of Wnt action in the adrenal cortex.[133] Recent data indicate that Wnt/beta-catenin signaling may additionally regulate adrenal homeostasis by inhibiting fasciculata differentiation, promoting the undifferentiated state of progenitor cells and priming progenitor cells for zG fate.[132,134]

Homeostasis of cortical zones
Homeostasis of the adrenal cortex also entails the maintenance of zonal structure and function in the context of continual centripetal cellular repopulation of the gland. Because stem/progenitor cells reside primarily in the outer/subcapsular zG, investigators have asked whether differentiated cells first adopt a zG fate and later transition to zF and zR, or alternatively whether the stem/progenitor cells differentiate directly into each of the 3 cell types.

As previously mentioned, lineage tracing studies using an inducible green fluorescent protein (GFP) marker to track the fate of Shh descendants revealed that GFP expression was more prevalent in zG cells initially following induction of Shh-GFP. However, at later times an increasing number of GFP-expressing zF cells were observed.[62] These results suggest that most progenitor cells become zG cells first and then transition to zF cells.

More direct evidence for this model comes from recently published work using a zG-specific *Cyp11b2* promoter–driven GFP knock-in mouse, wherein zG cell descendants are labeled by GFP.[135] In this model, GFP-positive cells are rare in the adrenal gland of newborn mice. However, within 3 months, the entire cortex becomes GFP-positive, suggesting that all cells within the zF and x-zone originated from the zG cells. Furthermore, treatment with dexamethasone, a cortisol analog used to repress ACTH, can prevent zG cells from transitioning to zF cells, manifesting in atrophy of the zF. These results implicate ACTH as an important mediator of zF homeostasis. However, when Sf1is ablated in zG cells, the mice are able to maintain a normal functional zF zone, despite the complete absence of zG-derived GFP cells within the zF, perhaps suggesting that progenitor cells can (although they usually do not) directly adopt a zF phenotype without first becoming *Cyp11b2*-expressing zG cells (see **Fig. 2**).

DEFECTS IN CORTICAL ZONAL DEVELOPMENT
Adrenal Hypoplasia

The term adrenal hypoplasia refers to distinct clinical conditions characterized by the underdevelopment or hypotrophism of the adrenal cortex. Patients with complete adrenal hypoplasia or aplasia characteristically develop adrenal insufficiency soon after birth or, less commonly, in a more insidious manner throughout childhood or even in young adulthood. Adrenal insufficiency is potentially life threatening if not promptly recognized and treated.

Based on its physiopathology, adrenal hypoplasia can be divided into 2 broad categories: primary and secondary. Primary adrenal hypoplasia is characterized by a hypotrophic (and hypofunctional) adrenal cortex in the presence of normal hypothalamic/pituitary function. The causes of primary adrenal hypoplasia can be further categorized into (1) defects of adrenal cortex formation or differentiation, a condition known as congenital adrenal hypoplasia (AHC); and (2) ACTH resistance and related conditions (also known as familial glucocorticoid deficiency). AHC is usually associated with a severe phenotype, which might also include disorders of sexual development caused by gonadal failure, and severe adrenal insufficiency associated with salt wasting and other developmental disorders.[136–139] The most common form of AHC is X-linked congenital adrenal hypoplasia caused by disruption of the nuclear receptor *DAX1* (OMIM 300200). Mutations of NR5A1 are a contributing cause of the autosomal form of AHC.[137–139] Rare autosomal forms of AHC include the intrauterine growth restriction, metaphyseal dysplasia, adrenal hypoplasia congenita, and genital anomalies (IMAGe) syndrome (OMIM 600856) and the SEx Reversion, Kidneys, Adrenal and Lung dysgenesis (SERKAL) syndrome (OMIM 603490), caused by mutations of *CDKN1C* and *WNT4*, respectively.[136,139] Familial isolated glucocorticoid deficiency syndromes (broadly known as ACTH resistance syndromes) are autosomal recessive diseases caused by mutations in genes that participate in ACTH signaling, including mutations in *MC2R* and *MRAP* (a gene that codes for an accessory protein of the ACTH receptor, essential for its targeting and function).[140,141] More recently, mutations in the *NNT* and *MCM4* genes were also associated with familial glucocorticoid deficiency.[141–143] Patients with ACTH resistance usually do not present with the salt-wasting phenotype because aldosterone-producing cells are not affected by these mutations.

Secondary adrenal hypoplasia is caused by a pituitary or hypothalamic dysfunction that results in the disruption of ACTH synthesis, processing, and/or release by the pituitary gland. Thus the adrenal zF becomes hypotrophic and hypofunctioning because of the lack of adequate stimulus. Causes of secondary adrenal hypoplasia include (1) developmental abnormalities of the CNS, such as anencephaly, septo-optic dysplasia (OMIM 182230), and holoprosencephaly/Pallister-Hall syndrome 2 spectrum (OMIM 615849), the last 2 being caused by mutations in *HESX1* and *GLI2*; (2) diseases of pituitary development, such as pituitary combined hormone deficiency syndromes (caused by mutations in *PROP1*, *POU1F1*, *OTX2*, *LHX3*, and *LHX4*); (3) isolated ACTH deficiency (OMIM 201400), caused by *TBX19* mutations; (4) defects in *POMC* and neuroendocrine convertase 1 (*PCSK1*), which leads to deficiencies in all POMC-related peptides[144,145]; and (5) miscellaneous nongenetic causes that lead to hypothalamic or pituitary dysfunction, such as with idiopathic conditions, intracranial tumors, infections, or birth-related traumatic injuries.[141,146–149]

Considerable progress has been made in the understanding of the genetic basis of many of these forms of adrenal hypoplasia in the past 20 years. These breakthroughs have been important to allow counseling of families and screening of other family members at risk of adrenal failure, as well to provide insight into the molecular mechanisms of adrenal development in humans. However, for a significant percentage of cases of primary adrenal hypoplasia, the underlying cause remains unknown.

Disorders of Excessive Growth

Adrenal hyperplasia

Disorders of the adrenal cortex characterized by excessive growth include hyperplasias and tumors. Hyperplasias are invariably polyclonal disorders defined by bilateral enlargement of the adrenal cortex. Adrenal hyperplasia can be secondary to ACTH overstimulation (also referred to as ACTH-dependent hyperplasia), such as in Cushing disease or congenital adrenal hyperplasia (CAH). The latter is a common denomination of a heterogeneous group of autosomal recessive disorders that affect the function of key enzymes of the steroidogenic cascade, resulting in deficient cortisol production. As a consequence, the pituitary produces higher amounts of ACTH, which leads to (1) accumulation of steroid precursors before the enzymatic defect, and (2) increase in adrenal size, ultimately leading to nodule formation. The symptoms depend on the level of the enzymatic blockage (which in turn determines the type of steroid precursors that accumulate) and the severity of the defect (how much it impairs cortisol production). The most common form of CAH is the 21-hydroxylase deficiency (*CYP21A2*), accounting for more than 95% of cases.[150] More than 100 mutations have been described in this disease and a strong genotype-phenotype correlation is observed.[151] The classic form is characterized by the presence of virilization at birth with genital ambiguity in female fetuses (because of androgen precursor accumulation) and severe adrenal insufficiency that can be aggravated by mineralocorticoid deficiency in the salt-wasting forms.[152] The nonclassic form is usually characterized by mild signs of hyperandrogenism that frequently go unnoticed until adulthood.[152] Other types of CAH (each of these with distinct clinical manifestations) may result from mutations in other genes that code for enzymes of the steroidogenesis cascade, including *STAR*, *CYP11A1*, *HSD3B2*, *CYP17A1*, *CYP11B1*, and *POR*.[153–155] Primary causes of adrenal hyperplasias are, by definition, ACTH independent. However, intra-adrenal ACTH production has recently been described in some cases of primary adrenal hyperplasia, suggesting that some of the growth might be mediated by paracrine/autocrine ACTH stimulation from the hyperplastic tissue.[156] Primary adrenal hyperplasias are often associated with a genetic syndrome. Some of these syndromes, such as multiple endocrine neoplasia type 1 (MEN1), Gardner syndrome, McCune-Albright syndrome, and Carney complex, are characterized by multiple organ involvement. In other syndromes, such as PMAH and isolated primary pigmented micronodular adrenal hyperplasia (PPNAD), the adrenals are the only organs affected.[157,158] Both PMAH and PPNAD have been described in familial and isolated forms. Recently, germline mutations in *ARMC5* were described in about half of the PMAH cases, being the most frequent genetic alteration associated with this disease. Remarkably, the prevalence of germline *ARMC5* mutations is high even among patients with apparent sporadic disease, suggesting that familial forms are much more prevalent than was previously appreciated. Regarding the endocrine manifestations, the adrenal hyperplasia can be either functioning or nonfunctioning. The most common endocrine manifestation is Cushing syndrome, but rare cases of mineralocorticoid and androgen production have been reported.[159,160] Abnormal activation of the protein kinase A (PKA) pathway by different molecular mechanisms, such as ectopic expression of G protein–coupled receptors by adrenal cells, activating somatic mutations in *GNAS*, inactivating mutations of *PRKAR1A* (the gene that codes for one of the regulatory subunits of the PKA complex), inactivating mutations of *PDE11A* and *PDE8B*, and gene amplification of a catalytic subunit of the PKA complex (*PRKACA*), is usually present in the hormonally active group (**Table 1**).[161,162]

Adrenal tumors

Adrenocortical tumors (ACTs) are common neoplasms, especially in older adults, in whom the prevalence can reach up to 6% of the population.[163] Unlike the hyperplasias, ACTs are usually unilateral, although bilateral tumors are a common finding.[163,164] Most of them are benign and nonfunctioning adenomas (adrenocortical adenoma [ACA]) and incidentally found during abdominal imaging for unrelated reasons (also designated incidentaloma in this setting). ACAs can also be hormonally active, being able to secrete cortisol (Cushing syndrome), aldosterone (Conn syndrome), or androgens.[163,164] Recently, the molecular mechanisms that lead to the formation of both aldosterone-producing adenomas (APA) and cortisol-producing adenomas have been elucidated by next-generation sequencing approaches. APAs are the second most common cause of idiopathic (nonfamilial) primary aldosteronism, accounting for ~30% of cases (hyperplasias are the leading cause, accounting for 70%).[152,165] APAs are characterized molecularly by somatic mutations in several genes involved in the regulation of the intracellular calcium concentration, leading to abnormal activation of the calcium-calmodulin–dependent protein kinase 1/2 (*CAMK1/2*), the main regulators of AngII and potassium-stimulated *CYP11B2* transcription.[152,153] Somatic mutations in *KCNJ5* have been identified in approximately 40% of the APAs.[166] Heterozygous germline *KCNJ5* mutations have also been described as the cause of familial primary aldosteronism type III.[167] This gene encodes an inward-rectifying potassium channel (GIRK4) localized at the plasma membrane, which is responsible for the maintenance of the resting membrane potential by regulating the potassium efflux. *KCNJ5* is highly expressed in normal adrenals, specifically at zG and outer ZF with its activity stimulated by AngII. Mutations in *KCNJ5* increase its permeability to potassium, favoring membrane depolarization (which in turn leads to the opening of membrane voltage-gated calcium channels, increasing the intracellular calcium concentrations and resulting in activation of *CAMK1/2*).[168,169] Mutations in other genes that regulate intracellular calcium concentrations have subsequently been described in APAs, including mutations of the sodium/potassium-transporting ATPase subunit alpha-1 (*ATP1A1*), the plasma membrane calcium-transporting ATPase 3 (*ATP2B3*), and the voltage-dependent L-type calcium channel subunit alpha-1D (*CACNA1D*). Taken together, somatic

Table 1
Genetic syndromes associated with adrenal hyperplasia/neoplasia

Syndrome	Heritage	Locus	Gene	Clinical Features	Adrenal Manifestations	Comments
Multiple endocrine neoplasia type 1	Autosomal dominant	11q13	MEN1	Primary hyperparathyroidism; gastric, pancreatic, and duodenal neuroendocrine tumors; pituitary adenomas; thymic carcinoid tumors	Nonfunctioning macronodular hyperplasia in up to 40% of patients. ACCs rarely described	Somatic MEN1 mutations have frequently been described in sporadic ACC; 11q LOH is a frequent finding
Carney complex	Autosomal dominant	17q22–24	PRKAR1A	Cutaneous lentigines, pituitary adenomas, cardiac myxomas, pancreatic and cutaneous tumors	Micronodular pigmented adrenal hyperplasia	Somatic PRKAR1A have been described in functioning ACAs; ACCs have been described in patients previously diagnosed with CC; 17q LOH frequently described in ACTs
McCune-Albright syndrome	Sporadic (postzygotic somatic mosaicism)	20q13.3	GNAS1	Polyostotic bone dysplasia, gonadotropin-independent precocious puberty, café-au-lait spots, pituitary adenomas	Cortisol-producing bilateral nodular hyperplasia	Activating GNAS1 mutations have been described in cortisol-producing ACAs and PMAH
Gardner syndrome	Autosomal dominant	5q21–q22	APC	Familial adenomatosis polyposis, increased risk for colon cancer, thyroid tumors, osteomas of the skull	Bilateral adrenocortical hyperplasia in 7%–13%	Somatic APC mutations have not been described in sporadic ACTs. Abnormal nuclear beta-catenin staining has been described in one-third of ACCs and ACAs

PMAH	Sporadic/autosomal dominant	16p11.2	ARMC5/	Bilateral macronodular enlargement of adrenal glands associated with Cushing syndrome	Intracranial meningiomas have been described in some patients, suggesting that these tumors are also a manifestation of the disease	Overexpression of GPCRs is virtually omnipresent; intra-adrenal ACTH production with paracrine/autocrine stimulation of cortisol production has been described in some cases
Li-Fraumeni syndrome	Autosomal dominant	17p13	TP53	ACCs in 5%	Increased risk for sarcomas, hematologic malignancies, lung tumors, breast tumors	Germline inactivating TP53 mutations are common in pediatric ACCs but rarely seen in adults. Somatic inactivating TP53 mutations are present in 30% of samples
Beckwith-Wiedemann syndrome	Autosomal dominant/ sporadic	11p15	IGF2	ACT in 1.5%	Organomegaly, omphalocele, microcephalia, mental retardation, fetal neoplasms (Wilms tumor, hepatoblastoma, ACC)	IGF2 overexpression and structural abnormalities of 11p15 are present in up to 90% of sporadic ACCs

Abbreviations: ACA, adrenocortical adenoma; ACC, adrenocortical carcinoma; ACT, adrenocortical tumors; CC, carney complex; LOH, loss of heterozygosity; GPCR, G protein-coupled receptor.

mutations in these genes are present in ~ 15% of APAs. Note that mutations in these genes are mutually exclusive, reinforcing their causative role in intracellular calcium homeostasis.[170] Cortisol-producing adenomas are characterized by abnormally high levels of PKA activation.[161] Recently, 3 different groups described the recurrent somatic activating mutations of a catalytic subunit of the PKA (*PRKACA*) in a large subset of cortisol-producing adenomas.[171–173] This mutation leads to a defective protein-protein interaction with the regulatory subunit (encoded by the gene *PRKAR1A*), causing its constitutive activation.

In contrast to ACAs, adrenocortical carcinomas (ACCs), are rare tumors with an incidence of 1 case per 0.5 million to 2 million per year.[174,175] A bimodal age distribution has been described, with a first peak occurring early in childhood and a second one around the fourth of fifth decades. Around 60% of ACCs are hormonally active and, unlike ACAs, they can secrete more than 1 class of steroids (eg, cortisol plus androgens).[176,177] ACC is a highly malignant tumor with few therapeutic options once surgical cure cannot be achieved. At the time of diagnosis, about 50% of patients present with stage III (locally advanced) and IV (metastatic) disease. Even after a complete surgical resection in early stage disease, the recurrence rates are high.[176–178] Compared with other types of tumor, little is known about the molecular pathogenesis of ACTs. Much of the current knowledge comes from the understanding of the molecular basis of rare cancer syndromes, of which ACC is one manifestation, although most ACCs are sporadic.[161]

Molecular pathways involved in adrenal tumorigenesis

The few studies focusing on the clonality of human ACTs have concluded that, although adenomas are either monoclonal or polyclonal, carcinomas are primarily monoclonal, indicating that they are derived from a single cell that undergoes transformation and clonal expansion after a set of mutational events.[179,180] Although there are no clear data to identify the origin of this initiating cell, whether it is a stem, progenitor, or even differentiated cell, it is reasonable to expect that mutations in genes involved in maintenance of stem cell properties are critical for the transformation process. As mentioned earlier, the IGF system and the Wnt pathway are of key importance for the maintenance and homeostasis of adrenal stem cell and progenitor cell populations. Abnormalities of the IGF system and of the Wnt pathway are present in a large subset of ACCs, as discussed later.

Wnt/beta-catenin Adrenal hyperplasia and tumors are manifestations of the Gardner syndrome.[181,182] This syndrome is caused by germline mutations of the *APC* gene, which is part of a multiprotein complex (destruction complex) that ubiquitinates cytoplasmic beta-catenin, targeting it for proteasomal degradation.[183] Without the proper function of the destruction complex, beta-catenin accumulates in the cytoplasm and is translocated to the nucleus where it activates Wnt pathway target genes. Thus, nuclear accumulation of beta-catenin, as observed by immunohistochemistry, is an indicator of pathway activation. Studies have shown that about a third of both ACAs and ACCs show nuclear beta-catenin immunostaining.[184] Accordingly, somatic activating *CTNNB1* mutations are also observed in both ACAs and ACCs, suggesting that some ACAs may be precursor lesions of ACCs.[184,185] Animal models further corroborate these observations. A study using a transgenic mouse model with constitutively active beta-catenin specifically expressed in adrenocortical cells shows increased Axin2 levels and beta-catenin scattered throughout the cortex and in clusters of cells at the cortical/medullary boundary.[129] Although differing in degree, these mutant mice all show adrenal hyperplasia and dysplasia, and disruption of normal adrenal zonation, with zG cells expanding into the zF. By 10 months of age, Sf1 expression can be found in the medulla region, suggesting that these abnormal cells are resistant to apoptosis. More importantly, all the mice between 5 and 10 months of age show increased vascular endothelial growth factor expression, and by 17 months some females develop large masses with malignant characteristics, such as high proliferation rate and decreased *Sf1* expression.[129]

These results suggest that abnormal activation of canonical Wnt signaling pathway can lead to an expansion of the stem/progenitor cell compartment. Alternatively, autonomous Wnt signaling in a differentiated cell results in the acquisition of stem/progenitor cell characteristics and coincident cellular expansion. Ultimately, imbalances in proliferation, differentiation, and apoptosis of these cells favor tumor formation. Further extending the importance of the Wnt pathway in adrenocortical tumorigenesis, biallelic inactivation of *ZNRF3* (an ubiquitin ligase that is a negative regulator of the Frizzled receptor) has been described as the most common change in a large cohort of ACCs.[186] These mutations are mutually exclusive with those of the *CTNNB1* gene, further suggesting that either mutation resulting in increased Wnt signaling can have a causative role in adrenocortical tumorigenesis.

Insulinlike growth factor 2 As discussed earlier, the IGF system has an important role in adrenal organogenesis and homeostasis. The link between abnormal activation of the IGF system and adrenocortical tumorigenesis came from observations of patients with the Beckwith-Wiedemann syndrome (BWS). BWS is an overgrowth disorder characterized by organomegaly, congenital malformations, and a predisposition to embryonic tumors and adrenocortical cancer.[187] The cause of this disorder is an imprinting defect at the 11p15 region that leads to high postnatal levels of *IGF2*.[187] Very high expression levels of IGF2 are observed in ~90% of adult ACC.[188–190] Somatic parental isodisomy of the 11p15 locus have been described in these tumors.[191] Mutant mice overexpressing Igf2 show a BWS-like phenotype, including adrenal hyperplasia and cytomegaly. However, these mice do not develop ACTs.[192] In a recent study, Igf2-overexpressing mice were crossed with mutant mice that had stabilized beta-catenin (*Apc* mutant). The offspring of these mice that show both abnormalities develop bigger tumors than those mice with stabilized beta-catenin alone. In addition, malignant transformation occurred at an earlier age in mice harboring both increased Igf2 and stabilized beta-catenin than in the single mutant mice.[193] Taken together, the data support the role of *IGF2* in tumorigenesis and provide a rationale for molecular targeted therapy. However, although preclinical studies indicate that blocking the IGF1R (one of the most important mediators of the IGF2 mitogenic effects) had antigrowth effects in vitro and in vivo, phase I and phase II clinical studies combining different agents showed low therapeutic efficacy.[194–198] However, long-term antitumor activity was observed in a small cohort of patients. Molecular markers that can predict which patients would respond to IGF1R blockage would be extremely useful for personalized medicine.[35,196,197]

TP53 The *TP53* tumor suppressor gene is a critical component of DNA repair and the senescence pathways. The clinical association between *TP53* and ACC was identified in patients with Li-Fraumeni syndrome. This syndrome is caused by germline inactivating mutations of the *TP53* and is characterized by various types of early-onset malignant tumors, such as breast cancer, brain tumors, and sarcomas.[199] ACC is also a manifestation of the syndrome, occurring in ~10% of patients.[200] In sporadic ACC, somatic inactivating mutations of *TP53* are present in a significant proportion of cases (~25%–30%), usually associated with a more aggressive phenotype.[201,202] Among patients with sporadic ACC, germline *TP53* mutations are estimated to account for

~5%.[203,204] However, unlike in adults, the prevalence of germline *TP53* mutations in the pediatric population is high, ranging from 50% to 90%.[205–207]

Telomere maintenance machinery One of the fundamental properties of stem/progenitor cells is self-renewal; the ability to give rise to 2 daughter cells, at least 1 of which is an exact copy of the stem/progenitor cell. With each cell division and coincident DNA replication, the telomeres at the end of each chromosome shorten. Unabated, the chromosomes become too short to engage in further DNA replication. Moreover, the protective cap on the end of the chromosome is disassembled, leaving the chromosome short and unprotected. Such DNA is recognized as damaged DNA and can initiate the DNA damage response with the cell ultimately undergoing apoptosis or senescence. Therefore, to perpetually engage in cell division/self-renewal, stem/progenitor cells must maintain telomere length and protect the naked telomere end.[208] This task is accomplished by increased telomerase activity and by maintaining the integrity of the shelterin complex. The shelterin complex is a set of proteins that caps and protects the ends of the chromosomes and regulates the activity of the repair mechanisms and telomerase.[209] Telomere dysfunction is a universal feature in cancer. In order to expand its replicative potential, many cancers overexpress telomerase.[210] A recent study has shown that *TERT*, a gene that codes for the catalytic subunit of the telomerase enzyme, is frequently amplified in ACC.[186] The importance of the telomere maintenance mechanisms for both normal stem cell function and cancer can be exemplified by a mouse model. The adrenocortical dysplasia mouse (*acd*) bears mutations in the *ACD/TPP1* gene, which codes for 1 component of the shelterin complex.[211] Because the shelterin complex is critical for protecting the ends of chromosomes and ensuing complete replication of coding sequences, loss of function promotes nonproliferative states and may explain some of the phenotypes seen in the *acd* mouse. These mice display early-onset adrenal failure, with dysplasia and cytomegaly of the cortex. Crossing the *acd* mutant mice with *Tp*53 null mice results in rescue of adrenal senescence and overall dysplasia, highlighting the role of the DNA repair mechanisms in removing cells with dysfunctional telomeres from the pool.[212] Both the *acd/acd* mice and the *Tp*53$^{-/-}$ mice develop a spectrum of cancers during their lifespan. The cross between the two strains results in offspring with earlier onset of a larger spectrum of tumors, including ACC, suggesting that mutations that affect genes involved in telomere maintenance together with cell cycle checkpoint genes may act by synergistic mechanisms.[212]

Development and stem cell implications for adrenal cancers
Genetic profiling indicates that most cancers are clonal (derived from a single cell) but cells within a given cancer are heterogeneous in terms of both differentiation state and proliferation potential. The significant heterogeneity within a cancer may be a result of secondary mutations in daughter cells. Two models have been proposed to explain cancer cell proliferation potentials. The stochastic model predicts that all cells in a tumor are biologically equivalent and any heterogeneity is caused by extrinsic/environmental factors; every cancer cell has the ability to proliferate and metastasize.[213] In contrast, the cancer stem cell model posits that only a distinct, generally rare subpopulation of tumor cells possess the so-called stem cell potential and the ability to differentiate into multiple cell types in a cancer and originate new metastatic lesions.[213] The properties of such cells theoretically have a profound impact on therapeutics, because they are able to repopulate the tumor if they are not targeted by a given treatment. Subsets of cancer cells with these unique properties have been identified in a variety of cancers, including hematologic malignancies and breast, brain,

colon, and pancreatic cancers.[213] However, the discovery of cancer stem cells does not rule out the stochastic model, which may be more appropriate for some tumor types. Alternatively, both models may coexist in the same tumor, depending on the context (ie, tumor cells may undergo a phenomenon called stem cell plasticity, in which they may fluctuate in a range of different degrees of differentiation and stemness when challenged).[214,215]

Studies have been directed at determining whether ACCs expand through the stochastic or cancer stem cell model. Lichtenauer and colleagues[216] took advantage of the multidrug-resistant properties of progenitor cells to study the side population of the H295R human ACC cell line. Cells that are able to efflux the Hoescht 33342 vital dye by increased activity of members of the ATP-binding cassette family have been shown to have stem cell properties in a wide variety of tissues and tumor samples. Based on these properties, these cells can be sorted by fluorescence activated cell sorting (FACS) after being treated with Hoescht 33342. These cells, which constitute a small fraction of the total cell pool, are consequently called side populations. Side populations derived from the H295R cells showed a less differentiated phenotype in terms of steroidogenic enzyme expression. However, in contrast with other cancer stem cells, these cells do not show a difference in growth potential or resistance to cytotoxic drugs compared with the predominant population.[216] Furthermore, after the side population cells are maintained for some time in culture, they give rise to a population of cells similar to the original H295R culture in terms of differentiation and the proportion of cells with properties of side populations. Although these observations argue against the existence of cancer stem cells in the H295R cell line, it does not completely rule out this possibility. In addition, because the study used a cell line rather than cells directly isolated from patients with ACC, it remains unclear whether the side population with multidrug resistance properties is a major contributor to ACC initiation and/or maintenance.

As detailed in this article, the most common mutated genes in both adrenocortical hypoplasia and adrenocortical tumors are also stem/progenitor cell factors critical for proper adrenal development and homeostasis. It is reasonable to hypothesize that defects in the adrenocortical stem cells serve as drivers for a spectrum of adrenal disorders of growth and differentiation. Future studies using novel genomic approaches in tumor samples and model systems should provide insight into the genetic and cellular defects underlying these diseases of the adrenal cortex.

REFERENCES

1. Gruenwald P. Embryonic and postnatal development of the adrenal cortex, particularly the zona glomerulosa and accessory nodules. Anat Rec 1946;95: 391–421.
2. Hatano O, Takakusu A, Nomura M, et al. Identical origin of adrenal cortex and gonad revealed by expression profiles of Ad4BP/SF-1. Genes Cells 1996;1(7): 663–71.
3. Luo X, Ikeda Y, Parker KL. A cell-specific nuclear receptor is essential for adrenal and gonadal development and sexual differentiation. Cell 1994;77(4):481–90.
4. Morohashi K. The ontogenesis of the steroidogenic tissues. Genes Cells 1997; 2(2):95–106.
5. Le Douarin NM, Teillet MA. Experimental analysis of the migration and differentiation of neuroblasts of the autonomic nervous system and of neurectodermal mesenchymal derivatives, using a biological cell marking technique. Dev Biol 1974;41(1):162–84.

6. Doupe AJ, Landis SC, Patterson PH. Environmental influences in the development of neural crest derivatives: glucocorticoids, growth factors, and chromaffin cell plasticity. J Neurosci 1985;5(8):2119–42.

7. Hillarp NA, Hokfelt B. Evidence of adrenaline and noradrenaline in separate adrenal medullary cells. Acta Physiol Scand 1953;30(1):55–68.

8. Ce K, Hammer GD. Recent insights into organogenesis of the adrenal cortex. Trends Endocrinol Metab 2002;13(5):200–8.

9. Ehrhart-Bornstein M, Hinson JP, Bornstein SR, et al. Intraadrenal interactions in the regulation of adrenocortical steroidogenesis. Endocr Rev 1998;19(2):101–43.

10. Seidl K, Unsicker K. The determination of the adrenal medullary cell fate during embryogenesis. Dev Biol 1989;136(2):481–90.

11. Finotto S, Krieglstein K, Schober A, et al. Analysis of mice carrying targeted mutations of the glucocorticoid receptor gene argues against an essential role of glucocorticoid signalling for generating adrenal chromaffin cells. Development 1999;126(13):2935–44.

12. Gut P, Huber K, Lohr J, et al. Lack of an adrenal cortex in Sf1 mutant mice is compatible with the generation and differentiation of chromaffin cells. Development 2005;132(20):4611–9.

13. Bland M, Fowkes RC, Ingraham HA. Differential requirement for steroidogenic factor-1 gene dosage in adrenal development versus endocrine function. Mol Endocrinol 2004;18(4):941–52.

14. Huber K, Combs S, Ernsberger U, et al. Generation of neuroendocrine chromaffin cells from sympathoadrenal progenitors: beyond the glucocorticoid hypothesis. Ann N Y Acad Sci 2002;971:554–9.

15. Unsicker K, Huber K, Schutz G, et al. The chromaffin cell and its development. Neurochem Res 2005;30(6–7):921–5.

16. Johannisson E. The foetal adrenal cortex in the human. Its ultrastructure at different stages of development and in different functional states. Acta Endocrinol (Copenh) 1968;58(130):7.

17. Goto M, Piper Hanley K, Marcos J, et al. In humans, early cortisol biosynthesis provides a mechanism to safeguard female sexual development. J Clin Invest 2006;116(4):953–60.

18. Hanley NA, Rainey WE, Wilson DI, et al. Expression profiles of SF-1, DAX1, and CYP17 in the human fetal adrenal gland: potential interactions in gene regulation. Mol Endocrinol 2001;15(1):57–68.

19. Achermann JC, Meeks JJ, Jameson JL. Phenotypic spectrum of mutations in DAX-1 and SF-1. Mol Cell Endocrinol 2001;185(1–2):17–25.

20. El-Khairi R, Martinez-Aguayo A, Ferraz-de-Souza B, et al. Role of DAX-1 (NR0B1) and steroidogenic factor-1 (NR5A1) in human adrenal function. Endocr Dev 2011;20:38–46.

21. Wong M, Ikeda Y, Luo X, et al. Steroidogenic factor 1 plays multiple roles in endocrine development and function. Recent Prog Horm Res 1997;52:167–82.

22. Doghman M, Karpova T, Rodrigues GA, et al. Increased steroidogenic factor-1 dosage triggers adrenocortical cell proliferation and cancer. Mol Endocrinol 2007;21(12):2968–87.

23. Val P, Martinez-Barbera JP, Swain A. Adrenal development is initiated by Cited2 and Wt1 through modulation of Sf-1 dosage. Development 2007;134(12):2349–58.

24. Bandiera R, Vidal VP, Motamedi FJ, et al. WT1 maintains adrenal-gonadal primordium identity and marks a population of AGP-like progenitors within the adrenal gland. Dev Cell 2013;27(1):5–18.

25. Zubair M, Ishihara S, Oka S, et al. Two-step regulation of Ad4BP/SF-1 gene transcription during fetal adrenal development: initiation by a Hox-Pbx1-Prep1 complex and maintenance via autoregulation by Ad4BP/SF-1. Mol Cell Biol 2006; 26(11):4111–21.

26. Zubair M, Parker KL, Morohashi KI. Developmental links between the fetal and adult zones of the adrenal cortex revealed by lineage tracing. Mol Cell Biol 2008;28(23):7030–40.

27. Ahmad I, Paterson WF, Lin L, et al. A novel missense mutation in DAX-1 with an unusual presentation of X-linked adrenal hypoplasia congenita. Horm Res 2007; 68(1):32–7.

28. Mantovani G, De Menis E, Borretta G, et al. DAX1 and X-linked adrenal hypoplasia congenita: clinical and molecular analysis in five patients. Eur J Endocrinol 2006;154(5):685–9.

29. Wood M, Hammer GD. Adrenocortical stem and progenitor cells: unifying model of two proposed origins. Mol Cell Endocrinol 2011;336(1–2):206–12.

30. Scheys JO, Heaton JH, Hammer GD. Evidence of adrenal failure in aging Dax1-deficient mice. Endocrinology 2011;152(9):3430–9.

31. Gummow BM, Scheys JO, Cancelli VR, et al. Reciprocal regulation of a glucocorticoid receptor-steroidogenic factor-1 transcription complex on the Dax-1 promoter by glucocorticoids and adrenocorticotropic hormone in the adrenal cortex. Mol Endocrinol 2006;20(11):2711–23.

32. Kelly VR, Hammer GD. LRH-1 and Nanog regulate Dax1 transcription in mouse embryonic stem cells. Mol Cell Endocrinol 2011;332(1–2):116–24.

33. Khalfallah O, Rouleau M, Barbry P, et al. Dax-1 knockdown in mouse embryonic stem cells induces loss of pluripotency and multilineage differentiation. Stem Cells 2009;27(7):1529–37.

34. Feek CM, Marante DJ, Edwards CR. The hypothalamic-pituitary-adrenal axis. Clin Endocrinol Metab 1983;12(3):597–618.

35. Janes M, Chu KM, Clark AJ, et al. Mechanisms of adrenocorticotropin-induced activation of extracellularly regulated kinase 1/2 mitogen-activated protein kinase in the human H295R adrenal cell line. Endocrinology 2008;149(4): 1898–905.

36. Pepe GJ, Albrecht ED. Regulation of the primate fetal adrenal cortex. Endocr Rev 1990;11(1):151–76.

37. Rainey W, Rehman KS, Carr BR. Fetal and maternal adrenals in human pregnancy. Obstet Gynecol Clin North Am 2004;31(4):817–35.

38. Beshay V, Carr BR, Rainey WE. The human fetal adrenal gland, corticotropin-releasing hormone, and parturition. Semin Reprod Med 2007;25(1):14–20.

39. Hornsby PJ. Regulation of adrenocortical cell proliferation in culture. Endocr Res 1984;10(3–4):259–81.

40. Simpson ER, Waterman MR. Regulation by ACTH of steroid hormone biosynthesis in the adrenal cortex. Can J Biochem Cell Biol 1983;61(7):692–707.

41. LeRoith D, Roberts CT Jr. The insulin-like growth factor system and cancer. Cancer Lett 2003;195(2):127–37.

42. Vale W, Spiess J, Rivier C, et al. Characterization of a 41-residue ovine hypothalamic peptide that stimulates secretion of corticotropin and beta-endorphin. Science 1981;213(4514):1394–7.

43. Spiess J, Rivier J, Rivier C, et al. Primary structure of corticotropin-releasing factor from ovine hypothalamus. Proc Natl Acad Sci U S A 1981;78(10):6517–21.

44. Takahashi K, Totsune K, Saruta M, et al. Expression of urocortin 3/stresscopin in human adrenal glands and adrenal tumors. Peptides 2006;27(1):178–82.

45. Karteris E, Randeva HS, Grammatopoulos DK, et al. Expression and coupling characteristics of the CRH and orexin type 2 receptors in human fetal adrenals. J Clin Endocrinol Metab 2001;86(9):4512–9.

46. Fukuda T, Takahashi K, Suzuki T, et al. Urocortin 1, urocortin 3/stresscopin, and corticotropin-releasing factor receptors in human adrenal and its disorders. J Clin Endocrinol Metab 2005;90(8):4671–8.

47. Dermitzaki E, Tsatsanis C, Minas V, et al. Corticotropin-releasing factor (CRF) and the urocortins differentially regulate catecholamine secretion in human and rat adrenals, in a CRF receptor type-specific manner. Endocrinology 2007;148(4):1524–38.

48. Sirinanni R, Rehman KS, Carr BR, et al. Corticotropin-releasing hormone directly stimulates cortisol and the cortisol biosynthetic pathway in human fetal adrenal cells. J Clin Endocrinol Metab 2005;90(1):279–85.

49. Andreis PG, Neri G, Nussdorfer GG. Corticotropin-releasing hormone (CRH) directly stimulates corticosterone secretion by the rat adrenal gland. Endocrinology 1991;128(2):1198–200.

50. Willenberg HS, Bornstein SR, Hiroi N, et al. Effects of a novel corticotropin-releasing-hormone receptor type I antagonist on human adrenal function. Mol Psychiatry 2000;5(2):137–41.

51. Schwartz J, Huo JS, Piwien-Pilipuk G. Growth hormone regulated gene expression. Minerva Endocrinol 2002;27(4):231–41.

52. Backlin C, Rastad J, Skogseid B, et al. Immunohistochemical expression of insulin-like growth factor 1 and its receptor in normal and neoplastic human adrenal cortex. Anticancer Res 1995;15(6B):2453–9.

53. Brice AL, Cheetham JE, Bolton VN, et al. Temporal changes in the expression of the insulin-like growth factor II gene associated with tissue maturation in the human fetus. Development 1989;106(3):543–54.

54. Coulter CL, Goldsmith PC, Mesiano S, et al. Functional maturation of the primate fetal adrenal in vivo: I. Role of insulin-like growth factors (IGFs), IGF-I receptor, and IGF binding proteins in growth regulation. Endocrinology 1996;137(10): 4487–98.

55. Bendall SC, Stewart MH, Menendez P, et al. IGF and FGF cooperatively establish the regulatory stem cell niche of pluripotent human cells in vitro. Nature 2007;448(7157):1015–21.

56. Jiang F, Frederick TJ, Wood TL. IGF-I synergizes with FGF-2 to stimulate oligodendrocyte progenitor entry into the cell cycle. Dev Biol 2001;232(2): 414–23.

57. Pitetti JL, Calvel P, Romero Y, et al. Insulin and IGF1 receptors are essential for XX and XY gonadal differentiation and adrenal development in mice. PLoS Genet 2013;9(1):e1003160.

58. Morohashi K, Zubair M. The fetal and adult adrenal cortex. Mol Cell Endocrinol 2011;336(1–2):193–7.

59. Zubair M, Oka S, Parker KL, et al. Transgenic expression of Ad4BP/SF-1 in fetal adrenal progenitor cells leads to ectopic adrenal formation. Mol Endocrinol 2009;23(10):1657–67.

60. Schulte D, Shapiro I, Reincke M, et al. Expression and spatio-temporal distribution of differentiation and proliferation markers during mouse adrenal development. Gene Expr Patterns 2007;7(1–2):72–81.

61. Guasti L, Paul A, Laufer E, et al. Localization of Sonic hedgehog secreting and receiving cells in the developing and adult rat adrenal cortex. Mol Cell Endocrinol 2011;336(1–2):117–22.

62. King P, Paul A, Laufer E. Shh signaling regulates adrenocortical development and identifies progenitors of steroidogenic lineages. Proc Natl Acad Sci U S A 2009;106(50):21185–90.
63. Wood MA, Acharya A, Finco I, et al. Fetal adrenal capsular cells serve as progenitor cells for steroidogenic and stromal adrenocortical cell lineages in *M. musculus*. Development 2013;140(22):4522–32.
64. Ishimoto H, Jaffe RB. Development and function of the human fetal adrenal cortex: a key component in the feto-placental unit. Endocr Rev 2011;32(3):317–55.
65. Havelock J, Auchus RJ, Rainey WE. The rise in adrenal androgen biosynthesis: adrenarche. Semin Reprod Med 2004;22(4):337–47.
66. Rosenfield RL, Lucky AW. Acne, hirsutism, and alopecia in adolescent girls. Clinical expressions of androgen excess. Endocrinol Metab Clin North Am 1993;22(3):507–32.
67. Corvalan C, Uauy R, Mericq V. Obesity is positively associated with dehydroepiandrosterone sulfate concentrations at 7 y in Chilean children of normal birth weight. Am J Clin Nutr 2013;97(2):318–25.
68. l'Allemand D, Schmidt S, Rousson V, et al. Associations between body mass, leptin, IGF-I and circulating adrenal androgens in children with obesity and premature adrenarche. Eur J Endocrinol 2002;146(4):537–43.
69. Saenger P, Dimartino-Nardi J. Premature adrenarche. J Endocrinol Invest 2001; 24(9):724–33.
70. Pintor C, Loche S, Faedda A, et al. Adrenal androgens in obese boys before and after weight loss. Horm Metab Res 1984;16(10):544–8.
71. Howard E. The effect of dietary factors on the adrenal X zone. Fed Proc 1947; 6(1 Pt 2):133.
72. Tanaka S, Matsuzawa A. What mouse contributed the first representation of the adrenal cortex X zone? Jikken Dobutsu 1993;42(3):305–16 [in Japanese].
73. Nishimoto K, Nakagawa K, Li D, et al. Adrenocortical zonation in humans under normal and pathological conditions. J Clin Endocrinol Metab 2010;95(5): 2296–305.
74. Nakamura Y, Maekawa T, Felizola SJ, et al. Adrenal CYP11B1/2 expression in primary aldosteronism: immunohistochemical analysis using novel monoclonal antibodies. Mol Cell Endocrinol 2014;392(1–2):73–9.
75. Gomez-Sanchez CE, Qi X, Velarde-Miranda C, et al. Development of monoclonal antibodies against human CYP11B1 and CYP11B2. Mol Cell Endocrinol 2014;383(1–2):111–7.
76. Chamoux E, Otis M, Gallo-Payet N. A connection between extracellular matrix and hormonal signals during the development of the human fetal adrenal gland. Braz J Med Biol Res 2005;38(10):1495–503.
77. Chamoux E, Narcy A, Lehoux JG, et al. Fibronectin, laminin, and collagen IV as modulators of cell behavior during adrenal gland development in the human fetus. J Clin Endocrinol Metab 2002;87(4):1819–28.
78. Chamoux E, Bolduc L, Lehoux JG, et al. Identification of extracellular matrix components and their integrin receptors in the human fetal adrenal gland. J Clin Endocrinol Metab 2001;86(5):2090–8.
79. Otis M, Campbell S, Payet MD, et al. Expression of extracellular matrix proteins and integrins in rat adrenal gland: importance for ACTH-associated functions. J Endocrinol 2007;193(3):331–47.
80. Cheng CY, Hornsby PJ. Expression of 11 beta-hydroxylase and 21-hydroxylase in long-term cultures of bovine adrenocortical cells requires extracellular matrix factors. Endocrinology 1992;130(5):2883–9.

81. Filippi L, Sardella B, Ciorra A, et al. Tumor thrombus in the renal vein from an adrenal metastasis of lung cancer: 18FDG PET/CT findings. Cancer Biother Radiopharm 2014;29(5):189–92.

82. Puech A, Pages A, Comelade P. Cutaneous metastases as the first manifestation of a cancer of the lungs; adrenal metastasis; terminal acute adrenal insufficiency. Montp Med 1955;47(6):565–6 [in French].

83. Onuigbo WI. Lung cancer metastasis to adrenal cortical adenomas. J Pathol Bacteriol 1963;86:541–3.

84. Lever JD. Observations on the adrenal blood vessels in the rat. J Anat 1952; 86(4):459–67.

85. Anson BJ, Cauldwell EW, Beaton LE, et al. The blood supply of the kidney, suprarenal gland, and associated structures. Surg Gynecol Obstet 1947; 84(3):313–20.

86. Johnstone FR. The suprarenal veins. Am J Surg 1957;94(4):615–20.

87. Monkhouse WS, Khalique A. The adrenal and renal veins of man and their connections with azygos and lumbar veins. J Anat 1986;146:105–15.

88. Gagnon R. The venous drainage of the human adrenal gland. Rev Can Biol 1956;14(4):350–9.

89. Engeland WC. Functional innervation of the adrenal cortex by the splanchnic nerve. Horm Metab Res 1998;30(6–7):311–4.

90. Hinson JP, Cameron LA, Purbrick A, et al. The role of neuropeptides in the regulation of adrenal vascular tone: effects of vasoactive intestinal polypeptide, substance P, neuropeptide Y, neurotensin, Met-enkephalin, and Leu-enkephalin on perfusion medium flow rate in the intact perfused rat adrenal. Regul Pept 1994; 51(1):55–61.

91. Li Q, Johansson H, Kjellman M, et al. Neuroendocrine differentiation and nerves in human adrenal cortex and cortical lesions. APMIS 1998;106(8):807–17.

92. Burnay MM, Python CP, Vallotton MB, et al. Role of the capacitative calcium influx in the activation of steroidogenesis by angiotensin-II in adrenal glomerulosa cells. Endocrinology 1994;135(2):751–8.

93. Johnson BB, Lieberman AH, Mulrow PJ. Aldosterone excretion in normal subjects depleted of sodium and potassium. J Clin Invest 1957;36(6 Part 1):757–66.

94. Laragh JH, Stoerk HC. A study of the mechanism of secretion of the sodium-retaining hormone (aldosterone). J Clin Invest 1957;36(3):383–92.

95. McCaa RE, Gillespie JB. Effects of captopril and enalapril on sodium excretion and blood pressure in sodium-deficient dogs. Fed Proc 1984;43(5):1336–41.

96. Deane HW, Bergner GE. Chemical and cytochemical studies of the rat's adrenal cortex following the administration of pituitary adrenocorticotropic hormone (ACTH). J Clin Endocrinol Metab 1947;7(6):457.

97. Hills AG, Thorn GW. An estimation of the quantity of 11–17-oxysteroid excretion by the human adrenal stimulated by ACTH. J Clin Endocrinol Metab 1948;8(7): 606.

98. Mason HL, Power MH, Rynearson EH, et al. Results of administration of anterior pituitary adrenocorticotropic hormone to a normal human being. J Biol Chem 1947;169(1):223.

99. Ingle DJ, Prestrud MC, Li CH. A further study of the essentiality of the adrenal cortex in mediating the metabolic effects of adrenocorticotrophic hormone. Endocrinology 1948;43(4):202–7.

100. Bellamy D, Leonard RA. The effect of cortisol on the activity of glutamate-pyruvate transaminase and the formation of glycogen and urea in starved rats. Biochem J 1964;93(2):331–6.

101. Sie HG, Hablanian A, Fishman WH. Solubilization of mouse liver glycogen synthetase and phosphorylase during starvation glycogenolysis and its reversal by cortisol. Nature 1964;201:393–4.
102. Bandy HE, Darrach M, Newsom SE, et al. Metabolism of adrenal steroids in the mouse. I. Observations on 20alpha-dihydrocorticosterone and corticosterone in the plasma of mice treated with corticotropin. Can J Biochem Physiol 1956; 34(5):913–8.
103. Halberg F, Albrecht PG, Bittner JJ. Corticosterone rhythm of mouse adrenal in relation to serum corticosterone and sampling. Am J Physiol 1959;197:1083–5.
104. Halberg F, Haus E. Corticosterone in mouse adrenal in relation to sex and heterotopic pituitary isografting. Am J Physiol 1960;199:859–62.
105. Ortega E, Rodriguez C, Strand LJ, et al. Effects of cloprednol and other corticosteroids on hypothalamic-pituitary-adrenal axis function. J Int Med Res 1976; 4(5):326–37.
106. Storrs FJ. Use and abuse of systemic corticosteroid therapy. J Am Acad Dermatol 1979;1(2):95–106.
107. Conley AJ, Pattison JC, Bird IM. Variations in adrenal androgen production among (nonhuman) primates. Semin Reprod Med 2004;22(4):311–26.
108. Davison B, Large DM, Anderson DC, et al. Basal steroid production by the zona reticularis of the guinea-pig adrenal cortex. J Steroid Biochem 1983;18(3): 285–90.
109. Hyatt PJ, Bhatt K, Tait JF. Steroid biosynthesis by zona fasciculata and zona reticularis cells purified from the mammalian adrenal cortex. J Steroid Biochem 1983;19(1C):953–9.
110. Kaufman FR, Stanczyk FZ, Matteri RK, et al. Dehydroepiandrosterone and dehydroepiandrosterone sulfate metabolism in human genital skin. Fertil Steril 1990; 54(2):251–4.
111. Rosenfield RL. Hirsutism and the variable response of the pilosebaceous unit to androgen. J Investig Dermatol Symp Proc 2005;10(3):205–8.
112. Pelletier G. Expression of steroidogenic enzymes and sex-steroid receptors in human prostate. Best Pract Res Clin Endocrinol Metab 2008;22(2):223–8.
113. Rege J, Nakamura Y, Satoh F, et al. Liquid chromatography-tandem mass spectrometry analysis of human adrenal vein 19-carbon steroids before and after ACTH stimulation. J Clin Endocrinol Metab 2013;98(3):1182–8.
114. Pabon JE, Li X, Lei ZM, et al. Novel presence of luteinizing hormone/chorionic gonadotropin receptors in human adrenal glands. J Clin Endocrinol Metab 1996;81(6):2397–400.
115. Jaffe RB, Seron-Ferre M, Crickard K, et al. Regulation and function of the primate fetal adrenal gland and gonad. Recent Prog Horm Res 1981;37: 41–103.
116. Vuorenoja S, Rivero-Muller A, Kiiveri S, et al. Adrenocortical tumorigenesis, luteinizing hormone receptor and transcription factors GATA-4 and GATA-6. Mol Cell Endocrinol 2007;269(1–2):38–45.
117. Lacroix A, Hamet P, Boutin JM. Leuprolide acetate therapy in luteinizing hormone–dependent Cushing's syndrome. N Engl J Med 1999;341(21):1577–81.
118. Baker BL. A comparison of the histological changes induced by experimental hyperadrenocorticalism and inanition. Recent Prog Horm Res 1952;7:331.
119. Zwemer RL, Wotton RM, Norkus MG. A study of corticoadrenal cells. Anat Rec 1938;72(2):249–63.
120. Salmon TN, Zwemer RL. A study of the life history of cortico-adrenal gland cells of the rat by means of trypan blue injections. Anat Rec 1941;80(4):421–9.

121. Malendowicz LK, Dembinska M. Proliferation and distribution of adrenocortical cells in ACTH treated female hamsters. Folia Histochem Cytobiol 1990;28(1–2):51–9.

122. Stachowiak A, Nussdorfer GG, Malendowicz LK. Proliferation and distribution of adrenocortical cells in the gland of ACTH- or dexamethasone-treated rats. Histol Histopathol 1990;5(1):25–9.

123. Sasano H, Imatani A, Shizawa S, et al. Cell proliferation and apoptosis in normal and pathologic human adrenal. Mod Pathol 1995;8(1):11–7.

124. Morley SD, Viard I, Chung BC, et al. Variegated expression of a mouse steroid 21-hydroxylase/beta- galactosidase transgene suggests centripetal migration of adrenocortical cells. Mol Endocrinol 1996;10(5):585–98.

125. Ching S, Vilain E. Targeted disruption of Sonic Hedgehog in the mouse adrenal leads to adrenocortical hypoplasia. Genesis 2009;47(9):628–37.

126. Huang C, Miyagawa S, Matsumaru D, et al. Progenitor cell expansion and organ size of mouse adrenal is regulated by sonic hedgehog. Endocrinology 2010; 151(3):1119–28.

127. Alex K, Barlaskar FM, Heaton JH, et al. In search of adrenocortical stem and progenitor cells. Endocr Rev 2009;30(3):241–63.

128. Kim AC, Reuter AL, Zubair M, et al. Targeted disruption of beta-catenin in Sf1-expressing cells impairs development and maintenance of the adrenal cortex. Development 2008;135(15):2593–602.

129. Berthon A, Sahut-Barnola I, Lambert-Langlais S, et al. Constitutive beta-catenin activation induces adrenal hyperplasia and promotes adrenal cancer development. Hum Mol Genet 2010;19:1561–76.

130. Assie G, Guillaud-Bataille M, Ragazzon B, et al. The pathophysiology, diagnosis and prognosis of adrenocortical tumors revisited by transcriptome analyses. Trends Endocrinol Metab 2010;21(5):325–34.

131. Schteingart DE, Doherty GM, Gauger PG, et al. Management of patients with adrenal cancer: recommendations of an international consensus conference. Endocr Relat Cancer 2005;12(3):667–80.

132. Berthon A, Drelon C, Ragazzon B, et al. WNT/beta-catenin signalling is activated in aldosterone-producing adenomas and controls aldosterone production. Hum Mol Genet 2014;23(4):889–905.

133. Mizusaki H, Kawabe K, Mukai T, et al. Dax-1 (dosage-sensitive sex reversal-adrenal hypoplasia congenita critical region on the X chromosome, gene 1) gene transcription is regulated by wnt4 in the female developing gonad. Mol Endocrinol 2003;17(4):507–19.

134. Walczak EM, Kuick R, Finco I, et al. Wnt signaling inhibits adrenal steroidogenesis by cell-autonomous and non-cell-autonomous mechanisms. Mol Endocrinol 2014;28(9):1471–86.

135. Freedman BD, Kempna PB, Carlone DL, et al. Adrenocortical zonation results from lineage conversion of differentiated zona glomerulosa cells. Dev Cell 2013;26(6):666–73.

136. Arboleda VA, Lee H, Parnaik R, et al. Mutations in the PCNA-binding domain of CDKN1C cause IMAGe syndrome. Nat Genet 2012;44:788–92.

137. Achermann JC, Ito M, Hindmarsh PC, et al. A mutation in the gene encoding steroidogenic factor-1 causes XY sex reversal and adrenal failure in humans. Nat Genet 1999;22(2):125–6.

138. Habiby RL, Boepple P, Nachtigall L, et al. Adrenal hypoplasia congenita with hypogonadotropic hypogonadism: evidence that DAX-1 mutations lead to combined hypothalmic and pituitary defects in gonadotropin production. J Clin Invest 1996;98(4):1055–62.

139. Mandel H, Shemer R, Borochowitz ZU, et al. SERKAL syndrome: an autosomal-recessive disorder caused by a loss-of-function mutation in WNT4. Am J Hum Genet 2008;82(1):39–47.
140. Clark AJ, McLoughlin L, Grossman A. Familial glucocorticoid deficiency associated with point mutation in the adrenocorticotropin receptor. Lancet 1993; 341(8843):461–2.
141. Gineau L, Cognet C, Kara N, et al. Partial MCM4 deficiency in patients with growth retardation, adrenal insufficiency, and natural killer cell deficiency. J Clin Invest 2012;122(3):821–32.
142. Hughes CR, Guasti L, Meimaridou E, et al. MCM4 mutation causes adrenal failure, short stature, and natural killer cell deficiency in humans. J Clin Invest 2012; 122(3):814–20.
143. Meimaridou E, Kowalczyk J, Guasti L, et al. Mutations in NNT encoding nicotinamide nucleotide transhydrogenase cause familial glucocorticoid deficiency. Nat Genet 2012;44:740–2.
144. Jackson RS, Creemers JW, Farooqi IS, et al. Small-intestinal dysfunction accompanies the complex endocrinopathy of human proprotein convertase 1 deficiency. J Clin Invest 2003;112(10):1550–60.
145. Krude H, Biebermann H, Luck W, et al. Severe early-onset obesity, adrenal insufficiency and red hair pigmentation caused by POMC mutations in humans. Nat Genet 1998;19(2):155–7.
146. Dattani MT, Martinez-Barbera JP, Thomas PQ, et al. Mutations in the homeobox gene HESX1/Hesx1 associated with septo-optic dysplasia in human and mouse. Nat Genet 1998;19:125–33.
147. Wu W, Cogan JD, Pfäffle RW, et al. Mutations in PROP1 cause familial combined pituitary hormone deficiency. Nat Genet 1998;18:147–9.
148. Wettstein M, Diez LF, Twohig M, et al. The role of birth injury and the consequences of inadequately treated hypogonadism in longstanding panhypopituitarism. Conn Med 1996;60(10):583–6.
149. Cohen LE. Genetic disorders of the pituitary. Curr Opin Endocrinol Diabetes Obes 2012;19(1):33–9.
150. Speiser PW, Azziz R, Baskin LS, et al. Congenital adrenal hyperplasia due to steroid 21-hydroxylase deficiency: an Endocrine Society clinical practice guideline. J Clin Endocrinol Metab 2010;95(9):4133–60.
151. Nimkarn S, New MI. Prenatal diagnosis and treatment of congenital adrenal hyperplasia. Horm Res 2007;67(2):53–60.
152. Nimkarn S, Lin-Su K, New MI. Steroid 21 hydroxylase deficiency congenital adrenal hyperplasia. Pediatr Clin North Am 2011;58(5):1281–300.
153. Hauffa B, Hiort O. P450 side-chain cleavage deficiency–a rare cause of congenital adrenal hyperplasia. Endocr Dev 2011;20:54–62.
154. Krone N, Arlt W. Genetics of congenital adrenal hyperplasia. Best Pract Res Clin Endocrinol Metab 2009;23(2):181–92.
155. Lekarev O, Mallet D, Yuen T, et al. Congenital lipoid adrenal hyperplasia (a rare form of adrenal insufficiency and ambiguous genitalia) caused by a novel mutation of the steroidogenic acute regulatory protein gene. Eur J Pediatr 2012; 171(5):787–93.
156. Louiset E, Duparc C, Young J, et al. Intraadrenal corticotropin in bilateral macronodular adrenal hyperplasia. N Engl J Med 2013;369(22):2115–25.
157. Groussin L, Jullian E, Perlemoine K, et al. Mutations of the PRKAR1A gene in Cushing's syndrome due to sporadic primary pigmented nodular adrenocortical disease. J Clin Endocrinol Metab 2002;87:4324–9.

158. Lacroix A. ACTH-independent macronodular adrenal hyperplasia. Best Pract Res Clin Endocrinol Metab 2009;23:245–59.
159. Ghayee HK, Rege J, Watumull LM, et al. Clinical, biochemical, and molecular characterization of macronodular adrenocortical hyperplasia of the zona reticularis: a new syndrome. J Clin Endocrinol Metab 2011;96:E243–50.
160. Hayashi Y, Takeda Y, Kaneko K, et al. A case of Cushing's syndrome due to ACTH-independent bilateral macronodular hyperplasia associated with excessive secretion of mineralocorticoids. Endocr J 1998;45:485–91.
161. Lerario AM, Moraitis A, Hammer GD. Genetics and epigenetics of adrenocortical tumors. Mol Cell Endocrinol 2014;386:67–84.
162. Espiard S, Ragazzon B, Bertherat J. Protein kinase A alterations in adrenocortical tumors. Horm Metab Res 2014;8:8.
163. Grumbach MM, Biller BM, Braunstein GD, et al. Management of the clinically inapparent adrenal mass ("incidentaloma"). Ann Intern Med 2003;138:424–9.
164. Arnaldi G, Boscaro M. Adrenal incidentaloma. Best Pract Res Clin Endocrinol Metab 2012;26:405–19.
165. Mulatero P, Stowasser M, Loh KC, et al. Increased diagnosis of primary aldosteronism, including surgically correctable forms, in centers from five continents. J Clin Endocrinol Metab 2004;89(3):1045–50.
166. Fernandes-Rosa FL, Williams TA, Riester A, et al. Genetic spectrum and clinical correlates of somatic mutations in aldosterone-producing adenoma. Hypertension 2014;64(2):354–61.
167. Choi M, Scholl UI, Yue P, et al. K+ channel mutations in adrenal aldosterone-producing adenomas and hereditary hypertension. Science 2011;331(6018): 768–72.
168. Krapivinsky G, Gordon EA, Wickman K, et al. The G-protein-gated atrial K+ channel IKACh is a heteromultimer of two inwardly rectifying K(+)-channel proteins. Nature 1995;374(6518):135–41.
169. Monticone S, Hattangady NG, Nishimoto K, et al. Effect of KCNJ5 mutations on gene expression in aldosterone-producing adenomas and adrenocortical cells. J Clin Endocrinol Metab 2012;97(8):2011–3132.
170. Monticone S, Else T, Mulatero P, et al. Understanding primary aldosteronism: impact of next generation sequencing and expression profiling. Mol Cell Endocrinol 2015;399:311–20.
171. Cao Y, He M, Gao Z, et al. Activating hotspot L205R mutation in PRKACA and adrenal Cushing's syndrome. Science 2014;344:913–7.
172. Goh G, Scholl UI, Healy JM, et al. Recurrent activating mutation in PRKACA in cortisol-producing adrenal tumors. Nat Genet 2014;46:613–7.
173. Sato Y, Maekawa S, Ishii R, et al. Recurrent somatic mutations underlie corticotropin-independent Cushing's syndrome. Science 2014;344:917–20.
174. Kebebew E, Reiff E, Duh QY, et al. Extent of disease at presentation and outcome for adrenocortical carcinoma: have we made progress? World J Surg 2006;30(5):872–8.
175. Kerkhofs TM, Verhoeven RH, Van der Zwan JM, et al. Adrenocortical carcinoma: a population-based study on incidence and survival in the Netherlands since 1993. Eur J Cancer 2013;49(11):2579–86.
176. Abiven G, Coste J, Groussin L, et al. Clinical and biological features in the prognosis of adrenocortical cancer: poor outcome of cortisol-secreting tumors in a series of 202 consecutive patients. J Clin Endocrinol Metab 2006;91:2650–5.
177. Wajchenberg BL, Albergaria Pereira MA, Medonca BB, et al. Adrenocortical carcinoma: clinical and laboratory observations. Cancer 2000;88:711–36.

178. Fassnacht M, Allolio B. Clinical management of adrenocortical carcinoma. Best Pract Res Clin Endocrinol Metab 2009;23:273–89.
179. Beuschlein F, Reincke M, Karl M, et al. Clonal composition of human adrenocortical neoplasms. Cancer Res 1994;54:4927–32.
180. Gicquel C, Leblond-Francillard M, Bertagna X, et al. Clonal analysis of human adrenocortical carcinomas and secreting adenomas. Clin Endocrinol 1994;40:465–77.
181. Kartheuser A, Walon C, West S, et al. Familial adenomatous polyposis associated with multiple adrenal adenomas in a patient with a rare 3' APC mutation. J Med Genet 1999;36:65–7.
182. Marshall WH, Martin FI, Mackay IR. Gardner's syndrome with adrenal carcinoma. Australas Ann Med 1967;16:242–4.
183. Kim W, Kim M, Jho EH. Wnt/β-catenin signalling: from plasma membrane to nucleus. Biochem J 2013;450:9–21.
184. Tissier F, Cavard C, Groussin L, et al. Mutations of beta-catenin in adrenocortical tumors: activation of the Wnt signaling pathway is a frequent event in both benign and malignant adrenocortical tumors. Cancer Res 2005;65:7622–7.
185. Tadjine M, Lampron A, Ouadi L, et al. Frequent mutations of beta-catenin gene in sporadic secreting adrenocortical adenomas. Clin Endocrinol 2008;68: 264–70.
186. Assié G, Letouzé E, Fassnacht M, et al. Integrated genomic characterization of adrenocortical carcinoma. Nat Genet 2014;46:607–12.
187. Choufani S, Shuman C, Weksberg R. Beckwith-Wiedemann syndrome. Am J Med Genet C Semin Med Genet 2010;154C:343–54.
188. Gicquel C, Bertagna X, Gaston V, et al. Molecular markers and long-term recurrences in a large cohort of patients with sporadic adrenocortical tumors. Cancer Res 2001;61:6762–7.
189. Giordano TJ, Kuick R, Else T, et al. Molecular classification and prognostication of adrenocortical tumors by transcriptome profiling. Clin Cancer Res 2009;15: 668–76.
190. Giordano TJ, Thomas DG, Kuick R, et al. Distinct transcriptional profiles of adrenocortical tumors uncovered by DNA microarray analysis. Am J Pathol 2003; 162:521–31.
191. Gicquel C, Raffin-Sanson ML, Gaston V, et al. Structural and functional abnormalities at 11p15 are associated with the malignant phenotype in sporadic adrenocortical tumors: study on a series of 82 tumors. J Clin Endocrinol Metab 1997; 82:2559–65.
192. Weber MM, Fottner C, Schmidt P, et al. Postnatal overexpression of insulin-like growth factor II in transgenic mice is associated with adrenocortical hyperplasia and enhanced steroidogenesis. Endocrinology 1999;140:1537–43.
193. Heaton JH, Wood MA, Kim AC, et al. Progression to adrenocortical tumorigenesis in mice and humans through insulin-like growth factor 2 and beta-catenin. Am J Pathol 2012;181(3):1017–33.
194. Almeida MQ, Fragoso MC, Lotfi CF, et al. Expression of insulin-like growth factor-II and its receptor in pediatric and adult adrenocortical tumors. J Clin Endocrinol Metab 2008;93:3524–31.
195. Barlaskar FM, Spalding AC, Heaton JH, et al. Preclinical targeting of the type I insulin-like growth factor receptor in adrenocortical carcinoma. J Clin Endocrinol Metab 2009;94:204–12.
196. Haluska P, Worden F, Olmos D, et al. Safety, tolerability, and pharmacokinetics of the anti-IGF-1R monoclonal antibody figitumumab in patients with refractory adrenocortical carcinoma. Cancer Chemother Pharmacol 2010;65:765–73.

197. Lerario AM, Worden FP, Ramm CA, et al. The combination of insulin-like growth factor receptor 1 (IGF1R) antibody cixutumumab and mitotane as a first-line therapy for patients with recurrent/metastatic adrenocortical carcinoma: a multi-institutional NCI-sponsored trial. Horm Cancer 2014;5:232–9.

198. Naing A, Lorusso P, Fu S, et al. Insulin growth factor receptor (IGF-1R) antibody cixutumumab combined with the mTOR inhibitor temsirolimus in patients with metastatic adrenocortical carcinoma. Br J Cancer 2013;108:826–30.

199. Li FP, Fraumeni JF, Mulvihill JJ, et al. A cancer family syndrome in twenty-four kindreds. Cancer Res 1988;48:5358–62.

200. Bougeard G, Sesboüé R, Baert-Desurmont S, et al. Molecular basis of the Li-Fraumeni syndrome: an update from the French LFS families. J Med Genet 2008;45(8):535–8.

201. Libè R, Groussin L, Tissier F, et al. Somatic TP53 mutations are relatively rare among adrenocortical cancers with the frequent 17p13 loss of heterozygosity. Clin Cancer Res 2007;13:844–50.

202. Waldmann J, Patsalis N, Fendrich V, et al. Clinical impact of TP53 alterations in adrenocortical carcinomas. Langenbecks Arch Surg 2012;397:209–16.

203. Herrmann LJ, Heinze B, Fassnacht M, et al. TP53 germline mutations in adult patients with adrenocortical carcinoma. J Clin Endocrinol Metab 2012;97:E476–85.

204. Raymond VM, Else T, Everett JN, et al. Prevalence of germline TP53 mutations in a prospective series of unselected patients with adrenocortical carcinoma. J Clin Endocrinol Metab 2013;98:E119–25.

205. Ribeiro RC, Sandrini F, Figueiredo B, et al. An inherited p53 mutation that contributes in a tissue-specific manner to pediatric adrenal cortical carcinoma. Proc Natl Acad Sci U S A 2001;98:9330–5.

206. Varley JM, McGown G, Thorncroft M, et al. Are there low-penetrance TP53 Alleles? evidence from childhood adrenocortical tumors. Am J Hum Genet 1999;65:995–1006.

207. Wagner J, Portwine C, Rabin K, et al. High frequency of germline p53 mutations in childhood adrenocortical cancer. J Natl Cancer Inst 1994;86:1707–10.

208. Choudhary B, Karande AA, Raghavan SC. Telomere and telomerase in stem cells: relevance in ageing and disease. Front Biosci 2012;4:16–30.

209. Ju Z, Rudolph KL. Telomeres and telomerase in stem cells during aging and disease. Genome Dyn 2006;1:84–103.

210. Kim NW, Piatyszek MA, Prowse KR, et al. Specific association of human telomerase activity with immortal cells and cancer. Science 1994;266:2011–5.

211. Keegan CE, Hutz JE, Else T, et al. Urogenital and caudal dysgenesis in adrenocortical dysplasia (acd) mice is caused by a splicing mutation in a novel telomeric regulator. Hum Mol Genet 2005;14:113–23.

212. Else T, Trovato A, Kim AC, et al. Genetic p53 deficiency partially rescues the adrenocortical dysplasia phenotype at the expense of increased tumorigenesis. Cancer Cell 2009;15(6):465–76.

213. Shackleton M, Quintana E, Fearon ER, et al. Heterogeneity in cancer: cancer stem cells versus clonal evolution. Cell 2009;138:822–9.

214. Gupta PB, Fillmore CM, Jiang G, et al. Stochastic state transitions give rise to phenotypic equilibrium in populations of cancer cells. Cell 2011;146:633–44.

215. Welte Y, Adjaye J, Lehrach HR, et al. Cancer stem cells in solid tumors: elusive or illusive? Cell communication and signaling. Cell Commun Signal 2010;8:6.

216. Lichtenauer UD, Shapiro I, Geiger K, et al. Side population does not define stem cell-like cancer cells in the adrenocortical carcinoma cell line NCI h295R. Endocrinology 2008;149(3):1314–22.

Adrenal Steroidogenesis and Congenital Adrenal Hyperplasia

Adina F. Turcu, MD[a], Richard J. Auchus, MD, PhD[a,b],*

KEYWORDS

- Steroidogenesis • Congenital adrenal hyperplasia • 21-Hydroxylase • Androgen
- Steroid hydroxylase • Adrenal insufficiency • Ambiguous genitalia
- Disorder of sex development

KEY POINTS

- Steroidogenesis in the adrenal gland reflects the zone-specific expression of enzymes, which comprise pathways to efficiently complete the biosynthesis of aldosterone, cortisol, and dehydroepiandrosterone sulfate.
- The most common form of congenital adrenal hyperplasia is 21-hydroxylase deficiency, in which a block in cortisol biosynthesis shifts precursors to pathways that make excess adrenal-derived androgens.
- Nonclassic 21-hydroxylase deficiency differs from the classic form in that cortisol deficiency and virilization of newborn girls are absent.
- Treatment of classic 21-hydroxylase deficiency consists of glucocorticoid and mineralocorticoid replacement, and for both classic and nonclassic disease, sufficient glucocorticoid is administered to correct the androgen excess.
- Patients with 21-hydroxylase deficiency are prone to developing adrenal cortical adenomas and myelolipomas as well as adrenal rest tumors in the testis or elsewhere.

ADRENAL STEROIDOGENESIS

Adrenal steroidogenesis is a dynamic process, reliant on de novo synthesis, with no presynthesized hormones stored for immediate release. Cholesterol is the common precursor for all steroids and is efficiently converted along a series of steps to the final product. To initiate steroidogenesis, cholesterol is mobilized from a pool in the outer

The authors have nothing to disclose.
[a] Division of Metabolism, Endocrinology, & Diabetes, Department of Internal Medicine, University of Michigan, Ann Arbor, MI 48109, USA; [b] Department of Pharmacology, University of Michigan, Room 5560A MSRBII, 1150 West Medical Center Drive, Ann Arbor, MI 48109, USA
* Corresponding author. Division of Metabolism, Endocrinology, & Diabetes, Department of Internal Medicine, University of Michigan, Room 5560A MSRBII, 1150 West Medical Center Drive, Ann Arbor, MI 48109.
E-mail address: rauchus@med.umich.edu

Endocrinol Metab Clin N Am 44 (2015) 275–296
http://dx.doi.org/10.1016/j.ecl.2015.02.002
0889-8529/15/$ – see front matter © 2015 Elsevier Inc. All rights reserved.
endo.theclinics.com

mitochondrial membrane (OMM),[1] which is replenished from cytosolic storage droplets of cholesterol esters. The steroidogenic acute regulatory (StAR) protein enables cholesterol transfer from the OMM to the inner mitochondrial membrane,[2] where the sidechain cleavage enzyme (CYP11A1, P450scc) catalyzes the first and rate-limiting step of steroidogenesis: the conversion of cholesterol to pregnenolone (**Fig. 1**A).[1,3]

Aldosterone Biosynthesis

Mineralocorticoid synthesis occurs in the zona glomerulosa (ZG) and requires the subsequent action of 3 enzymes: (1) 3β-hydroxysteroid dehydrogenase type 2 (HSD3B2), which performs the irreversible conversion of the hydroxyl group to a keto group on carbon 3 and simultaneous isomerization of the double bond from the Δ^5 to the Δ^4 position[4]; (2) 21-hydroxylase (CYP21A2, P450c21), which converts progesterone into 11-deoxycosticosterone; (3) aldosterone synthase (CYP11B2, P450c11AS), which catalyzes the final 3 steps of aldosterone synthesis: 11β-hydroxylation, 18-hydroxylation, and 18-methyl oxidation. The 18-aldehyde group, from which the name "aldosterone" derives, forms an intramolecular cyclic hemiacetal using the 11β-hydroxyl group, with loss of water.

The ZG is optimized for aldosterone synthesis: it is the only zone that has CYP11B2 and, in contrast, has little 17α-hydroxylase/17,20-lyase (CYP17A1, P450c17), an enzyme that directs steroids substrates toward cortisol and androgens synthesis (see **Fig. 1**B).[5] Angiotensin 2 and high extracellular potassium are the main stimulators of aldosterone synthesis, via increased intracellular calcium.[6]

Cortisol Biosynthesis

The glucocorticoid cortisol is synthesized in the zona fasciculata (ZF) under the regulation of adrenocorticotropin (ACTH). CYP17A1 catalyzes the 17α-hydroxylation of pregnenolone and progesterone with roughly equal efficiency, and this reaction leads to cortisol production. In addition, CYP17A1 subsequently cleaves the C17-C20 bond of 17-hydroxypregnenolone and to a much lesser degree of 17-hydroxyprogesterone (17OHP), which leads to 19-carbon (C_{19}) steroids (see **Fig. 1**A). Both reactions occur in a single active site, but with different regulation, as discussed later. With the activities of HDS3B2 and CYP21A2, which perform reactions similar to those on the mineralocorticoid pathway, 17-hydroxysteroids are converted to 11-deoxycortisol. Last, 11β-hydroxylase (CYP11B1, P450c11β), an enzyme closely related to CYP11B2, completes the synthesis of cortisol. In rodents and many small animals, the ZF lacks CYP17A1. Consequently, nascent progesterone is 21-hydroxylated and 11β-hydroxylated to yield corticosterone, which is the dominant glucocorticoid in these species, but it is ordinarily a minor product of the human adrenal.

Adrenal Androgen Biosynthesis

Adrenal C_{19} steroids are synthesized in the zona reticularis (ZR). Dehydroepiandrosterone (DHEA) is converted to its sulfate (DHEAS), which is the most abundant adrenal steroid. CYP17A1 is the only enzyme required for DHEA synthesis from pregnenolone and for androstenedione (AD) synthesis from progesterone. Although CYP17A1 is present in both ZF and ZR, its 17,20-lyase reaction is enhanced approximately 10 times by the cofactor cytochrome b_5 (CYB5A), which is absent in the ZF (see **Fig. 1**B).[7] Sulfotransferase SULT2A1 conjugates DHEA to DHEAS, a steroid with an important role in the regulation of adrenal androgen synthesis.[8] The adrenal synthesizes small amounts of testosterone, by the action of 17β-hydroxysteroid dehydrogenase type 5 (17βHSD5, AKR1C3) on AD (see **Fig. 1**A).

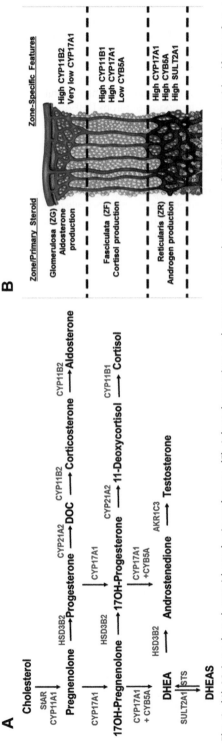

Fig. 1. (A) Major adrenal steroid synthesis pathways. (B) Adrenal zonation and enzyme expression pattern. SULTA1/STS, steroid sulfotransferase type 2A1.

ACTH is the primary stimulus of steroidogenesis in the ZR and is required for ZR development.[9,10] Additional growth factors have been postulated to regulate adrenal androgen synthesis and to control the development of the ZR, but these remain poorly understood. The ZR resembles the fetal adrenal, which provides the C_{19} substrate for estrogen synthesis during pregnancy but involutes at birth. The ZR is only a few cells thick at birth but expands during childhood, leading to an increase in circulating DHEAS and the phenomenon of adrenarche, which manifests as the development of axillary and pubic hair. ZR function and serum DHEAS peak about age 25 and then gradually decline, falling to childhood values in the seventh or eighth decade of life.

CONGENITAL ADRENAL HYPERPLASIA
Definition and Classification

Congenital adrenal hyperplasia (CAH) refers to a group of inherited enzymatic defects in cortisol biosynthesis. Impaired cortisol production relieves negative feedback to the hypothalamus and the pituitary gland, which in response amplify the secretion of corticotropin-releasing hormone (CRH) and ACTH, respectively, resulting in hyperplasia of the adrenal cortex. The spectrum of enzymatic deficiencies ranges from mild to complete and from a single activity to several activities. Steroid 21-hydroxylase deficiency (21OHD) accounts for greater than 90% of CAH cases.[11] Conventionally, 21OHD is dichotomized into classic and nonclassic forms, based on the presence or absence of cortisol insufficiency. The classic forms of 21OHD are further grouped into "salt wasting" and "simple virilizing" subtypes, depending on whether mineralocorticoid synthesis is sufficiently impaired to cause spontaneous hypotensive crises in the infant.

Other forms of CAH are summarized in **Table 1**. For additional information, the reader is directed to recent reviews and articles on deficiencies in CYP17A1,[12] CYP11B1,[13] HSD3B2,[14] lipoid CAH,[15] cholesterol side-cleavage enzyme (P450scc),[16] and P450-oxidoreductase (POR).[17] This review further expands the discussion of 21OHD.

Epidemiology

Classic 21OHD occurs in 1 of 16,000 live births worldwide.[18] Nonclassic 21OHD is much more frequent, occurring in approximately 1 of 1000 Caucasians and more commonly in certain ethnic groups, such as Ashkenazi Jews (1:27), Hispanics (1:53), Yugoslavs (1:62), and Italians (1:300).[19] The reason classic 21OHD has a similar prevalence throughout most of the world is related to the structure of the RCCX locus, which contains the tandemly arranged RP protein kinase, C4, CYP21, and tenascin X genes, which are duplicated together, as a discrete genetic unit.

Genetics

All forms of CAH are inherited in a monogenic, autosomal-recessive pattern. Human CYP21A2 is encoded by the *CYP21A2* gene, on chromosome 6p21.3, within the HLA major histocompatibility complex and adjacent to the genes for the fourth component of complement.[20–22] Only 30 kb away resides the nonfunctional *CYP21A1P* pseudogene, which encodes a truncated, inactive enzyme. Both *CYP21A2* and *CYP21A1P* contain 10 exons, and the 2 genes share 98% homology. Most mutant 21OHD alleles result from intergenic recombinations and gene conversion events between the 2 CYP21A genes.[23] Complete deletions, large gene conversions, and nonsense or frame-shift mutations that completely ablate CYP21A2 activity typically result in salt-wasting forms of CAH. Mutations resulting in even 1% to 2% residual enzyme activity allow sufficient aldosterone production and lead to simple virilizing forms of CAH. Nonclassic 21OHD patients retain up to 20% of the enzyme

Table 1
Rare forms of congenital adrenal hyperplasia

Defective Enzyme	Gene/Chromosome	Incidence and Populations	Clinical Features	Laboratory Findings
CYP11B1 (P450c11β)	CYP11B1/8q24.3	1:200,000 newborns High prevalence in Moroccan Jews	Hypertension in most patients; hypokalemia; hyperandrogenemia and virilization	↑: 11DOC, 11-deoxycortisol, AD, T ↓: aldosterone, cortisol
17-Hyroxylase/17,20-lyase (P450c17)	CYP17A1/10q21-q22	1:50,000 newborns; 2nd most common CAH form in Brazil	Hypertension, hypokalemia, and hypogonadism; 46,XX: primary amenorrhea and absence of secondary sexual characteristics 46,XY: undervirilization, abdominal testes	↑: progesterone, 11DOC, corticosterone; LH and FSH ↓: cortisol, DHEA, DHEAS, AD, T
HSD3B2	HSD3B2/1p13.1	Rare	Volume depletion, hyponatremia, and hyperkalemia 46,XX: mild clitoromegaly 46,XY: undervirilization from hypospadias to female-appearing	↑: Δ5 steroids-pregnenolone, 17OH-pregnenolone, DHEA, DHEAS ↓: cortisol, aldosterone
Steroidogenic acute regulatory protein (StAR, Lipoid CAH)	STAR/8p11.2	More frequent in Japanese, Palestinians, Koreans	Adrenal insufficiency; enlarged, lipid-laden adrenal glands. Female phenotype of external genitalia in both sexes	All steroids decreased
Cholesterol side-chain cleavage enzyme (P450scc)	CYP11A1/15q23-q24	Isolated cases reported	Adrenal insufficiency; adrenal glands may appear absent	All steroids decreased
POR	POR/7q11.2	Rare; more common in Japan and Korea	Volume depletion, skeletal malformations (Antley-Bixler); maternal virilization 46,XX: mild-to-moderate virilization 46,XY: undervirilization from hypospadias to female-appearing	Highly variable profiles, multiple partial defects ↑: progesterone; 11DOC, corticosterone, 17OHP variably high ↓: cortisol, aldosterone, androgens, and estrogens

Abbreviations: 11DOC, 11-deoxycorticosterone; AD, androstenedione; CYP11B1, 11β-hydroxylase; DHEA, dehydroepiandrosterone; DHEAS, DHEA sulfate; FSH, follicle-stimulating hormone; HSD3B2, 3β-hydroxysteroid dehydrogenase type 2; LH, luteinizing hormone; POR, P450-oxidoreductase deficiency; T, testosterone.

activity and do not have adrenal insufficiency. Nonclassic 21OHD patients may be either compound heterozygotes (with one classic allele and one nonclassic allele) or heterozygotes with 2 nonclassic alleles. Although the most severe and mildest forms of the disease tend to maintain some genotype-phenotype correlation, the intermediate forms are often poorly linked with specific gene defects, suggesting other contributors (genetic or environmental) to the phenotypical expression.[23]

Biochemistry of 21-Hydroxylase Deficiency

As a result of 21-hydroxylase dysfunction, upstream steroid precursors accumulate and are diverted toward accessible pathways to form potent androgens (**Fig. 2**). Elevations of 17OHP, the main substrate of CYP21A2, are a hallmark of 21OHD, and 17OHP has traditionally been used for both diagnosis and monitoring of the disease. In addition, the CYP21A2 blockage promotes the buildup of other C_{21} steroids. Human CYP17A1 hydroxylates pregnenolone and progesterone in position 17 with equal efficiencies, but also 16α-hydroxylates up to 30% of progesterone.[24] In the normal pathways to aldosterone and cortisol, progesterone and 17OHP are first hydroxylated at position 21 by CYP21A2, and subsequently at other positions. In 21OHD, progesterone and 17OHP accumulate and are substrates for CYP11B1, leading to 11β-hydroxyprogesterone and 21-deoxycortisol (21dF), respectively.

The excess 17OHP resulting from CYP21A2 deficiency is diverted through the pathways left accessible, to form potent androgens, such as testosterone and 5α-dihydrotestosterone (DHT). CYP17A1 mediates the conversion of 17-hydroxypregnenolone to DHEA (Δ^5 pathway) and of 17OHP to AD (Δ^4 pathway). The catalytic efficiency of the

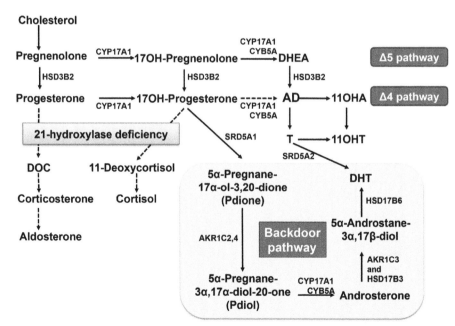

Fig. 2. Pathways of steroid hormone synthesis in 21-OHD, including backdoor pathway and 11-oxygenated androgens. AD, androstenedione; AKR1C2,4, aldo-keto reductase types 1C2 and 1C4; CYB5A, cytochrome b₅; CYP17A1, 17α-hydroxylase/17,20-lyase; DHEA, dehydroepiandrosterone; HSD17B6, 17β-hydroxysteroid dehydrogenase type 6 (an oxidative 3α-HSD); SRD5A1/2, 5α-reductase, types 1 and 2; T, testosterone; 11OHA, 11β-hydroxyandrostenedione; 11OHT, 11β-hydroxytestosterone.

human 17,20-lyase, however, is approximately 100 times greater for the Δ^5 reaction, as compared with the Δ^4 reaction,[25] explaining the enormous 17OHP accumulation in 21OHD. In patients with 21OHD, significant AD synthesis might still occur via the Δ^4 pathway due to very high intra-adrenal 17OHP.

More recently, a third potential fate of 17OHP has been suggested in patients with 21OHD: androgen synthesis via the "backdoor pathway" (see **Fig. 2**). This pathway was initially described a decade ago in tammar wallabies, whose testes produce 5α-androstane-3α,17β-diol (5αAdiol) rather than testosterone.[26] The 17OHP is first 5α-reduced, then 3α-reduced, and only subsequently undergoes 17,20-lyase cleavage, to form androsterone. After 17β-reduction to 5αAdiol, circulating 5αAdiol is 3α-oxidized to produce DHT in target tissues such as genital skin and prostate, thus bypassing the conventional androgens AD and testosterone as intermediates. This pathway might contribute to the virilization of female fetuses with CAH.[27] Kamrath and colleagues[28] were the first to demonstrate increased excretion of 5α-reduced products and intermediates of the backdoor pathway in 142 patients with CAH between 1 and 25 years old, compared with 138 similarly aged controls. Using gas chromatography/mass spectrometry (MS), they found significantly increased urinary excretion of 5α-pregnane-3α,17α-diol-20-one, the critical intermediate and a specific marker of the backdoor pathway, in patients with 21OHD. Furthermore, they reported 7-fold elevations of urinary androsterone, the dominant 5α-reduced C_{19} steroid derived from both classical and backdoor pathways, in children and young adults with 21OHD. In contrast, they found only a 2-fold elevation in etiocholanolone, the 5β-reduced C_{19} derived only from the classical pathways. Importantly, 5α-/5β-reduced cortisol metabolites ratios were not different in controls and 21OHD, excluding a general increase in 5α-reductase activity to explain their data.[28]

Diagnosis

Diagnosis of 21OHD relies on elevated 17OHP, one of the direct substrates of the deficient enzyme. The 17OHP levels are reflective of disease severity. Most patients with classic 21OHD have 17OHP levels consistently greater than 10,000 ng/dL, whereas unaffected patients typically have baseline 17OHP values less than 200 ng/dL.[29] In nonclassic 21OHD, a random 17OHP is often equivocal, and post-cosyntropin values greater than 1000 ng/dL are required to make the diagnosis. A few nonclassic 21OHD patients who are compound heterozygotes for classic and nonclassic alleles will have stimulated 17OHP values greater than 10,000 ng/dL, but by definition, they lack clinically significant adrenal insufficiency, with stimulated cortisol values greater than 14 μg/dL.

Newborn screening

Screening of newborns for CAH is performed in all 50 states of the United States. Screening decreases time to diagnosis and improves morbidity and mortality,[30–33] particularly by preventing salt wasting crises. Male newborns with CAH are more likely to not be diagnosed early clinically, because they do not exhibit genital ambiguity at birth.

First-tier screening uses dried blood spots on standard screening cards and measures 17OHP by immunofluorometric assay (DELFIA). A very high random 17OHP (>20,000 ng/dL) is diagnostic of 21OHD. False-positive results, however, are common in premature and severely ill infants.[34,35] Thus, weight and gestational age-adjusted cutoffs for 17OHP improve the positive predictive value of screening.[36–38] False negative rates of up to 22% have been reported in infant screening,[39,40] particularly when mothers had been exposed to glucocorticoids prenatally. Although false negative results are reportedly more common in girls,[40] it is possible that missed boys remained unidentified, while the diagnosis was more likely to be pursued in girls, who are born with ambiguous genitalia.

Some of the limitations of immunoassay-based screening can be overcome by adjudicating positive tests with a second-tier assay using liquid chromatography/tandem MS(LC-MS/MS).[41–43] In addition to increased specificity, LC-MS/MS can also quantify multiple steroids with one measurement. Elevated 21dF by LC-MS/MS has been shown to increase the sensitivity of newborn screening[42] and better discriminate heterozygote carriers.[44] LC-MS/MS assays, however, are not widely available, are often time-consuming, and are prohibitively expensive for screening purposes currently.

Diagnosis of 21-hydroxylase deficiency beyond infancy

Patients evaluated for clinical evidence of inappropriate androgen excess initially undergo testing of 17OHP in an early morning serum sample.[29] The gold standard for diagnosing any form of CAH in patients with indeterminate values is a cosyntropin stimulation test, which maximizes the ratio between the steroids upstream and downstream the enzymatic blockage.[45] **Fig. 3** shows suggested cutoff baseline and stimulated 17OHP values in patients with 21OHD. Genetic testing of *CYP21A2* detects 90% to 95% of mutant alleles[46] and is useful when steroid results are equivocal[47] or unreliable (hypopituitarism) and for genetic counseling, particularly in nonclassic 21OHD. Because other forms of CAH are not tested, the cost is high, and management is rarely changed, genetic testing is not routinely recommended.

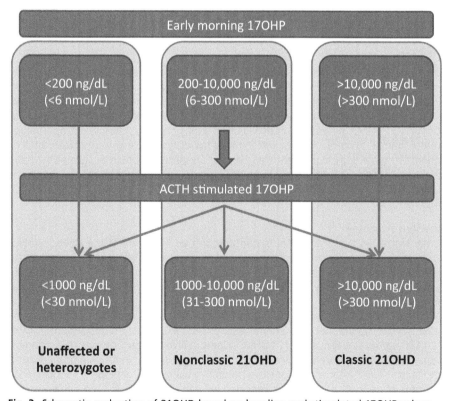

Fig. 3. Schematic evaluation of 21OHD based on baseline and stimulated 17OHP values.

Clinical Features

Salt wasting

Approximately three-quarters of patients with classic 21OHD have aldosterone deficiency and thus are prone to volume depletion and hyperkalemia.[48] Where neonatal screening is not performed, undiagnosed male infants might present with failure to thrive and dehydration in the first 2 weeks of life, which can lead to death if not appropriately recognized and treated. All untreated classic 21OHD patients waste salt during illness, but spontaneous volume depletion in a well infant defines "salt-wasting" disease, a term that has little utility beyond childhood.

Ambiguous genitalia and prenatal virilization

Girls with classic 21OHD of all severities are born with varying degrees of genital ambiguity. Prenatal exposure to adrenal androgens activates the androgen receptors in genital skin, favors clitoral enlargement and labial fusion, and interferes with the urogenital sinus septation, which normally occurs at 7 weeks of gestation in girls. The degree of virilization is classified according to the 5-point Prader scale (**Fig. 4**). If virilization is severe (Prader 4–5), assignment to male sex of rearing might inadvertently occur, and in rare cases, parents choose to raise the child as a boy knowing the diagnosis.

Boys with classic 21OHD typically have normal male genitalia (Prader 5). Subtle findings, such as hyperpigmentation of the scrotum and enlarged phallus, might be present at birth.

Postanatal virilization

In inadequately treated classic 21OHD, the adrenal androgen excess promotes further clitoral growth in girls and phallus enlargement in boys. Children with nonclassic 21OHD may exhibit evidence of androgen excess at various ages, such as premature pubarche and oily skin, but not genital virilization. Poorly controlled adolescent girls might experience hirsutism, acne, and irregular menses, similarly with patients with polycystic ovarian syndrome (PCOS).[48]

Growth

Both male and female infants with classic 21OHD are longer than average at birth.[49] Increased circulating levels of sex steroids promote accelerated linear growth and bone maturation early in life, which results in below average final height, due to

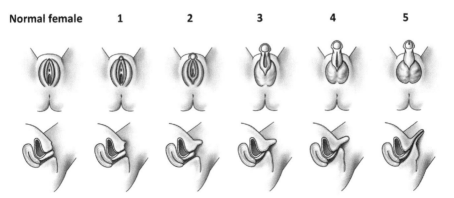

Fig. 4. Prader scale, female external genitalia viewed from above (*top*) and in cross-section (*bottom*).

premature epiphyseal closure. In addition, glucocorticoid treatment, especially when excessive, suppresses growth. A meta-analysis of data from 35 centers concluded that the near-final height of patients with classic 21OHD was −1.38 SD below the population mean and −1 SD below the predicted mid-parental height.[50] A multitude of factors influence adult height, including severity of disease,[51] age at diagnosis,[49] treatment regimen,[52,53] and compliance. These known factors, however, failed to prove significant individually in pooled data, possibly because of heterogeneity and inconsistent reporting between studies. Both boys and girls can experience central precocious puberty when control is poor or erratic, thought to be due to adrenal-derived sex steroid "priming" and withdrawal, which further compromises adult height.

Psychosexual development

Girls with classic 21OHD show more male-pattern play, activities, and career preferences.[54,55] In addition, some studies have found that affected girls display more aggressive behaviors and lower maternal drive as compared with their unaffected sisters.[56,57] Exposure to higher than normal androgens prenatally and in childhood is thought to "imprint" the brain, leading to masculine behavior but rarely to male gender identity if treated from birth.

Some studies suggest that female patients with 21OHD, particularly those with more severe forms, undergo malelike cognitive development, with higher visuospatial and logic performance and lower verbal abilities.[58–60] Data regarding the overall intelligence coefficient (IQ) of patients with 21OHD have been conflicting. It has been suggested that salt-wasting 21OHD might result in lower IQs, possibly because of electrolyte imbalances in infancy.[61] Conversely, other authors found no overall IQ or cross-gender performance differences between 21OHD patients and unaffected controls.[62]

Female reproduction

Women with 21OHD have lower fertility rates, which correlate inversely with disease severity.[63,64] The live-birth rates in salt-wasting classic 21OHD have been reported to be only up to 10%, 33% to 50% in simple virilizing forms, and 63% to 90% in nonclassic 21OHD, the latter rate being similar to that observed in the general population.[65–69] Hormonal, anatomic, and psychosocial factors have been suggested to contribute to impaired fertility.[64] Adrenal androgen overproduction can inhibit ovarian folliculogenesis and disturb the normal gonadotropin secretion pattern.[69,70] Elevated adrenal-derived progesterone in the follicular phase interferes with the normal menstrual cycle and impairs sperm penetration.[66,71,72] Women with 21OHD may also have excessive ovarian androgen production[73,74] and secondary PCOS.[75]

Nonhormonal contributors to decreased fertility in 21OHD women include distorted genital anatomy, such as vaginal stenosis and reduced clitoral sensitivity, as well as decreased sexual motivation[67,76] and lower maternal interest.[54] Nevertheless, in women with classical 21OHD who attempt pregnancy under skilled management, fecundity rates are normal.[77]

In contrast with the frequent development of adrenal rest tumors in the testes of men with 21OHD, ovarian adrenal rest tumors have only sporadically been reported in affected women.[78–81] This difference could be due to several factors, including more difficult distinction of ectopic adrenal tissue from theca cells in the heterogeneous ovary, the position of the ovaries in the pelvis, and possibly better control in most women, in whom undesirable clinical manifestations of androgen excess might provide motivation for compliance.

Male reproduction

Fertility in men with 21OHD has not been studied as extensively as in women. In the absence of newborn screening, boys with simple-virilizing 21OHD might remain undiagnosed, until they present with sexual precocity, accelerated growth, adrenal crisis during an infection, or rarely, after fathering an affected girl. Studies from the United Kingdom and Finland suggest that male fertility is well below that of the normal population.[82,83] The 2 main contributors to male infertility in 21OHD are hypogonadotropic hypogonadism, due to gonadal axis suppression from adrenal-derived androgens, and testicular adrenal rest tumors (TARTs).[84,85]

TARTs are typically bilateral masses, arising in the rete testes, thus often nonpalpable when small.[84] Ultrasound studies have identified TARTs in greater than 20% of boys[86,87] and up to 94% of adults with classic 21OHD.[84,85,88] Some, but not all TARTs, regress following intensified glucocorticoid treatment.[89] The variable response might be in part due to fibrotic changes[90] and to the number of adrenal-lineage cells, which migrated to the gonad during embryologic development.[91] TARTs may lead to obstruction of seminiferous tubules, gonadal dysfunction, and infertility.[84] Surgery to remove TARTs gives good long-term control of tumor growth and mass effect,[92,93] but rarely restores fertility or testicular testosterone production.[93,94] For this reason, medical therapy is continued as primary treatment as long as the luteinizing hormone (LH) is in the normal range, the rests are shrinking, and the testosterone is increasing, for at least 6 months and longer if tolerated. An increase in follicle-stimulating hormone (FSH) and a decrease in inhibin B indicate loss of Sertoli cell function and poor prognosis for restoration of testicular function. Abrupt resumption of tight disease control in patients with TARTs and suppressed testicular function will lower serum testosterone into the hypogonadal range. To enhance compliance, the patient should be warned of these changes, and a gradual increase in medication should be considered. TARTs rarely if ever occur in men with nonclassic 21OHD. Little is known about fertility in men with nonclassic 21OHD, because few are ever diagnosed, and men with unexplained infertility are rarely tested for 21OHD.

Adrenal masses

A high prevalence of benign adrenal masses has been reported in patients with 21OHD. Greater than 80% of homozygous and 45% of heterozygous patients had adrenal tumors in one study,[95] although no correlation between tumor size and serum 17OHP concentrations was found. Most tumors had a diameter of less than 2 cm, but several giant myelolipomas have also been reported, typically in patients who are chronically undertreated.[96–98]

Metabolic abnormalities

In a prospective cross-sectional study that followed 203 patients with CAH, 41% were obese, 46% had hypercholesterolemia, 29% were insulin-resistant, 40% had osteopenia, and 7% had osteoporosis.[82] Similar findings have been reported in smaller studies[99–101] and have been mostly attributed to glucocorticoid overtreatment.

Management

Medical treatment

Glucocorticoids and mineralocorticoids are the mainstays of treatment of 21OHD. Glucocorticoids exert 2 principal actions: replacement of the deficient cortisol and suppression of the adrenal androgen overproduction, by exerting negative feedback on the hypothalamus and the pituitary, which subsequently decreases CRH production and ACTH stimulation.

Glucocorticoid replacement Patients with classic 21OHD require chronic glucocorticoid replacement. Hydrocortisone is preferred in children and adolescents, until growth is completed, because of its short action, which limits the potential to suppress growth. A total of 10 to 17 mg/m² daily divided in 2 to 3 doses is typically recommended,[29] although it remains unclear if a specific dose distribution throughout the day has a significant clinical impact.[102] The lowest possible dose should be used to avoid growth suppression.[51,53,103,104]

Hydrocortisone also serves as replacement therapy for adults, but long-acting synthetic glucocorticoids are often preferred, owing to less frequent dosing. The longer duration of action and higher potency of drugs like prednisolone and dexamethasone, however, might increase the risk of detrimental effects, including weight gain, dermal atrophy, poor sleep, and bone loss.[82,105–108]

Available treatment options and suggested doses are shown in **Table 2**. Stress doses of steroids should be given in patients with classic 21OHD during surgery, physical illness, labor, and delivery.[29] In women attempting to conceive and during pregnancy, a glucocorticoid that is inactivated by placental 11β-hydroxysteroid dehydrogenase type 2 (eg, hydrocortisone, prednisone, and prednisolone) should be used, to avoid fetal exposure.

Asymptomatic patients with nonclassic 21OHD do not require treatment, and stress doses of steroids are rarely needed. Glucocorticoid treatment is primarily given to children with sexual precocity and advanced bone age or to women with infertility due to this condition. For other consequences of androgen excess, including acne, hirsutism, or body odor, alternative therapies include antiandrogens (spironolactone), oral contraceptives, and mechanical depilation. When treated, replacement regimens are similar to those prescribed to classic 21OHD patients with lower doses. One retrospective series found high rates of pregnancy loss in women with nonclassic 21OHD, but this rate was lower in women who were treated with glucocorticoids.[109] For this reason, glucocorticoids (hydrocortisone) are often continued throughout gestation, particularly in women who conceive while taking glucocorticoids.

The goals of therapy for classic 21OHD are to replace the hormonal deficits, while adequately suppressing the androgen excess. This balance is often hard to achieve without causing iatrogenic Cushing syndrome. Near-normalization of AD in both men and women and of testosterone in women indicates adequate control in most circumstances. Conversely, the 17OHP should not be consistently in the normal range: values of 1000 to 3000 ng/dL are acceptable if androgen production is controlled.[110] An exception is women attempting pregnancy, in whom treatment needs to be intensified to keep the follicular-phase progesterone suppressed (<0.6 ng/mL). Men with TARTs require at least one dose of a long-acting glucocorticoid to keep the ACTH suppressed and to allow regression.

Table 2
Available corticoid formulations and suggested doses for adults

Type of Steroid	Total Daily Dose (mg)	Number of Doses/d
Hydrocortisone	15–25	2–3
Prednisone	5–7.5	2
Prednisolone	4–6	2
Dexamethasone	0.25–0.5	1
Fludrocortisone	0.05–0.2	1

Mineralocorticoid replacement Mineralocorticoid replacement (fludrocortisone acetate, 0.1–0.3 mg daily) is necessary in patients with classic 21OHD. Infants with the most severe (salt-wasting) forms of disease need higher mineralocorticoid doses and additionally require supplementation with sodium chloride (1–2 g sodium chloride daily) while the renal function matures.[111] Mineralocorticoid replacement is generally maintained but occasionally becomes unnecessary in adults, possibly because of extra-adrenal 21-hydroxylation of adrenal-derived progesterone.[112,113] Mineralocorticoid replacement and restoration of euvolemia decrease vasopressin and ACTH secretion, which often lowers the dose of glucocorticoid required to achieve adequate control of androgen production.[50,103] The dose of fludrocortisone is titrated to achieve normal sitting and standing blood pressure without an orthostatic drop, plasma renin activity near the lower limit of the normal range, and normal serum potassium; reevaluations should occur periodically.

Experimental therapy Addition of the antiandrogen flutamide and the aromatase inhibitor testolactone allowed the use of lower doses of hydrocortisone and fludrocortisone acetate and normalized linear growth and bone maturation in children followed for 2 years.[114,115] Growth hormone, with or without a GnRH agonist, improved final height in some studies.[116,117] In addition, GnRH antagonist has been successful in improving height in children with 21OHD and precocious puberty.[117] Abiraterone acetate, a potent CYP17A1 inhibitor indicated for testosterone suppression in patients with prostate cancer, when added to physiologic doses of hydrocortisone and fludrocortisone acetate, normalizes AD in adult women with classic 21OHD and elevated androgens.[118] Extended-release hydrocortisone preparations, which might improve compliance and limit the need for more potent glucocorticoids, are being studied.[119] Long-term safety data on all of these agents are lacking, and large, randomized controlled studies are yet needed.

Surgical treatment
Reconstructive surgery For girls with virilized genitalia, surgery has been used to normalize voiding and to enable vaginal intercourse, but no good evidence to support a specific timing for surgical correction exists. A multidisciplinary team gathering expertise from pediatric endocrinologists, surgeons, social workers, and psychologists should support the family into making an individualized decision. Advantages of early surgery include tissue malleability[120] and decreased psychological impact on both affected girls and parents.[63,121] A potential benefit of delaying surgery until adolescence or young adulthood is incorporating patient autonomy in the decision-making process.

A 2-step neurovascular-sparing clitoroplasty and vaginoplasty using total or partial urogenital mobilization is the preferred surgical approach, for minimizing clitoral insensitivity and urinary incontinence.[29,122] Good long-term outcomes data are difficult to obtain, due to the variations in surgical approach, baseline anatomy, hormonal control, and other mitigating factors. Postsurgical complications, such as urethra-vaginal fistulae, impaired sensation, and vaginal stenosis, have been described, and current procedures strive to minimize these complications. The evolution of urogenital function following these procedures is particularly critical for young women contemplating pregnancy.

Elective adrenalectomy Bilateral adrenalectomy has been performed in selected patients with severe forms of 21OHD, in whom hyperandrogenism was difficult to control despite generous glucocorticoid replacement or to avoid their associated side effects.[123–125] The ensuing primary adrenal insufficiency, however, is more tenuous than 21OHD and mandates strict adherence to lifelong glucocorticoid and mineralocorticoid replacement, to prevent potentially fatal adrenal crises.[125,126] Complete absence of epinephrine and DHEA are additional theoretic concerns, but the consequences of these deficiencies remain unknown.

Prenatal diagnosis and treatment

The goal of prenatal treatment is to prevent virilization of external genitalia in female fetuses with classic 21OHD. Administration of a glucocorticoid that is not degraded by the placenta, such as dexamethasone, suppresses fetal ACTH and the adrenal hyperandrogenism. Because virilization of affected female fetuses starts as soon as the sixth week of gestation,[127] treatment has to be initiated as soon as pregnancy is documented.[128–131] Treatment initiated after 9 weeks of gestation will be incompletely effective[132]; therefore, early diagnosis is required if prenatal treatment is desired. Chorionic villus sampling and rapid genotypic of fetal cells is performed at 11 weeks of gestation,[133] and treatment is discontinued if genetic testing reveals a male or unaffected female fetus. Screening for the most common *CYP21A2* mutations identifies approximately 90% of the affected patients,[46] but screening does not detect other forms of CAH. These procedures and treatments are costly and involve some risk to the mother. Earlier diagnosis appears to be possible by targeted massively parallel sequencing performed on cell-free fetal DNA circulating in maternal plasma at 5 weeks gestation,[134,135] and this approach might facilitate the decision of whom to treat.

Dexamethasone prevents or reduces virilization in greater than 85% of prenatally treated girls.[132] On the other hand, data regarding maternal and fetal long-term safety are scarce.[136] In the absence of a diagnosis when treatment must commence, 7 unaffected children receive treatment to prevent virilization in one affected female child on average. Parents should receive counseling regarding potential side effects and give informed consent to treatment. If elected, treatment from an experienced team in research centers that monitor outcomes is recommended.[29]

SUMMARY AND FUTURE DIRECTIONS

Adrenal biosynthesis of mineralocorticoids, glucocorticoids, and androgen precursors follow specific enzymatic cascades in distinct, concentric adrenal zones, a design that optimizes steroid production efficiency. CAH results from autosomal-recessive enzymatic defects in cortisol biosynthesis. The most common form is 21OHD, accounting for greater than 90% of CAH cases. The clinical spectrum ranges from severe or classic forms, of which 75% have both mineralocorticoid and glucocorticoid deficiency, to mild, nonclassic 21OHD, in which ACTH overstimulation compensates for the partial block in cortisol production. All forms are characterized by excessive adrenal androgen production, which parallels the severity of the enzymatic defect. Diagnosis of 21OHD is based on elevations of 17OHP and is included in standard newborn screening throughout the United States and many other countries. Although this approach is excellent in distinguishing the classic forms and unaffected individuals, it suffers from false positive and negative results and poorer discrimination of intermediate severity cases from heterozygote carriers. Incorporation of other steroids upstream the enzymatic defect, such as 21dF in the diagnostic panel, as well as wider use of second-tier MS assays, might increase sensitivity and specificity in future.

Glucocorticoids and, when needed, mineralocorticoids, are the mainstay of treatment in 21OHD. These treatments serve in replacing the deficient steroids as well as in suppressing the excessive adrenal androgen production. New treatments under study include sustained-release hydrocortisone and inhibitors of androgen biosynthesis. Balancing and accurately monitoring treatment remain clinically challenging. 17OHP, AD, and, in women, testosterone have been used for treatment adjustment, but they do not always correlate well with clinical evidence of androgen excess. The identification and validation of adrenal-specific steroids and other molecules, which can be used clinically as biomarkers of adrenal-derived androgen production, would be of major clinical utility to facilitate treatment monitoring.

REFERENCES

1. Miller WL, Auchus RJ. The molecular biology, biochemistry, and physiology of human steroidogenesis and its disorders. Endocr Rev 2011;32(1):81–151.
2. Clark BJ, Wells J, King SR, et al. The purification, cloning, and expression of a novel luteinizing hormone-induced mitochondrial protein in MA-10 mouse Leydig tumor cells. Characterization of the steroidogenic acute regulatory protein (StAR). J Biol Chem 1994;269(45):28314–22.
3. Koritz SB, Kumar AM. On the mechanism of action of the adrenocorticotrophic hormone. The stimulation of the activity of enzymes involved in pregnenolone synthesis. J Biol Chem 1970;245(1):152–9.
4. Lachance Y, Luu-The V, Labrie C, et al. Characterization of human 3 β-hydroxysteroid dehydrogenase/Δ5-Δ4-isomerase gene and its expression in mammalian cells. J Biol Chem 1990;265(33):20469–75.
5. White PC. Disorders of aldosterone biosynthesis and action. N Engl J Med 1994; 331(4):250–8.
6. Wang XL, Bassett M, Zhang Y, et al. Transcriptional regulation of human 11β-hydroxylase (hCYP11B1). Endocrinology 2000;141(10):3587–94.
7. Auchus RJ, Lee TC, Miller WL. Cytochrome b_5 augments the 17,20-lyase activity of human P450c17 without direct electron transfer. J Biol Chem 1998;273(6): 3158–65.
8. Noordam C, Dhir V, McNelis JC, et al. Inactivating PAPSS2 mutations in a patient with premature pubarche. N Engl J Med 2009;360(22):2310–8.
9. Reiter EO, Fuldauer VG, Root AW. Secretion of the adrenal androgen, dehydroepiandrosterone sulfate, during normal infancy, childhood, and adolescence, in sick infants, and in children with endocrinologic abnormalities. J Pediatr 1977; 90(5):766–70.
10. Rosenfield RL, Grossman BJ, Ozoa N. Plasma 17-ketosteroids and testosterone in prepubertal children before and after ACTH administration. J Clin Endocrinol Metab 1971;33(2):249–53.
11. Speiser PW, White PC. Congenital adrenal hyperplasia. N Engl J Med 2003; 349(8):776–88.
12. Auchus RJ. Genetic deficiencies of cytochrome P450c17 (CYP17A1): combined 17-hydroxylase/17,20-lyase and isolated 17,20-lyase deficiency. In: New M, editor. Genetic steroid disorders. Waltham (MA): Elsevier; 2014. p. 111–23.
13. Krone N, Riepe FG, Gotze D, et al. Congenital adrenal hyperplasia due to 11-hydroxylase deficiency: functional characterization of two novel point mutations and a three-base pair deletion in the CYP11B1 gene. J Clin Endocrinol Metab 2005;90(6):3724–30.
14. Pang S. Congenital adrenal hyperplasia owing to 3β-hydroxysteroid dehydrogenase deficiency. Endocrinol Metab Clin North Am 2001;30(1):81–99, vi–vii.
15. Bose HS, Sugawara T, Strauss JF 3rd, et al. International congenital lipoid adrenal hyperplasia C. The pathophysiology and genetics of congenital lipoid adrenal hyperplasia. N Engl J Med 1996;335(25):1870–8.
16. Parajes S, Chan AO, But WM, et al. Delayed diagnosis of adrenal insufficiency in a patient with severe penoscrotal hypospadias due to two novel P450 side-

change cleavage enzyme (CYP11A1) mutations (p.R360W; p.R405X). Eur J Endocrinol 2012;167(6):881–5.

17. Krone N, Dhir V, Ivison HE, et al. Congenital adrenal hyperplasia and P450 oxidoreductase deficiency. Clin Endocrinol 2007;66(2):162–72.

18. Therrell BL. Newborn screening for congenital adrenal hyperplasia. Endocrinol Metab Clin North Am 2001;30(1):15–30.

19. Speiser PW, Dupont B, Rubinstein P, et al. High frequency of nonclassical steroid 21-hydroxylase deficiency. Am J Hum Genet 1985;37(4):650–67.

20. Carroll MC, Campbell RD, Porter RR. Mapping of steroid 21-hydroxylase genes adjacent to complement component C4 genes in HLA, the major histocompatibility complex in man. Proc Natl Acad Sci U S A 1985;82(2):521–5.

21. White PC, Grossberger D, Onufer BJ, et al. Two genes encoding steroid 21-hydroxylase are located near the genes encoding the fourth component of complement in man. Proc Natl Acad Sci U S A 1985;82(4):1089–93.

22. White PC, New MI, Dupont B. Structure of human steroid 21-hydroxylase genes. Proc Natl Acad Sci U S A 1986;83(14):5111–5.

23. White PC, Speiser PW. Congenital adrenal hyperplasia due to 21-hydroxylase deficiency. Endocr Rev 2000;21(3):245–91.

24. Swart AC, Storbeck KH, Swart P. A single amino acid residue, Ala 105, confers 16α-hydroxylase activity to human cytochrome P450 17α-hydroxylase/17,20 lyase. J Steroid Biochem Mol Biol 2010;119(3–5):112–20.

25. Fluck CE, Miller WL, Auchus RJ. The 17, 20-lyase activity of cytochrome P450c17 from human fetal testis favors the Δ^5 steroidogenic pathway. J Clin Endocrinol Metab 2003;88(8):3762–6.

26. Wilson JD, Auchus RJ, Leihy MW, et al. 5α-androstane-3α,17β-diol is formed in tammar wallaby pouch young testes by a pathway involving 5α-pregnane-3α,17α-diol-20-one as a key intermediate. Endocrinology 2003;144(2):575–80.

27. Auchus RJ. The backdoor pathway to dihydrotestosterone. Trends Endocrinol Metab 2004;15(9):432–8.

28. Kamrath C, Hochberg Z, Hartmann MF, et al. Increased activation of the alternative "backdoor" pathway in patients with 21-hydroxylase deficiency: evidence from urinary steroid hormone analysis. J Clin Endocrinol Metab 2012;97(3):E367–75.

29. Speiser PW, Azziz R, Baskin LS, et al. Congenital adrenal hyperplasia due to steroid 21-hydroxylase deficiency: an Endocrine Society clinical practice guideline. J Clin Endocrinol Metab 2010;95(9):4133–60.

30. Balsamo A, Cacciari E, Piazzi S, et al. Congenital adrenal hyperplasia: neonatal mass screening compared with clinical diagnosis only in the Emilia-Romagna region of Italy, 1980-1995. Pediatrics 1996;98(3 Pt 1):362–7.

31. Brosnan PG, Brosnan CA, Kemp SF, et al. Effect of newborn screening for congenital adrenal hyperplasia. Arch Pediatr Adolesc Med 1999;153(12):1272–8.

32. Therrell BL Jr, Berenbaum SA, Manter-Kapanke V, et al. Results of screening 1.9 million Texas newborns for 21-hydroxylase-deficient congenital adrenal hyperplasia. Pediatrics 1998;101(4 Pt 1):583–90.

33. Thil'en A, Nordenstrom A, Hagenfeldt L, et al. Benefits of neonatal screening for congenital adrenal hyperplasia (21-hydroxylase deficiency) in Sweden. Pediatrics 1998;101(4):E11.

34. Cavarzere P, Samara-Boustani D, Flechtner I, et al. Transient hyper-17-hydroxyprogesteronemia: a clinical subgroup of patients diagnosed at neonatal screening for congenital adrenal hyperplasia. Eur J Endocrinol 2009;161(2):285–92.

35. Coulm B, Coste J, Tardy V, et al. Efficiency of neonatal screening for congenital adrenal hyperplasia due to 21-hydroxylase deficiency in children born in

mainland France between 1996 and 2003. Arch Pediatr Adolesc Med 2012; 166(2):113–20.

36. Steigert M, Schoenle EJ, Biason-Lauber A, et al. High reliability of neonatal screening for congenital adrenal hyperplasia in Switzerland. J Clin Endocrinol Metab 2002;87(9):4106–10.

37. Olgemoller B, Roscher AA, Liebl B, et al. Screening for congenital adrenal hyperplasia: adjustment of 17-hydroxyprogesterone cut-off values to both age and birth weight markedly improves the predictive value. J Clin Endocrinol Metab 2003;88(12):5790–4.

38. van der Kamp HJ, Oudshoorn CG, Elvers BH, et al. Cutoff levels of 17α-hydroxyprogesterone in neonatal screening for congenital adrenal hyperplasia should be based on gestational age rather than on birth weight. J Clin Endocrinol Metab 2005;90(7):3904–7.

39. Sarafoglou K, Banks K, Kyllo J, et al. Cases of congenital adrenal hyperplasia missed by newborn screening in Minnesota. JAMA 2012;307(22):2371–4.

40. Varness TS, Allen DB, Hoffman GL. Newborn screening for congenital adrenal hyperplasia has reduced sensitivity in girls. J Pediatr 2005;147(4):493–8.

41. Schwarz E, Liu A, Randall H, et al. Use of steroid profiling by UPLC-MS/MS as a second tier test in newborn screening for congenital adrenal hyperplasia: the Utah experience. Pediatr Res 2009;66(2):230–5.

42. Janzen N, Peter M, Sander S, et al. Newborn screening for congenital adrenal hyperplasia: additional steroid profile using liquid chromatography-tandem mass spectrometry. J Clin Endocrinol Metab 2007;92(7):2581–9.

43. Janzen N, Sander S, Terhardt M, et al. Fast and direct quantification of adrenal steroids by tandem mass spectrometry in serum and dried blood spots. J Chromatogr B Analyt Technol Biomed Life Sci 2008;861(1):117–22.

44. Costa-Barbosa FA, Tonetto-Fernandes VF, Carvalho VM, et al. Superior discriminating value of ACTH-stimulated serum 21-deoxycortisol in identifying heterozygote carriers for 21-hydroxylase deficiency. Clin Endocrinol 2010;73(6): 700–6.

45. New MI, Lorenzen F, Lerner AJ, et al. Genotyping steroid 21-hydroxylase deficiency: hormonal reference data. J Clin Endocrinol Metab 1983;57(2):320–6.

46. Finkielstain GP, Chen W, Mehta SP, et al. Comprehensive genetic analysis of 182 unrelated families with congenital adrenal hyperplasia due to 21-hydroxylase deficiency. J Clin Endocrinol Metab 2011;96(1):E161–72.

47. Nordenstrom A, Thilen A, Hagenfeldt L, et al. Genotyping is a valuable diagnostic complement to neonatal screening for congenital adrenal hyperplasia due to steroid 21-hydroxylase deficiency. J Clin Endocrinol Metab 1999;84(5): 1505–9.

48. White PC, Bachega TA. Congenital adrenal hyperplasia due to 21 hydroxylase deficiency: from birth to adulthood. Semin Reprod Med 2012;30(5):400–9.

49. Jaaskelainen J, Voutilainen R. Growth of patients with 21-hydroxylase deficiency: an analysis of the factors influencing adult height. Pediatr Res 1997; 41(1):30–3.

50. Muthusamy K, Elamin MB, Smushkin G, et al. Clinical review: adult height in patients with congenital adrenal hyperplasia: a systematic review and metaanalysis. J Clin Endocrinol Metab 2010;95(9):4161–72.

51. Manoli I, Kanaka-Gantenbein C, Voutetakis A, et al. Early growth, pubertal development, body mass index and final height of patients with congenital adrenal hyperplasia: factors influencing the outcome. Clin Endocrinol 2002;57(5): 669–76.

52. Kirkland RT, Keenan BS, Holcombe JH, et al. The effect of therapy on mature height in congenital adrenal hyperplasia. J Clin Endocrinol Metab 1978;47(6):1320–4.

53. Grigorescu-Sido A, Bettendorf M, Schulze E, et al. Growth analysis in patients with 21-hydroxylase deficiency influence of glucocorticoid dosage, age at diagnosis, phenotype and genotype on growth and height outcome. Horm Res 2003; 60(2):84–90.

54. Dittmann RW, Kappes MH, Kappes ME, et al. Congenital adrenal hyperplasia. I: gender-related behavior and attitudes in female patients and sisters. Psychoneuroendocrinology 1990;15(5–6):401–20.

55. Berenbaum SA. Effects of early androgens on sex-typed activities and interests in adolescents with congenital adrenal hyperplasia. Horm Behav 1999;35(1): 102–10.

56. Berenbaum SA, Resnick SM. Early androgen effects on aggression in children and adults with congenital adrenal hyperplasia. Psychoneuroendocrinology 1997;22(7):505–15.

57. Mathews GA, Fane BA, Conway GS, et al. Personality and congenital adrenal hyperplasia: possible effects of prenatal androgen exposure. Horm Behav 2009;55(2):285–91.

58. Helleday J, Bartfai A, Ritzen EM, et al. General intelligence and cognitive profile in women with congenital adrenal hyperplasia (CAH). Psychoneuroendocrinology 1994;19(4):343–56.

59. Kelso WM, Nicholls ME, Warne GL, et al. Cerebral lateralization and cognitive functioning in patients with congenital adrenal hyperplasia. Neuropsychology 2000;14(3):370–8.

60. Mueller SC, Temple V, Oh E, et al. Early androgen exposure modulates spatial cognition in congenital adrenal hyperplasia (CAH). Psychoneuroendocrinology 2008;33(7):973–80.

61. Johannsen TH, Ripa CP, Reinisch JM, et al. Impaired cognitive function in women with congenital adrenal hyperplasia. J Clin Endocrinol Metab 2006; 91(4):1376–81.

62. Malouf MA, Migeon CJ, Carson KA, et al. Cognitive outcome in adult women affected by congenital adrenal hyperplasia due to 21-hydroxylase deficiency. Horm Res 2006;65(3):142–50.

63. Nordenskjold A, Holmdahl G, Frisen L, et al. Type of mutation and surgical procedure affect long-term quality of life for women with congenital adrenal hyperplasia. J Clin Endocrinol Metab 2008;93(2):380–6.

64. Stikkelbroeck NM, Hermus AR, Braat DD, et al. Fertility in women with congenital adrenal hyperplasia due to 21-hydroxylase deficiency. Obstet Gynecol Surv 2003;58(4):275–84.

65. Jaaskelainen J, Hippelainen M, Kiekara O, et al. Child rate, pregnancy outcome and ovarian function in females with classical 21-hydroxylase deficiency. Acta Obstet Gynecol Scand 2000;79(8):687–92.

66. Helleday J, Siwers B, Ritzen EM, et al. Subnormal androgen and elevated progesterone levels in women treated for congenital virilizing 21-hydroxylase deficiency. J Clin Endocrinol Metab 1993;76(4):933–6.

67. Mulaikal RM, Migeon CJ, Rock JA. Fertility rates in female patients with congenital adrenal hyperplasia due to 21-hydroxylase deficiency. N Engl J Med 1987; 316(4):178–82.

68. Klingensmith GJ, Garcia SC, Jones HW, et al. Glucocorticoid treatment of girls with congenital adrenal hyperplasia: effects on height, sexual maturation, and fertility. J Pediatr 1977;90(6):996–1004.

69. Feldman S, Billaud L, Thalabard JC, et al. Fertility in women with late-onset adrenal hyperplasia due to 21-hydroxylase deficiency. J Clin Endocrinol Metab 1992;74(3):635–9.
70. Hughes IA, Read GF. Menarche and subsequent ovarian function in girls with congenital adrenal hyperplasia. Horm Res 1982;16(2):100–6.
71. Holmes-Walker DJ, Conway GS, Honour JW, et al. Menstrual disturbance and hypersecretion of progesterone in women with congenital adrenal hyperplasia due to 21-hydroxylase deficiency. Clin Endocrinol 1995;43(3): 291–6.
72. Rosenfield RL, Bickel S, Razdan AK. Amenorrhea related to progestin excess in congenital adrenal hyperplasia. Obstet Gynecol 1980;56(2):208–15.
73. Barnes RB, Rosenfield RL, Ehrmann DA, et al. Ovarian hyperandrogynism as a result of congenital adrenal virilizing disorders: evidence for perinatal masculinization of neuroendocrine function in women. J Clin Endocrinol Metab 1994; 79(5):1328–33.
74. Ghizzoni L, Virdis R, Vottero A, et al. Pituitary-ovarian responses to leuprolide acetate testing in patients with congenital adrenal hyperplasia due to 21-hydroxylase deficiency. J Clin Endocrinol Metab 1996;81(2):601–6.
75. Hague WM, Adams J, Rodda C, et al. The prevalence of polycystic ovaries in patients with congenital adrenal hyperplasia and their close relatives. Clin Endocrinol 1990;33(4):501–10.
76. Kuhnle U, Bullinger M, Schwarz HP. The quality of life in adult female patients with congenital adrenal hyperplasia: a comprehensive study of the impact of genital malformations and chronic disease on female patients life. Eur J Pediatr 1995;154(9):708–16.
77. Casteras A, De Silva P, Rumsby G, et al. Reassessing fecundity in women with classical congenital adrenal hyperplasia (CAH): normal pregnancy rate but reduced fertility rate. Clin Endocrinol 2009;70(6):833–7.
78. Al-Ahmadie HA, Stanek J, Liu J, et al. Ovarian 'tumor' of the adrenogenital syndrome: the first reported case. Am J Surg Pathol 2001;25(11):1443–50.
79. Russo G, Paesano P, Taccagni G, et al. Ovarian adrenal-like tissue in congenital adrenal hyperplasia. N Engl J Med 1998;339(12):853–4.
80. Zaarour MG, Atallah DM, Trak-Smayra VE, et al. Bilateral ovary adrenal rest tumor in a congenital adrenal hyperplasia following adrenalectomy. Endocr Pract 2014;20(4):e69–74.
81. Tiosano D, Vlodavsky E, Filmar S, et al. Ovarian adrenal rest tumor in a congenital adrenal hyperplasia patient with adrenocorticotropin hypersecretion following adrenalectomy. Horm Res Paediatr 2010;74(3):223–8.
82. Arlt W, Willis DS, Wild SH, et al. Health status of adults with congenital adrenal hyperplasia: a cohort study of 203 patients. J Clin Endocrinol Metab 2010; 95(11):5110–21.
83. Jaaskelainen J, Kiekara O, Hippelainen M, et al. Pituitary gonadal axis and child rate in males with classical 21-hydroxylase deficiency. J Endocrinol Invest 2000; 23(1):23–7.
84. Stikkelbroeck NM, Otten BJ, Pasic A, et al. High prevalence of testicular adrenal rest tumors, impaired spermatogenesis, and Leydig cell failure in adolescent and adult males with congenital adrenal hyperplasia. J Clin Endocrinol Metab 2001;86(12):5721–8.
85. Stikkelbroeck NM, Suliman HM, Otten BJ, et al. Testicular adrenal rest tumours in postpubertal males with congenital adrenal hyperplasia: sonographic and MR features. Eur Radiol 2003;13(7):1597–603.

86. Martinez-Aguayo A, Rocha A, Rojas N, et al. Testicular adrenal rest tumors and Leydig and Sertoli cell function in boys with classical congenital adrenal hyperplasia. J Clin Endocrinol Metab 2007;92(12):4583–9.
87. Claahsen-van der Grinten HL, Sweep FC, Blickman JG, et al. Prevalence of testicular adrenal rest tumours in male children with congenital adrenal hyperplasia due to 21-hydroxylase deficiency. Eur J Endocrinol 2007;157(3):339–44.
88. Falhammar H, Nystrom HF, Ekstrom U, et al. Fertility, sexuality and testicular adrenal rest tumors in adult males with congenital adrenal hyperplasia. Eur J Endocrinol 2012;166(3):441–9.
89. Rutgers JL, Young RH, Scully RE. The testicular "tumor" of the adrenogenital syndrome. A report of six cases and review of the literature on testicular masses in patients with adrenocortical disorders. Am J Surg Pathol 1988; 12(7):503–13.
90. Claahsen-van der Grinten HL, Otten BJ, Stikkelbroeck MM, et al. Testicular adrenal rest tumours in congenital adrenal hyperplasia. Best Pract Res Clin Endocrinol Metab 2009;23(2):209–20.
91. Reisch N, Rottenkolber M, Greifenstein A, et al. Testicular adrenal rest tumors develop independently of long-term disease control: a longitudinal analysis of 50 adult men with congenital adrenal hyperplasia due to classic 21-hydroxylase deficiency. J Clin Endocrinol Metab 2013;98(11):E1820–6.
92. Ashley RA, McGee SM, Isotaolo PA, et al. Clinical and pathological features associated with the testicular tumor of the adrenogenital syndrome. J Urol 2007;177(2):546–9 [discussion: 549].
93. Walker BR, Skoog SJ, Winslow BH, et al. Testis sparing surgery for steroid unresponsive testicular tumors of the adrenogenital syndrome. J Urol 1997; 157(4):1460–3.
94. Claahsen-van der Grinten HL, Otten BJ, Takahashi S, et al. Testicular adrenal rest tumors in adult males with congenital adrenal hyperplasia: evaluation of pituitary-gonadal function before and after successful testis-sparing surgery in eight patients. J Clin Endocrinol Metab 2007;92(2):612–5.
95. Jaresch S, Kornely E, Kley HK, et al. Adrenal incidentaloma and patients with homozygous or heterozygous congenital adrenal hyperplasia. J Clin Endocrinol Metab 1992;74(3):685–9.
96. Nermoen I, Rorvik J, Holmedal SH, et al. High frequency of adrenal myelolipomas and testicular adrenal rest tumours in adult Norwegian patients with classical congenital adrenal hyperplasia because of 21-hydroxylase deficiency. Clin Endocrinol 2011;75(6):753–9.
97. German-Mena E, Zibari GB, Levine SN. Adrenal myelolipomas in patients with congenital adrenal hyperplasia: review of the literature and a case report. Endocr Pract 2011;17(3):441–7.
98. McGeoch SC, Olson S, Krukowski ZH, et al. Giant bilateral myelolipomas in a man with congenital adrenal hyperplasia. J Clin Endocrinol Metab 2012;97(2): 343–4.
99. Reisch N, Arlt W, Krone N. Health problems in congenital adrenal hyperplasia due to 21-hydroxylase deficiency. Horm Res Paediatr 2011;76(2):73–85.
100. Falhammar H, Filipsson H, Holmdahl G, et al. Metabolic profile and body composition in adult women with congenital adrenal hyperplasia due to 21-hydroxylase deficiency. J Clin Endocrinol Metab 2007;92(1):110–6.
101. Mooij CF, Kroese JM, Claahsen-van der Grinten HL, et al. Unfavourable trends in cardiovascular and metabolic risk in paediatric and adult patients with congenital adrenal hyperplasia? Clin Endocrinol 2010;73(2):137–46.

102. German A, Suraiya S, Tenenbaum-Rakover Y, et al. Control of childhood congenital adrenal hyperplasia and sleep activity and quality with morning or evening glucocorticoid therapy. J Clin Endocrinol Metab 2008;93(12):4707–10.

103. Balsamo A, Cicognani A, Baldazzi L, et al. CYP21 genotype, adult height, and pubertal development in 55 patients treated for 21-hydroxylase deficiency. J Clin Endocrinol Metab 2003;88(12):5680–8.

104. Bonfig W, Pozza SB, Schmidt H, et al. Hydrocortisone dosing during puberty in patients with classical congenital adrenal hyperplasia: an evidence-based recommendation. J Clin Endocrinol Metab 2009;94(10):3882–8.

105. Horrocks PM, London DR. Effects of long term dexamethasone treatment in adult patients with congenital adrenal hyperplasia. Clin Endocrinol 1987;27(6):635–42.

106. Young MC, Hughes IA. Dexamethasone treatment for congenital adrenal hyperplasia. Arch Dis Child 1990;65(3):312–4.

107. El-Maouche D, Collier S, Prasad M, et al. Cortical bone mineral density in patients with congenital adrenal hyperplasia due to 21-hydroxylase deficiency. Clin Endocrinol 2014;82(3):330–7.

108. Falhammar H, Filipsson Nystrom H, Wedell A, et al. Bone mineral density, bone markers, and fractures in adult males with congenital adrenal hyperplasia. Eur J Endocrinol 2013;168(3):331–41.

109. Bidet M, Bellanne-Chantelot C, Galand-Portier MB, et al. Fertility in women with nonclassical congenital adrenal hyperplasia due to 21-hydroxylase deficiency. J Clin Endocrinol Metab 2010;95(3):1182–90.

110. Auchus RJ. Congenital adrenal hyperplasia in adults. Curr Opin Endocrinol Diabetes Obes 2010;17(3):210–6.

111. Mullis PE, Hindmarsh PC, Brook CG. Sodium chloride supplement at diagnosis and during infancy in children with salt-losing 21-hydroxylase deficiency. Eur J Pediatr 1990;150(1):22–5.

112. Gomes LG, Huang N, Agrawal V, et al. Extraadrenal 21-hydroxylation by CYP2C19 and CYP3A4: effect on 21-hydroxylase deficiency. J Clin Endocrinol Metab 2009;94(1):89–95.

113. Speiser PW, Agdere L, Ueshiba H, et al. Aldosterone synthesis in salt-wasting congenital adrenal hyperplasia with complete absence of adrenal 21-hydroxylase. N Engl J Med 1991;324(3):145–9.

114. Laue L, Merke DP, Jones JV, et al. A preliminary study of flutamide, testolactone, and reduced hydrocortisone dose in the treatment of congenital adrenal hyperplasia. J Clin Endocrinol Metab 1996;81(10):3535–9.

115. Merke DP, Keil MF, Jones JV, et al. Flutamide, testolactone, and reduced hydrocortisone dose maintain normal growth velocity and bone maturation despite elevated androgen levels in children with congenital adrenal hyperplasia. J Clin Endocrinol Metab 2000;85(3):1114–20.

116. Quintos JB, Vogiatzi MG, Harbison MD, et al. Growth hormone therapy alone or in combination with gonadotropin-releasing hormone analog therapy to improve the height deficit in children with congenital adrenal hyperplasia. J Clin Endocrinol Metab 2001;86(4):1511–7.

117. Lin-Su K, Vogiatzi MG, Marshall I, et al. Treatment with growth hormone and luteinizing hormone releasing hormone analog improves final adult height in children with congenital adrenal hyperplasia. J Clin Endocrinol Metab 2005;90(6):3318–25.

118. Auchus RJ, Buschur EO, Chang AY, et al. Abiraterone acetate to lower androgens in women with classic 21-hydroxylase deficiency. J Clin Endocrinol Metab 2014;99(8):2763–70.

119. Verma S, Vanryzin C, Sinaii N, et al. A pharmacokinetic and pharmacodynamic study of delayed- and extended-release hydrocortisone (Chronocort) vs conventional hydrocortisone (Cortef) in the treatment of congenital adrenal hyperplasia. Clin Endocrinol 2010;72(4):441–7.
120. Bernbaum JC, Umbach DM, Ragan NB, et al. Pilot studies of estrogen-related physical findings in infants. Environ Health Perspect 2008;116(3):416–20.
121. Wisniewski AB, Migeon CJ, Malouf MA, et al. Psychosexual outcome in women affected by congenital adrenal hyperplasia due to 21-hydroxylase deficiency. J Urol 2004;171(6 Pt 1):2497–501.
122. Pena A. Total urogenital mobilization–an easier way to repair cloacas. J Pediatr Surg 1997;32(2):263–7 [discussion: 267–8].
123. Gunther DF, Bukowski TP, Ritzen EM, et al. Prophylactic adrenalectomy of a three-year-old girl with congenital adrenal hyperplasia: pre- and postoperative studies. J Clin Endocrinol Metab 1997;82(10):3324–7.
124. Bruining H, Bootsma AH, Koper JW, et al. Fertility and body composition after laparoscopic bilateral adrenalectomy in a 30-year-old female with congenital adrenal hyperplasia. J Clin Endocrinol Metab 2001;86(2):482–4.
125. Van Wyk JJ, Ritzen EM. The role of bilateral adrenalectomy in the treatment of congenital adrenal hyperplasia. J Clin Endocrinol Metab 2003;88(7):2993–8.
126. Ogilvie CM, Rumsby G, Kurzawinski T, et al. Outcome of bilateral adrenalectomy in congenital adrenal hyperplasia: one unit's experience. Eur J Endocrinol 2006; 154(3):405–8.
127. Witchel SF, Miller WL. Prenatal treatment of congenital adrenal hyperplasia-not standard of care. J Genet Couns 2012;21(5):615–24.
128. Forest MG, Betuel H, David M. Prenatal treatment in congenital adrenal hyperplasia due to 21-hydroxylase deficiency: up-date 88 of the French multicentric study. Endocr Res 1989;15(1–2):277–301.
129. Mercado AB, Wilson RC, Cheng KC, et al. Prenatal treatment and diagnosis of congenital adrenal hyperplasia owing to steroid 21-hydroxylase deficiency. J Clin Endocrinol Metab 1995;80(7):2014–20.
130. Evans MI, Chrousos GP, Mann DW, et al. Pharmacologic suppression of the fetal adrenal gland in utero. Attempted prevention of abnormal external genital masculinization in suspected congenital adrenal hyperplasia. JAMA 1985; 253(7):1015–20.
131. David M, Forest MG. Prenatal treatment of congenital adrenal hyperplasia resulting from 21-hydroxylase deficiency. J Pediatr 1984;105(5):799–803.
132. New MI, Carlson A, Obeid J, et al. Prenatal diagnosis for congenital adrenal hyperplasia in 532 pregnancies. J Clin Endocrinol Metab 2001;86(12):5651–7.
133. New MI, Abraham M, Yuen T, et al. An update on prenatal diagnosis and treatment of congenital adrenal hyperplasia. Semin Reprod Med 2012;30(5):396–9.
134. Barinaga M. Technical advances power neuroscience. Science 1990;250(4983): 908–9.
135. New MI, Tong YK, Yuen T, et al. Noninvasive prenatal diagnosis of congenital adrenal hyperplasia using cell-free fetal DNA in maternal plasma. J Clin Endocrinol Metab 2014;99(6):E1022–30.
136. Merce Fernandez-Balsells M, Muthusamy K, Smushkin G, et al. Prenatal dexamethasone use for the prevention of virilization in pregnancies at risk for classical congenital adrenal hyperplasia because of 21-hydroxylase (CYP21A2) deficiency: a systematic review and meta-analyses. Clin Endocrinol 2010; 73(4):436–44.

Animal Models of Adrenocortical Tumorigenesis

Sara Galac, DVM, PhD[a], David B. Wilson, MD, PhD[b],*

KEYWORDS

- Adrenal cortex • Cushing syndrome • Dog • Endocrine tumor • Ferret
- Gonadectomy • Mouse

KEY POINTS

- The high incidence of adrenocortical neoplasia in certain species (mice, ferrets, dogs) can facilitate genetic approaches to elucidate the molecular basis for tumorigenesis in humans.
- Targeted mutagenesis in animal models can be used to verify the functional significance of a given gene or signaling pathway for adrenocortical tumorigenesis.
- Animal models can be used for preclinical testing of novel therapies for adrenocortical neoplasia.

INTRODUCTION

The genetic basis of adrenocortical neoplasia has been the subject of intense study over the last decade.[1] Through molecular profiling of tissue specimens and characterization of heritable tumor predisposition syndromes, investigators have identified key genes and signaling pathways that are dysregulated in human adrenocortical tumors (ACTs).[1–3] Naturally occurring and genetically engineered animal models provide a complementary means to investigate the mechanisms underlying adrenocortical tumorigenesis and to develop novel therapeutics. This article provides an overview of experimental models useful for either mechanistic studies or preclinical screening.

Dr D.B. Wilson has received a grant from the American Heart Association (13GRNT16850031).
Dr D.B. Wilson has nothing to disclose.
[a] Department of Clinical Sciences of Companion Animals, Faculty of Veterinary Medicine, Utrecht University, Yalelaan 108, Utrecht 3508 TD, The Netherlands; [b] Departments of Pediatrics and Developmental Biology, St. Louis Children's Hospital, Washington University, 660 South Euclid Avenue, Box 8208, St Louis, MO 63110, USA
* Corresponding author.
E-mail address: wilson_d@wustl.edu

Endocrinol Metab Clin N Am 44 (2015) 297–310
http://dx.doi.org/10.1016/j.ecl.2015.02.003
0889-8529/15/$ – see front matter © 2015 Elsevier Inc. All rights reserved.

endo.theclinics.com

Three model organisms—mouse, ferret, and dog—are discussed in detail, and their relevance to ACTs in humans is reviewed.

COMPARATIVE ANATOMY AND PHYSIOLOGY OF THE ADRENAL CORTEX

The adrenal cortex of humans and most domestic animals is composed of 3 principal layers: the zona glomerulosa (zG), zona fasciculata (zF), and zona reticularis (zR) (**Fig. 1**). The zG contains cells that secrete mineralocorticoids under the control of the renin-angiotensin system. The zF and zR function together to produce glucocorticoids as part of the hypothalamic-pituitary-adrenal axis. In some species, including humans, the zR secretes adrenal androgens such as dehydroepiandrosterone (DHEA) and DHEA-sulfate (DHEA-S). The mouse adrenal cortex contains a zG and zF, but there is no discernable zR. The adrenal cortex of the young mouse contains an additional juxtamedullary layer, the X-zone, that is a remnant of the fetal adrenal cortex.[4] The ferret adrenal cortex contains a less-prominent layer, the zona intermedia (zI), located between the zG and zF[5]; an analogous layer in the rat, the undifferentiated zone, has been implicated in adrenocortical homeostasis and remodeling.[6,7]

Mice, ferrets, dogs, and humans differ in the gamut of steroidogenic enzymes and cofactors expressed in the adrenal cortex, and these differences have functional ramifications (see **Fig. 1**). Two key proteins that are differentially expressed among species are CYP17A1 and its allosteric regulator, cytochrome b_5 (CYB₅). CYP17A1 catalyzes both the 17α-hydroxylation reaction required for the synthesis of cortisol and the 17,20-lyase reaction required for the production of androgens.[8] The latter activity is enhanced by CYB₅.[8] Cells in the zF and zR of ferrets, dogs, and humans possess the 17α-hydroxylase activity, so cortisol is the principal glucocorticoid secreted by the adrenal gland of these species.[9] In humans, the adrenal cortex begins

Species	Mouse	Spiny Mouse	Ferret	Dog	Human
Anatomy	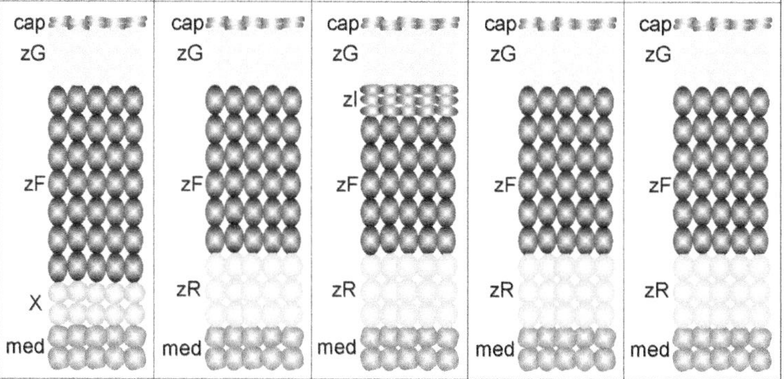 cap, zG, zF, X, med	cap, zG, zF, zR, med	cap, zG, zI, zF, zR, med	cap, zG, zF, zR, med	cap, zG, zF, zR, med
CYP17A1 expressed	No	Yes	Yes	Yes	Yes
Major glucocorticoid	Corticosterone	Cortisol	Cortisol	Cortisol	Cortisol
Adrenal androgens	No	Yes	Minimal	Minimal	Yes

Fig. 1. Comparative anatomy and physiology of the adrenal cortex. cap, capsule; med, medulla; X, X-zone.

to produce DHEA and DHEA-S at adrenarche, contemporaneous with increased expression of CYB_5 in the zR.[8] Under physiologic conditions, the adrenal glands of ferrets and dogs produce only limited amounts of androgens.[9] In the case of ferrets, this low adrenocortical androgen production has been attributed to low CYB_5 expression,[10] but the biochemical basis for limited androgen production by the dog adrenal cortex is unknown. Adrenocortical cells in the adult mouse lack Cyp17a1, so corticosterone is the principal glucocorticoid secreted by the mouse adrenal cortex, and adrenal androgens are not produced.[9]

Recently, the spiny mouse (genus *Acomys*) has garnered attention as another useful rodent model. In contrast to the laboratory mouse, the adrenal cortex of the spiny mouse contains a zR, expresses CYP17A1 and CYB5, and produces cortisol plus DHEA.[11] In this respect, the adrenal gland of the spiny mouse is similar to that of humans (see **Fig. 1**).

Adrenocortical cell differentiation, growth, and function are controlled by a diverse array of signaling factors, including adrenocorticotropic hormone (ACTH), angiotensin-II, insulin-related growth factors (IGFs), sonic hedgehog, and wingless-related integration site (Wnt) proteins.[5,12] Hormones traditionally associated with reproductive function, including luteinizing hormone (LH), activin, inhibin, and prolactin, also influence the differentiation and function of adrenocortical cells in animal models and humans.[5,13,14] Many of the aforementioned hormones bind and activate G-protein–coupled receptors on the surface of adrenocortical cells. Signaling through these receptors is mediated in part via the cyclic adenosine monophosphate (cAMP)-dependent protein kinase A signaling pathway, which culminates in the phosphorylation of transcription factors and enhanced expression of steroidogenic genes.[15]

MICE AS MODELS OF ADRENOCORTICAL NEOPLASIA
Xenograft Models

Normal bovine and human adrenocortical cells can be genetically modified and then implanted into nude mice to investigate the molecular underpinnings of tumorigenesis. For example, to model the role of illicit expression of hormone receptors in adrenocortical tumorigenesis, bovine adrenal cells were transduced with either gastric inhibitory polypeptide receptor or the LH/human chorionic gonadotropin (hCG) receptor (LHCGR) and then transplanted beneath the kidney capsule of mice.[16,17] The grafted cells developed into adenomas that caused ACTH-independent hypercortisolism.

Xenografts are also useful for preclinical drug testing.[18] One widely used model entails subcutaneous injection of nude mice with NCI-H295R cells, a human adrenocortical carcinoma (ACC) cell line that retains the capacity to produce all of the major classes of adrenocorticoids. The resultant subcutaneous tumors exhibit dysregulation of the insulinlike growth factor (IGF) system, a hallmark of human ACCs.[19] Treatment of with inhibitors of the type 1 insulinlike growth factor receptor (IGF1R) is found to ameliorate tumor growth and improve survival in mice harboring NCI-H295R xenografts.[20] The same model was used to show an effect of rosiglitazone, a peroxisome proliferator-activated receptor-γ agonist, on ACC growth and survival.[21] More recently, this experimental system has been used to assess the effects of other drugs on ACC growth, including NVP-BEZ235, an inhibitor of signaling through phosphatidylinositol 3-kinase and mTOR, the mammalian target of rapamycin.[22] Additionally, NCI-H295R xenografts have been used to show that liposomal preparations of certain chemotherapeutic agents (cisplatin, doxorubicin) may have enhanced efficacy against ACC.[23]

Although xenograft models offer many benefits, there are limitations to this methodology. Short-term xenografts do not recapitulate certain features of human carcinogenesis, such as tumor heterogeneity, genomic instability, and contributions of the immune system and tumor microenvironment.[24] Indeed, subcutaneous or renal xenografts represent a nonphysiologic niche for ACC. Another caveat to the NCI-H295R xenograft model is that it may not reflect the in vivo responsiveness of primary human ACCs to certain agents such as mitotane.[25] In the era of personalized medicine, improvements in xenograft technology are needed, so tumor specimens from individual patients can be efficiently and accurately screened for sensitivity to specific drugs, as was recently reported for a case of pediatric ACC.[26]

Gonadectomy-Induced Adrenocortical Tumors in Inbred Mice

Gonadectomy (GDX) and the ensuing changes in plasma hormone levels induce sex steroid–producing ACTs in certain inbred mouse strains, including DBA/2J.[5] This phenomenon is thought to reflect gonadotropin-induced metaplasia of stem/progenitor cells in the periphery of the adrenal gland, but the term *neoplasia* is used more often than the term *metaplasia* to describe the process. The neoplastic tissue expresses gonadal-like differentiation markers, including *Lhcgr*, enzymes required for sex steroid biosynthesis (*Cyp17a1*, *Cyp19a1*), and *Gata4*, a zinc finger transcription factor known to regulate genes involved in gonadal development and function.[5,27]

Hypophysectomy, transplantation, and parabiosis (surgical joining of the circulatory systems of a pair of animals) experiments have found that the adrenal glands of susceptible strains of mice exhibit an inherent predisposition to develop neoplasms in response to LH stimulation.[5,28] Linkage analysis of crosses between susceptible and nonsusceptible strains has established that GDX-induced adrenocortical neoplasia is a complex trait driven by epistatic loci.[29] Targeted mutagenesis of *Gata4* attenuates GDX-induced adrenocortical tumor formation in susceptible strains,[30] and enforced expression of *Gata4* enhances adrenocortical neoplasia in a nonsusceptible strain.[31] In addition to genetic changes, preexisting epigenetic alterations, such as DNA methylation, may impact the phenotypic plasticity of tumor progenitor cells in the adrenal cortex, allowing cells to respond to the hormonal changes associated with GDX or increasing the likelihood of subsequent genetic alterations.[2,32]

GDX-induced adrenocortical tumorigenesis has been reported in other species, including hamsters, ferrets (see later discussion), and goats,[9,33] but the relevance of this phenomenon to ACTs in humans has been questioned. There are anecdotal reports of ACTs with histologic features resembling luteinized ovarian stroma in postmenopausal women and men with acquired testicular atrophy.[5]

Genetically Engineered Mouse Models of Adrenocortical Neoplasia

Transgenic and knockout mouse models afford a means to test the roles of specific genes and signaling pathways in adrenocortical tumorigenesis. Additionally, these models can be harnessed for preclinical testing of drugs.

Simian virus 40 large T-antigen (TAg), a potent oncogene, has been found to elicit ACTs in transgenic mice when expressed under the control of the promoters of certain genes, including *inhibin-α* (*Inha*; **Fig. 2**), *CYP11A*, and *Akr1b7*.[34,35] In the case of the *Inha* promoter-TAg mouse, ACCs are induced by GDX via a signaling loop involving *Lhcgr* and *Gata4*.[36] Gonadectomized *Inha* promoter-TAg animals have been used in preclinical studies of LHCGR-targeted therapy.[37]

Like *Inha* promoter-TAg mice, inhibin-α knockout (*Inha[-/-]*) mice develop ACTs in response to GDX.[38] The GDX-induced tumors in *Inha[-/-]* mice are characterized by increased expression of *Gata4* and other gonadal-like markers.[39] Enforced expression of LH enhances adrenocortical neoplasia in *Inha[-/-]* mice.[40] In contrast, ablation of *Smad3*, which is essential for activin signaling, has been shown to attenuate ACT growth in this model.[41]

Gata4   Lhcgr

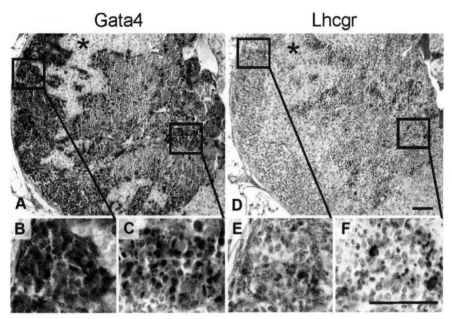

Fig. 2. Transgenic mouse model of ACC. Adjacent sections of adrenal tissue from a gonad-ectomized *Inha* promoter-TAg mouse were subjected to immunoperoxidase staining for (*A–C*) Gata4 or Lhcgr (*D–F*). The lower panels are higher magnification views of the boxed areas in the upper panels. Asterisks indicate normal adrenal cortex. Bars = 100 μm (original magnifications: 40× [*A,D*], 400× [*B,C,E,F*]).

Another important transgenic mouse model harbors multiple copies of the steroido-genic factor-1 (*Sf1*) genetic locus, mimicking the amplification and overexpression of *Sf1* seen in childhood ACC.[42,43] These mice develop age-dependent macronodular adrenocortical disease. Recently, genetic ablation the SF1 target gene *Vnn1*, encod-ing Vanin-1, was found to reduce the severity of neoplastic lesions in the *Sf1* trans-genic mice.[44] Vanin-1 has pantetheinase activity, which releases cysteamine in tissues and regulates the response to oxidative stress by modulating glutathione production. Based on these experiments, it has been proposed that alterations of intracellular redox mechanisms contribute to the pathogenesis of adrenocortical neoplasia induced by SF1 overexpression.

The Wnt/β-catenin signaling pathway is essential for cell renewal in the adrenal cor-tex,[7] and activation of this pathway has been documented in human ACTs.[3,45] Acti-vating β-catenin (*CTNNB1*) mutations occur with similar frequency in human adrenocortical adenomas and carcinomas.[45] Constitutive activation of β-catenin in the adrenal cortex of genetically engineered mice results in progressive adrenocortical cellular hyperplasia/dysplasia, which progresses toward malignancy in a subset of animals.[46] This phenotype is associated with autonomous production of aldoste-rone.[46] Decreased expression of the gene encoding secreted frizzled-related protein 2 (SFRP2), a Wnt inhibitor, may contribute to deregulated Wnt signaling and aldosterone-producing adenoma development in patients, as supported by both patient studies and a genetically engineered mouse model.[47]

In approximately 85% of human ACCs, *IGF2* is overexpressed compared with adenomas or normal adrenocortical tissue. Although IGF2 is an established marker of ACC, its role in ACT initiation and progression has been difficult to show using animal models.[48] Enforced expression of *Igf2* in transgenic mice does not elicit ACT formation by itself and only mildly accelerates the tumor progression associated with constitutive β-catenin activation.[49,50] Lending further credence to this notion that Igf2 is not a major driver of carcinogenesis, spontaneous ACCs in dogs do not exhibit *Igf2* overexpression (see later discussion).[9] Rather than functioning as classic oncogene, human *IGF2* may function as a tumor-progenitor gene.[51] The normal function of tumor-progenitor genes is to promote pluripotency and replication of stem/progenitor cells. According to one model of oncogenesis,[51] overexpression of tumor-progenitor genes leads to expansion of the stem/progenitor cell compartment, which, in turn, increases the probability of neoplasia through secondary genetic or epigenetic events. Hence, *IGF2* overexpression in human ACCs may reflect the cell of origin of these tumors rather than dependence on this signaling pathway per se. In keeping with this premise, drugs that inhibit *IGF2* signaling, such as cixutumumab, have shown limited efficacy in the treatment of patients with ACC.[52]

Many of the mutations associated with human adrenocortical hyperplasias and adenomas result in dysregulation of cAMP signaling.[15] For example, certain benign multinodular adrenocortical hyperplasias have been linked to activating mutations in the gene encoding $G_s\alpha$ or inactivating mutations in the gene encoding $G_i2\alpha$, both of which cause excess cAMP production.[15] Acquired gain-of-function mutations in *PRKACA*, encoding the catalytic subunit of cAMP-dependent protein kinase A, have been observed in patients with ACTH-independent Cushing syndrome caused by unilateral adenomas.[53] Inactivating mutations in the protein kinase A regulatory subunit (*PRKAR1A*) cause Carney complex, a multiple endocrine neoplasia syndrome associated with primary pigmented adrenocortical disease and pituitary-independent Cushing syndrome. Conditional mutagenesis of *Prkar1a* in the adrenal cortex of mice leads to disrupted stem/progenitor cell differentiation, excess cell proliferation, and impaired apoptosis. Interestingly, fetal-like adrenocortical cells that express *Cyp17a1* and secrete cortisol accumulate in these mice.[54] Analysis of these mice has yielded insights into the role of cAMP in the regulation of adrenocortical differentiation, tumor development, and steroidogenesis.[55]

Although extensively studied, there are drawbacks to genetically engineered mouse models of adrenocortical tumorigenesis. For instance, disparities in adrenocortical anatomy and physiology between mice and humans limit the utility of these models (see **Fig. 1**). Additionally, mouse and human cells exhibit differences in certain key biological processes. For example, telomerase, an enzyme often activated during malignant transformation of human cells, is functionally active in most normal mouse cells, and the telomeres of mouse cells are extremely long compared with their human counterparts.[24] Consequently, the role of telomere maintenance in oncogenesis is difficult to model with mice.

FERRETS AS MODELS OF ADRENOCORTICAL NEOPLASIA

Domestic ferrets, like certain inbred and genetically engineered strains of mice, get GDX-induced adrenocortical neoplasia.[9] In countries in which prepubertal ferrets are routinely gonadectomized, the incidence of adrenocortical neoplasia is about 20%.[5] The average age of diagnosis of adrenocortical neoplasia in ferrets is approximately 4.5 years (the average lifespan of a ferret is about 7 years), and there is no sex predilection.[5] The neoplastic cells that accumulate in the adrenal glands of gonadectomized ferrets express markers characteristic of gonadal steroidogenic cells (eg, Lhcgr, Gata4) and secrete sex steroids rather than adrenocorticoids.[5,56] In contrast to normal adrenocortical tissue, ferret ACTs express CYB_5, which enhances the 17,20-lyase activity of CYP17A1 and favors the production of androgens over cortisol in these tumors.[10]

The ectopic production of sex steroids by neoplastic adrenocortical tissue causes a syndrome known as adrenal-associated endocrinopathy (AAE), characterized by alopecia, vulvar enlargement, stranguria, and resumption of mating behavior (**Fig. 3**).[5] The diagnosis is confirmed by documenting elevated plasma concentrations of 17α-hydroxyprogesterone, androstenedione, DHEA-S, or estradiol.[57] In most ferrets with AAE, only one adrenal gland is enlarged.[5] Histologic examination of the adrenal cortex may find nodular hyperplasia, adenoma, or carcinoma.

As in mice, the chronic elevation in circulating LH that follows GDX is thought to be essential for neoplastic transformation of the ferret adrenal cortex.[5] Inhibition of LH secretion with gonadotropin-releasing hormone (GnRH) agonists can temporarily ameliorate signs of AAE.[58,59] Another effective treatment for AAE is GonaCon, a gonadotropin-releasing hormone vaccine originally developed to reduce the fertility of wildlife species.[60] Importantly, treatment of young, asymptomatic gonadectomized ferrets with GonaCon reduces the incidence of ACT development later in life.

GDX-induced adrenocortical tumorigenesis in ferrets is hypothesized to involve genetic and epigenetic alterations that act in concert with LH signaling. As noted earlier, analyses of human ACTs have documented alterations in hormone receptors (eg, LHCGR, gastric inhibitory polypeptide receptor), their downstream effectors (eg, PRKAR1A), or developmental signaling pathways (eg, Wnt/β-catenin) that impact tumor development.[2] Whether such genetic changes contribute to ACTs in gonadectomized ferrets is unknown. Preliminary studies suggest that the Wnt/β-catenin signaling pathway is not activated in ferret ACTs.[61]

Although the domestic ferret is an established model for studies of reproductive endocrinology and pulmonary diseases, it is not standardized with regard to genotype and, therefore, not ideal for studies of tumor genetics. The recent sequencing of the ferret genome, coupled with the expanding database of genomic DNA sequences and single nucleotide polymorphisms in the mouse and other species, should facilitate the characterization of alleles and genetic modifiers influencing GDX-induced adrenocortical tumorigenesis.

DOGS AS MODELS OF ADRENOCORTICAL NEOPLASIA

Spontaneous tumors in dogs often share biological and clinical features with human tumors, making the dog an attractive model for oncology research.[24] The incidence of functional ACTs is about 1000-fold higher in dogs than in humans.[9] Most functional canine ACTs secrete cortisol.[62] Such tumors account for approximately 15% of cases of spontaneous Cushing syndrome, which has an overall incidence of about 1 in 1000

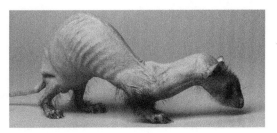

Fig. 3. Gonadectomized ferret with severe alopecia caused by a sex steroidogenic ACT.

dogs per year.[63] Most canine adrenocortical adenomas and carcinomas are unilateral, but bilateral ACTs occur in about 10% of cases. Functional ACTs occur without breed predilection, and GDX does not impact the incidence of ACTs in dogs.

In dogs, the typical clinical signs and symptoms of a functional ACT are those of glucocorticoid excess, including abdominal obesity, weight gain, muscle atrophy, skin changes, fatigue, polyuria, and polyphagia (**Fig. 4**).[64] The diagnosis of canine adrenal Cushing syndrome relies on the determination of elevated circulating or urinary cortisol concentrations, which cannot be suppressed by administration of high-dose dexamethasone, and on the demonstration of suppressed basal circulating ACTH concentrations.[62] Serum inhibin levels are higher in gonadectomized dogs with ACTs or pituitary-dependent Cushing syndrome than in healthy neutered controls.[65]

The treatment of choice for canine ACT is adrenalectomy,[66,67] which can generate substantial amounts of primary canine ACT tissue for in vitro research purposes. In cases of inoperable or metastatic ACTs, medical treatment with mitotane is used.[68] If neither adrenalectomy nor adrenocortical destruction with mitotane is feasible, a competitive inhibitor of 3β-hydroxysteroid dehydrogenase (trilostane) can be considered as a palliative treatment.[9]

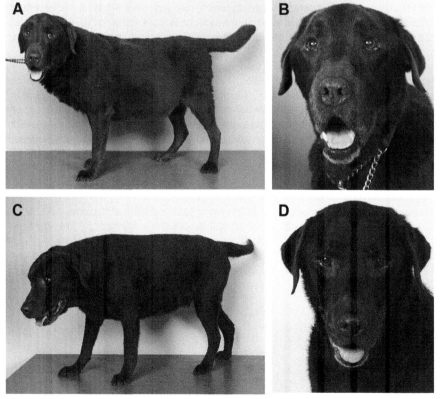

Fig. 4. (*A, B*) Dog with clinical signs of Cushing syndrome including abdominal obesity, muscle atrophy, and skin changes. (*C, D*) The same dog after surgical removal of a cortisol-secreting ACT.

The hormonal autonomy of canine ACTs has been investigated through expression profiling. Steroidogenic enzyme gene expression does not differ significantly among adrenocortical carcinomas, adenomas, and normal adrenocortical tissue.[69] One distinguishing feature of canine ACCs is the lower expression of *MC2R* compared with that of adenomas.[69] Consequently, ACTH administration elicits a clear increase in serum cortisol levels in dogs with adrenocortical adenomas but not carcinomas. Recent studies suggest that increased SF-1 expression in ACCs is associated with early tumor recurrence in dogs.[70]

Constitutive activation of cAMP signaling is a frequent event in canine cortisol-secreting ACTs and may contribute to ACTH-independent cortisol production and tumorigenesis.[71] Mutational analysis found that approximately 30% of these ACTs harbor activating mutations in the gene encoding $G_s\alpha$.[71] No functional mutations have been reported in *MC2R* or *PRKAR1A*.

Additionally, the expression of angiogenesis-related genes has been studied in canine cortisol-secreting ACTs.[72] Both angiopoietin-2 (ANGPT2) and the splice variant ANGPT2443 were expressed at higher levels in adenomas and carcinomas than in normal adrenal glands. This enhanced ANGPT2 expression was associated with a concomitant shift toward a proangiogenic state.

Several tools are now available to interrogate the canine genome, including a publically available genome assembly and various high-throughput techniques.[73] Given the homology between the genomes of dogs and humans and the overlap in the biological behavior of ACTs in these 2 species, the dog may prove to be a particularly valuable model for the study of adrenocortical neoplasia. Compared with the mouse or ferret models discussed earlier, spontaneous ACTs in dogs more accurately reflect the tumor heterogeneity seen in a population of human patients, which is important for therapeutic studies. In addition, because pet dogs share the same environment as their owners, the ACTs in this animal model include external interactions responsible for the development of adrenal cancer.

The Canine Comparative Oncology and Genomics Consortium is currently performing comprehensive analysis of other types of canine tumors (eg, lymphoma, osteosarcoma) to gain insight into the pathogenesis and treatment of the corresponding tumors in humans.[74] Canine models have become a proving ground for the delivery of personalized medicine to humans. Pilot studies have found that it is possible to expeditiously diagnose and molecularly characterize tumor specimens from dogs, facilitating the prompt initiation of experimental therapies using crossover-design clinical trials.[74] Thus, dogs with cancer now fill an important niche in translational oncology.

The molecular profiling of canine ACTs is still in its infancy. By systematically characterizing the molecular abnormalities in resected canine ACTs, it should be possible to leverage the dog model to improve therapy for humans.

SUMMARY

Over the last decade, research on human adrenocortical neoplasia has been dominated by gene expression profiling of tumor specimens and by analysis of genetic disorders associated with a predisposition to these tumors. Although these studies have identified key signaling pathways that are dysregulated in ACTs, these observations have not translated yet into substantive improvements in clinical outcome. Adrenocortical tumorigenesis is a complex biological process that requires comprehensive and complementary experimental systems for its study. Animal models have many desired characteristics that can bridge the gap between molecular profiling and enhancements in clinical care.

ACKNOWLEDGMENTS

The authors thank Sanne Kiiveri, Nafis Rahman, and Ilpo Huhtaniemi for providing the photomicrograph of the transgenic mouse tissue and Nico Schoemaker for providing the photograph of the ferret.

REFERENCES

1. Lerario AM, Moraitis A, Hammer GD. Genetics and epigenetics of adrenocortical tumors. Mol Cell Endocrinol 2014;386(1–2):67–84.
2. Bielinska M, Parviainen H, Kiiveri S, et al. Review paper: origin and molecular pathology of adrenocortical neoplasms. Vet Pathol 2009;46(2):194–210.
3. Assie G, Letouze E, Fassnacht M, et al. Integrated genomic characterization of adrenocortical carcinoma. Nat Genet 2014;46(6):6.
4. Morohashi K, Zubair M. The fetal and adult adrenal cortex. Mol Cell Endocrinol 2011;336(1–2):193–7.
5. Bielinska M, Kiiveri S, Parviainen H, et al. Gonadectomy-induced adrenocortical neoplasia in the domestic ferret (*Mustela putorius furo*) and laboratory mouse. Vet Pathol 2006;43(2):97–117.
6. Guasti L, Cavlan D, Cogger K, et al. Dlk1 upregulates Gli1 expression in male rat adrenal capsule cells through the activation of beta1 integrin and ERK1-2. Endocrinology 2013;154(12):4675–84.
7. Pihlajoki M, Heikinheimo M, Wilson DB. Never underestimate the complexity of remodeling. Endocrinology 2013;154(12):4446–9.
8. Miller WL, Auchus RJ. The molecular biology, biochemistry, and physiology of human steroidogenesis and its disorders. Endocr Rev 2011;32(1):81–151.
9. Beuschlein F, Galac S, Wilson DB. Animal models of adrenocortical tumorigenesis. Mol Cell Endocrinol 2012;351(1):78–86.
10. Wagner S, Kiupel M, Peterson RA, et al. Cytochrome b5 expression in gonadectomy-induced adrenocortical neoplasms of the domestic ferret (Mustela putorius furo). Vet Pathol 2008;45(4):439–42.
11. Quinn TA, Ratnayake U, Dickinson H, et al. Ontogeny of the adrenal gland in the spiny mouse, with particular reference to production of the steroids cortisol and dehydroepiandrosterone. Endocrinology 2013;154(3):1190–201.
12. Laufer E, Kesper D, Vortkamp A, et al. Sonic hedgehog signaling during adrenal development. Mol Cell Endocrinol 2012;351(1):19–27.
13. Bernichtein S, Peltoketo H, Huhtaniemi I. Adrenal hyperplasia and tumours in mice in connection with aberrant pituitary-gonadal function. Mol Cell Endocrinol 2009;300(1–2):164–8.
14. Bernichtein S, Alevizaki M, Huhtaniemi I. Is the adrenal cortex a target for gonadotropins? Trends Endocrinol Metab 2008;19(7):231–8.
15. de Joussineau C, Sahut-Barnola I, Levy I, et al. The cAMP pathway and the control of adrenocortical development and growth. Mol Cell Endocrinol 2012;351(1):28–36.
16. Mazzuco TL, Chabre O, Sturm N, et al. Ectopic expression of the gastric inhibitory polypeptide receptor gene is a sufficient genetic event to induce benign adrenocortical tumor in a xenotransplantation model. Endocrinology 2006;147(2):782–90.
17. Mazzuco TL, Chabre O, Feige JJ, et al. Aberrant expression of human luteinizing hormone receptor by adrenocortical cells is sufficient to provoke both hyperplasia and Cushing's syndrome features. J Clin Endocrinol Metab 2006;91(1):196–203.

18. Luconi M, Mannelli M. Xenograft models for preclinical drug testing: implications for adrenocortical cancer. Mol Cell Endocrinol 2012;351(1):71–7.
19. Ribeiro TC, Latronico AC. Insulin-like growth factor system on adrenocortical tumorigenesis. Mol Cell Endocrinol 2012;351(1):96–100.
20. Barlaskar FM, Spalding AC, Heaton JH, et al. Preclinical targeting of the type I insulin-like growth factor receptor in adrenocortical carcinoma. J Clin Endocrinol Metab 2009;94(1):204–12.
21. Luconi M, Mangoni M, Gelmini S, et al. Rosiglitazone impairs proliferation of human adrenocortical cancer: preclinical study in a xenograft mouse model. Endocr Relat Cancer 2010;17(1):169–77.
22. Doghman M, Lalli E. Efficacy of the novel dual PI3-kinase/mTOR inhibitor NVP-BEZ235 in a preclinical model of adrenocortical carcinoma. Mol Cell Endocrinol 2012;364(1–2):101–4.
23. Hantel C, Jung S, Mussack T, et al. Liposomal polychemotherapy improves adrenocortical carcinoma treatment in a preclinical rodent model. Endocr Relat Cancer 2014;21(3):383–94.
24. Pinho SS, Carvalho S, Cabral J, et al. Canine tumors: a spontaneous animal model of human carcinogenesis. Transl Res 2012;159(3):165–72.
25. Doghman M, Lalli E. Lack of long-lasting effects of mitotane adjuvant therapy in a mouse xenograft model of adrenocortical carcinoma. Mol Cell Endocrinol 2013;381(1–2):66–9.
26. Pinto EM, Morton C, Rodriguez-Galindo C, et al. Establishment and characterization of the first pediatric adrenocortical carcinoma xenograft model identifies topotecan as a potential chemotherapeutic agent. Clin Cancer Res 2013;19(7):1740–7.
27. Schillebeeckx M, Pihlajoki M, Gretzinger E, et al. Novel markers of gonadectomy-induced adrenocortical neoplasia in the mouse and ferret. Mol Cell Endocrinol 2015;399:122–30.
28. Bielinska M, Genova E, Boime I, et al. Gonadotropin-induced adrenocortical neoplasia in NU/J nude mice. Endocrinology 2005;146(9):3975–84.
29. Bernichtein S, Petretto E, Jamieson S, et al. Adrenal gland tumorigenesis after gonadectomy in mice is a complex genetic trait driven by epistatic loci. Endocrinology 2007;149(2):651–61.
30. Krachulec J, Vetter M, Schrade A, et al. GATA4 is a critical regulator of gonadectomy-induced adrenocortical tumorigenesis in mice. Endocrinology 2012;153(6):2599–611.
31. Chrusciel M, Vuorenoja S, Mohanty B, et al. Transgenic GATA-4 expression induces adrenocortical tumorigenesis in C57Bl/6 mice. J Cell Sci 2013;126(Pt 8):1845–57.
32. Schillebeeckx M, Schrade A, Lobs AK, et al. Laser capture microdissection-reduced representation bisulfite sequencing (LCM-RRBS) maps changes in DNA methylation associated with gonadectomy-induced adrenocortical neoplasia in the mouse. Nucleic Acids Res 2013;41(11):e116.
33. Altman NH, Streett CS, Terner JY. Castration and its relationship to tumors of the adrenal gland in the goat. Am J Vet Res 1969;30(4):583–9.
34. Kananen K, Markkula M, Mikola M, et al. Gonadectomy permits adrenocortical tumorigenesis in mice transgenic for the mouse inhibin à-subunit promoter/simian virus 40 T-antigen fusion gene: evidence for negative autoregulation of the inhibin à-subunit gene. Mol Endocrinol 1996;10(12):1667–77.
35. Sahut-Barnola I, Lefrancois-Martinez AM, Jean C, et al. Adrenal tumorigenesis targeted by the corticotropin-regulated promoter of the aldo-keto reductase AKR1B7 gene in transgenic mice. Endocr Res 2000;26(4):885–98.

36. Vuorenoja S, Rivero-Muller A, Kiiveri S, et al. Adrenocortical tumorigenesis, luteinizing hormone receptor and transcription factors GATA-4 and GATA-6. Mol Cell Endocrinol 2007;269(1–2):38–45.
37. Vuorenoja S, Rivero-Muller A, Ziecik AJ, et al. Targeted therapy for adrenocortical tumors in transgenic mice through their LH receptor by Hecate-human chorionic gonadotropin beta conjugate. Endocr Relat Cancer 2008;15(2):635–48.
38. Matzuk MM, Finegold MJ, Su JG, et al. Alpha-inhibin is a tumour-suppressor gene with gonadal specificity in mice. Nature 1992;360(6402):313–9.
39. Looyenga BD, Hammer GD. Origin and identity of adrenocortical tumors in inhibin knockout mice: implications for cellular plasticity in the adrenal cortex. Mol Endocrinol 2006;20(11):2848–63.
40. Beuschlein F, Looyenga BD, Bleasdale SE, et al. Activin induces x-zone apoptosis that inhibits luteinizing hormone-dependent adrenocortical tumor formation in inhibin-deficient mice. Mol Cell Biol 2003;23(11):3951–64.
41. Looyenga BD, Hammer GD. Genetic removal of Smad3 from inhibin-null mice attenuates tumor progression by uncoupling extracellular mitogenic signals from the cell cycle machinery. Mol Endocrinol 2007;21(10):18.
42. Figueiredo BC, Cavalli LR, Pianovski MA, et al. Amplification of the steroidogenic factor 1 gene in childhood adrenocortical tumors. J Clin Endocrinol Metab 2005; 90(2):615–9.
43. Doghman M, Karpova T, Rodrigues GA, et al. Increased steroidogenic factor-1 dosage triggers adrenocortical cell proliferation and cancer. Mol Endocrinol 2007;21(12):2968–87.
44. Latre de Late P, Wakil AE, Jarjat M, et al. Vanin-1 inactivation antagonizes the development of adrenocortical neoplasia in Sf-1 transgenic mice. Endocrinology 2014;155(7):16.
45. Tissier F, Cavard C, Groussin L, et al. Mutations of beta-catenin in adrenocortical tumors: activation of the Wnt signaling pathway is a frequent event in both benign and malignant adrenocortical tumors. Cancer Res 2005;65(17):7622–7.
46. Berthon A, Sahut-Barnola I, Lambert-Langlais S, et al. Constitutive beta-catenin activation induces adrenal hyperplasia and promotes adrenal cancer development. Hum Mol Genet 2010;19(8):1561–76.
47. Berthon A, Drelon C, Ragazzon B, et al. WNT/beta-catenin signalling is activated in aldosterone-producing adenomas and controls aldosterone production. Hum Mol Genet 2014;23(4):889–905.
48. Drelon C, Berthon A, Val P. Adrenocortical cancer and IGF2: is the game over or our experimental models limited? J Clin Endocrinol Metab 2013;98(2):505–7.
49. Drelon C, Berthon A, Ragazzon B, et al. Analysis of the role of Igf2 in adrenal tumour development in transgenic mouse models. PLoS One 2012;7(8):e44171.
50. Heaton JH, Wood MA, Kim AC, et al. Progression to adrenocortical tumorigenesis in mice and humans through insulin-like growth factor 2 and beta-catenin. Am J Pathol 2012;181(3):1017–33.
51. Feinberg AP, Ohlsson R, Henikoff S. The epigenetic progenitor origin of human cancer. Nat Rev Genet 2006;7(1):21–33.
52. Lerario AM, Worden FP, Ramm CA, et al. the combination of insulin-like growth factor receptor 1 (IGF1R) antibody cixutumumab and mitotane as a first-line therapy for patients with recurrent/metastatic adrenocortical carcinoma: a multi-institutional NCI-sponsored trial. Horm Cancer 2014;5(4):232–9.
53. Beuschlein F, Fassnacht M, Assie G, et al. Constitutive activation of PKA catalytic subunit in adrenal Cushing's syndrome. N Engl J Med 2014;370(11): 1019–28.

54. Sahut-Barnola I, de Joussineau C, Val P, et al. Cushing's syndrome and fetal features resurgence in adrenal cortex-specific Prkar1a knockout mice. PLoS Genet 2010;6(6):e1000980.

55. de Joussineau C, Sahut-Barnola I, Tissier F, et al. mTOR pathway is activated by PKA in adrenocortical cells and participates in vivo to apoptosis resistance in primary pigmented nodular adrenocortical disease (PPNAD). Hum Mol Genet 2014; 23(20):5418–28.

56. Schoemaker NJ, Teerds KJ, Mol JA, et al. The role of luteinizing hormone in the pathogenesis of hyperadrenocorticism in neutered ferrets. Mol Cell Endocrinol 2002;197(1–2):117–25.

57. Rosenthal KL, Peterson ME. Evaluation of plasma androgen and estrogen concentrations in ferrets with hyperadrenocorticism. J Am Vet Med Assoc 1996; 209(6):1097–102.

58. Wagner RA, Bailey EM, Schneider JF, et al. Leuprolide acetate treatment of adrenocortical disease in ferrets. J Am Vet Med Assoc 2001;218(8):1272–4.

59. Zeeland YR, Pabon M, Roest J, et al. Use of a GnRH agonist implant as alternative for surgical neutering in pet ferrets. Vet Rec 2014;175(3):66.

60. Miller LA, Fagerstone KA, Wagner RA, et al. Use of a GnRH vaccine, GonaCon, for prevention and treatment of adrenocortical disease (ACD) in domestic ferrets. Vaccine 2013;31:4619–23.

61. de Jong MK, Schoemaker NJ, Mol JA. Expression of sfrp1 and activation of the Wnt pathway in the adrenal glands of healthy ferrets and neutered ferrets with hyperadrenocorticism. Vet J 2013;196(2):176–80.

62. Galac S, Reusch CE, Kooistra HS, et al. Adrenals. In: Rijnberk A, Kooistra HS, editors. Clinical endocrinology of dogs and cats. 2nd edition. Hannover (Germany): Schluetersche; 2010. p. 93–154.

63. Willeberg P, Priester WA. Epidemiological aspects of clinical hyperadrenocorticims in dogs (canine Cushing's syndrome). J Am Anim Hosp Assoc 1982;18: 717–24.

64. de Bruin C, Meij BP, Kooistra HS, et al. Cushing's disease in dogs and humans. Horm Res 2009;71(Suppl 1):140–3.

65. Bromel C, Nelson RW, Feldman EC, et al. Serum inhibin concentration in dogs with adrenal gland disease and in healthy dogs. J Vet Intern Med 2013;27(1): 76–82.

66. van Sluijs FJ, Sjollema BE, Voorhout G, et al. Results of adrenalectomy in 36 dogs with hyperadrenocorticism caused by adreno-cortical tumour. Vet Q 1995;17(3): 113–6.

67. Kyles AE, Feldman EC, De Cock HE, et al. Surgical management of adrenal gland tumors with and without associated tumor thrombi in dogs: 40 cases (1994-2001). J Am Vet Med Assoc 2003;223(5):654–62.

68. Kintzer PP, Peterson ME. Mitotane treatment of 32 dogs with cortisol-secreting adrenocortical neoplasms. J Am Vet Med Assoc 1994;205(1):54–61.

69. Galac S, Kool MM, Naan EC, et al. Expression of the ACTH receptor, steroidogenic acute regulatory protein, and steroidogenic enzymes in canine cortisol-secreting adrenocortical tumors. Domest Anim Endocrinol 2010; 39(4):259–67.

70. Galac S, Kool MM, van den Berg MF, et al. Expression of steroidogenic factor 1 in canine cortisol-secreting adrenocortical tumors and normal adrenals. Domest Anim Endocrinol 2014;49:6.

71. Kool MM, Galac S, Spandauw CG, et al. Activating mutations of GNAS in canine cortisol-secreting adrenocortical tumors. J Vet Intern Med 2013;27(6):1486–92.

72. Kool MM, Galac S, Kooistra HS, et al. Expression of angiogenesis-related genes in canine cortisol-secreting adrenocortical tumors. Domest Anim Endocrinol 2014;47:73–82.
73. Hoeppner MP, Lundquist A, Pirun M, et al. An improved canine genome and a comprehensive catalogue of coding genes and non-coding transcripts. PLoS One 2014;9(3):e91172.
74. Paoloni M, Webb C, Mazcko C, et al. Prospective molecular profiling of canine cancers provides a clinically relevant comparative model for evaluating personalized medicine (PMed) trials. PLoS One 2014;9(3):e90028.

The Genetics of Adrenocortical Tumors

Stéphanie Espiard, MD[a,b,c], Jérôme Bertherat, MD, PhD[a,b,c,d],*

KEYWORDS

- Adrenal cortex • Cancer • Cushing syndrome • PKA • TP53 • IGF2 • Wnt/β-catenin
- ARMC5

KEY POINTS

- Cushing's syndrome due to primary bilateral adrenal hyperplasias is mainly due to germline alterations leading to cAMP/PKA pathway activation or *ARMC5* inactivation.
- Cortisol-secreting adenomas are caused by somatic mutations of genes controlling the cAMP/protein kinase A (PKA) pathway, mainly the PKA catalytic subunit alpha.
- The most frequent somatic genetics alterations in adrenocortical carcinomas are mutations or deletions of *TP53* and *CTNNB1* or *ZNRF3*, altering the p53 and the Wnt/β-catenin pathways, respectively.

INTRODUCTION

Tumors of the adrenal cortex can be diagnosed by the investigation of clinical signs of steroid excess or incidentally on medical imaging. Most tumors are unilateral and can be classified as benign adrenocortical adenoma (ACA) or adrenocortical cancer (ACC). Benign adenomas can be nonsecretory or be responsible for various degrees of cortisol or aldosterone excess. ACAs are frequent in the general population, because it is the most frequent tumor found in adrenal incidentalomas that are present in 1% to 7 % of the general population. By contrast ACC is a rare tumor with an estimated

The authors' work is supported in part by the ENSAT-CANCER Health-F2-2010-259735 (FP7 program), the Institut national de la santé et de la recherche médicale (S. Espiard is receiving a Poste Accueil), the E-rare # O1GM1407G from the European Community (Genomics of cAMP signaling alterations in adrenal Cushing), and the Conny-Maeva Charitable Foundation.
^a Cochin Institut, INSERM U1016, 24 rue du Faubourg Saint Jacques, Paris 75014, France;
^b Cochin Institut, CNRS UMR8104, 24 rue du Faubourg Saint-Jacques, Paris 75014, France;
^c Paris Descartes University, 12 rue de l'Ecole de Médecine, Paris 75006, France;
^d Endocrinology Department, Center for Rare Adrenal Diseases, Hôpital Cochin, Assistance Publique Hôpitaux de Paris, 27 Rue du Fg-St-Jacques, Paris F-75014, France
* Corresponding author. Endocrinology Department, Hôpital Cochin, 27 Rue du Fg-St-Jacques, Paris F-75014, France.
E-mail address: jerome.bertherat@cch.aphp.fr

Endocrinol Metab Clin N Am 44 (2015) 311–334
http://dx.doi.org/10.1016/j.ecl.2015.02.004
0889-8529/15/$ – see front matter © 2015 Elsevier Inc. All rights reserved.

endo.theclinics.com

prevalence between 4 and 12 cases per million. Bilateral tumors are less common and can be classified in 2 groups according to the size of the multiples nodules that develop in both adrenals: primary bilateral macronodular adrenal hyperplasia (PBMAH) and micronodular adrenocortical adrenal hyperplasia.

The current knowledge regarding the development of adrenal cortical tumors (ACTs) suggests that molecular alterations stimulating the proliferation of adrenocortical cells are drivers of this disorder. In this perspective, a genetic or/and epigenetic alteration would occur initially, followed by subsequent secondary events leading to tumor development. The molecular alterations initially described in ACT were identified by the study of rare familial tumor syndrome in which ACA or ACC were observed.[1] These candidate gene approaches are based on the hypothesis that a germline alteration of a gene causing a hereditary familial tumor syndrome also occurs as a somatic event limited to a sporadic tumor. This approach was indeed very successful in identifying TP53 mutation or insulin-like growth factor 2 (IGF2) overexpression in ACC, and protein kinase A (PKA) regulatory subunit 1-alpha (PRKAR1A) mutations in ACA.[2–5] However, using this approach, only genes that are already identified can be investigated. More recently, the development of pan-genomic approaches to study the genome and epigenome allowed for the identification of many new alterations in cancer.[6] The application of these genomic tools to the study of ACT resulted in major advances in our understanding of the molecular genetics of these tumors. In particular, the use of next-generation sequencing in the past 2 years led to the identification of several new gene alterations in various types of ACT. This review describes the current knowledge on the genetics of ACT with a special emphasis on these recent advances (**Table 1**). Because alterations vary depending on the type of ACT, the review first describes bilateral tumors causing Cushing syndrome (CS), followed by cortisol-secreting adenomas and adrenal cancer.

GENETICS OF BILATERAL ADRENOCORTICAL TUMORS

Bilateral tumors of the adrenal cortex are primary adrenal diseases causing CS characterized by the development of multiples nodules in both adrenals. In the micronodular forms (micronodular adrenocortical hyperplasia [MiAH]), the diameter of most adrenal nodules is less than 1 cm. MiAH is usually diagnosed in children and young adults. Primary pigmented nodular adrenocortical disease (PPNAD) represents the most frequent form of MiAH and is characterized by the pigmented aspect of the nodules. In the macronodular form (PBMAH), the nodules are greater than 1 cm and the total adrenal weight can reach more than 10 times the normal adrenal weight. Apart from very rare pediatric cases in patients with McCune-Albright, PBMAH is usually diagnosed in adults between 50 and 70 years of age. Illegitimate membrane receptors expression as well as intra-adrenal synthesis of adrenocorticotropic hormone (ACTH) have been identified in the pathophysiology of this disease.[7–9] The bilateral nature of these tumors might lead to speculation that germline genetic or epigenetic factors play an important role in their development. Indeed many cases of PPNAD are part of a familial syndrome, and some families with PBMAH have been reported as discussed later.

Micronodular Adrenocortical Hyperplasia and Primary Pigmented Nodular Adrenocortical Disease

Protein kinase A regulatory subunit 1–alpha
PPNAD is most often part of a multiple tumors syndrome termed *Carney complex* (CNC: Online Mendelian Inheritance in Man [OMIM] No. 160980), but it can be

isolated in 12% of cases. CNC is transmitted in an autosomal dominant mode. A PPNAD is detected in 60% of patients with CNC.[10,11] The nonendocrine manifestations of CNC are mainly cardiac myxomas, pigmented skin lesions (lentiginosis and nevi), and melanocytic schwannomas. The tumors of endocrine glands observed in CNC include somatotroph-pituitary adenomas, testicular Sertoli cell calcified tumors, benign thyroid nodules, differentiated thyroid cancer, and PPNAD.[12,13] Genetic linkage analysis identified 2 loci in chromosome 2p16 and 17p22-24. Loss of heterozygosity (LOH) and copy number gains have been described in chromosome 2, but no causative gene at this locus has been found to date.[14] At the 17p locus, inactivating mutations of the *PRKAR1A* gene have been identified[10,15,16] that may explain more than two-thirds of patients with CNC and probably more in typical familial forms of the disease.[10,17] Germline mutations of *PRKAR1A* lead to the inactivation of the protein and overactivation of the cAMP/PKA pathway (**Fig. 1**). The mutations are mainly unique because usually each family has its own mutation and that mutation's hot spots are very limited. The mutations are spread along the whole coding sequence and the adjacent intronic sequences. Eighty percent of the mutations lead to a premature stop codon by nonsense or frame shift, and the mutant mRNA is degraded by the mechanism of nonsense-mediated mRNA decay (NMD).[17] The other mutations escape NMD but lead to the production of defective proteins (longer, shorter, or with modified sequence).[17,18] The longest proteins could be degraded by the proteasome leading to haploinsufficiency.[19] Additional somatic events in *PRKAR1A*, such as mutations or LOH in the nodules of PPNAD, suggest that it is a tumor suppressor gene.[17,18] Genotype/phenotype correlations have been established: isolated PPNAD is associated with the hot-spot c.709-7_709-2del,[20] whereas mutations escaping NMD or exonic mutations lead to the occurrence of more manifestations of the CNC.[10] Mice models confirmed that inactivation of *PRKAR1A* leads to tumorigenesis.[13] Particularly, mice with specific inactivation of this gene in the adrenal cortex (AdKO mice) develop adrenal cortex hyperactivity and bilateral hyperplasia as observed in PPNAD.[21] However, the role of additive effects of other pathways on the occurrence of tumors is suggested. Several studies have reported an activation of the Wnt/β-catenin signaling, mitogen-activated protein kinase (MAPK) signaling, or the mammalian target of rapamycin (mTOR) pathways and dysregulation of cyclins and the E2F family.[22] In particular, PPNAD macronodules can harbor somatic secondary mutations of *CTNNB1*[23,24] and overexpression of the Wnt/β-catenin signaling pathway targets is observed in PPNAD,[25] suggesting a role of this pathway.

Phosphodiesterases

The phosphodiesterases (PDEs) hydrolyze cAMP and/or cGMP, decreasing cAMP levels after stimulation of the cAMP/PKA pathway (see **Fig. 1**). Pan-genomic single nucleotide polymorphism (SNP) analysis on DNA chips led to the identification of the 2q31-2q35 locus. Study of candidate genes in this region identified germline-inactivating mutations of *PDE11A* in patients with MiAH/PPNAD.[26] Additionally, *PDE11A* rare variants with reduced enzymatic activity may play a role in the genetic predisposition to PPNAD; the frequency of these rare *PDE11A* variants is higher among patients with CNC with *PRKAR1A* mutations that develop PPNAD.[27] An association of these rare variants with PBMAH has also been observed.[28,29]

A germline-inactivating mutation of *PDE8B* on chromosome 5 has been described in a young girl who had a CS at 2 years of age.[30] Somatic mutations of *PDE8B* have been described in PPNAD, PBMAH, and nonsecreting adenomas.[31] *PDE8B* knockout mice present with increased corticosterone production.[32]

Table 1
Main genes associated with adrenocortical tumors

Gene	Locus	Action	Alteration	Tumors and Associated Conditions
TP53	17q13	Regulation of genes involved in cell cycle, apoptosis, senescence, DNA repair	Germ mutation	Li-Fraumeni syndrome (soft tissue sarcoma, breast cancers, brain tumors, ACC) Pediatric sporadic ACC
			Som mutation Som LOH	Sporadic ACC
ZNRF3	22q12.1	Inhibition of Wnt receptors, inhibition of Wnt/β-catenin pathway	Som mutation Som LOH	Sporadic ACC
CTNNB1	3q21	Cytoplasmic/nuclear β-catenin regulates genes expression involved in proliferation and differentiation	Som mutation	Sporadic ACC Nonfunctional ACA
IGFII	11p15	Growth factor involved in development and growth	Germ LOH/Epi-genetic alteration (overexpression)	Beckwith-Wiedemann syndrome (organomegaly, hemihypertrophy, Wilms tumor, ACC)
			Som LOH/Epi-genetic alteration (overexpression)	Sporadic ACC
Menin	11q13	Regulation of genes involved in cell proliferation	Germ mutation	Multiple endocrine neoplasia type 1 (hyperparathyroidism, pituitary adenomas, ACA or adrenal hyperplasia, ACC)
			Som mutation/LOH	Sporadic ACC
GNAS1	20q13	Stimulation of adenylate cyclase, activation of the cAMP/PKA pathway	Postzygotic mutation	McCune-Albright syndrome (fibrous dysplasia, café-au-lait spots, hyperfunction of endocrine glands, CPA) PBMAH, ACA
			Som mutation	Sporadic ACC

Gene	Locus	Function	Mutation	Associated conditions
MC2R	18p11	ACTH receptor, activation of PKA pathway	Germ mutation	*PBMAH*
APC	5q12-22	Prevent β-catenin accumulation, inhibition of Wnt/β-catenin pathway	Germ mutation	Familial adenomatous polyposis (colon adenomas and carcinomas, pigmented retinal lesions, desmoids tumors, other malignant tumors, PBMAH, CPA, and ACC)
			Som mutation	*Sporadic ACC*
PRKAR1A	17q22-24	Inhibition of the catalytic subunit of PKA, inhibition of the cAMP/PKA pathway	Germ mutation	Carney complex (miAH, pituitary adenoma, testicular tumors, cardiac myxomas, lentiginosis)
				Isolated MiAH
			Som mutation/LOH	*Sporadic CPA*
PDE11A	2q31-35	Hydrolysis of cAMP, inhibition of the cAMP/PKA pathway	Germ mutation	MiAH
PDE8B	5q13	Hydrolysis of cAMP, inhibition of the cAMP/PKA pathway	Germ mutation	*MiAH*
			Som mutation	*MiAH, PBMAH, nonfunctional ACA*
ARMC5	16p11	Regulation of apoptosis	Germ mutation	PBMAH
			Germ deletion	
FH	1q42	Krebs cycle, amino acid metabolism	Germ mutation	PBMAH
PRKACA	19p13	Catalytic subunit of PKA, activation of PKA pathway targets	Som mutation	CPA
			Germ amplification	*MiAH, PBMAH*

Italic font style: rare feature.

Abbreviations: ACA, adrenocortical adenomas; ACC, adrenocortical carcinoma; CPA, cortisol-producing adenoma; Germ, germline; LOH, loss of heterozygosity; MiAH, micronodular adrenal hyperplasia; PBMAH, primary bilateral macronodular adrenal hyperplasia; Som, somatic.

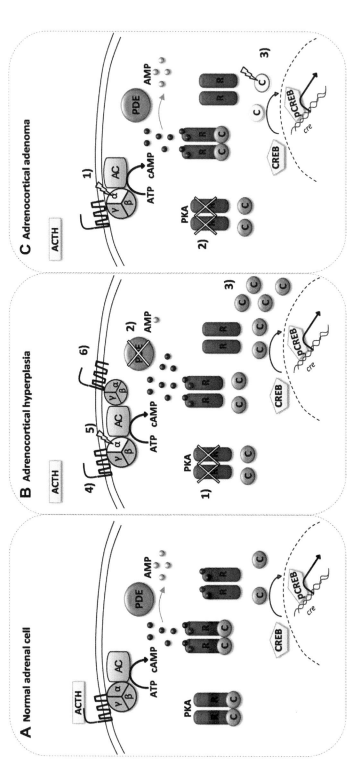

Fig. 1. Normal and abnormal activation of the PKA pathway in adrenocortical cells. (A) In normal adrenocortical cells, the ligand ACTH binds to its 7-transmembrane G protein–coupled receptor resulting in the activation of Gs protein, activation of adenylyl cyclase (AC), and cAMP production. Four cAMP molecules bind to the dimer of regulatory subunits (R) that set free catalytic subunits (C). Free catalytic subunits phosphorylate a series of targets, including the transcription factor CREB, which then activate the transcription of cAMP-regulated genes. The phosphodiesterases (PDE) regulate the pathway by degrading the cAMP. (B) In adrenocortical hyperplasia, (1) inactivating mutations of the regulatory subunit 1 alpha of the PKA (PRKAR1A) lead to the dissociation of the catalytic subunits in the absence of cAMP; (2) inactivation of phosphodiesterase by mutation leads to an accumulation of cAMP; (3) duplication of PRKACA gene activates the PKA by overexpression of catalytic subunits alpha; mutations of (4) the ACTH receptor gene and (5) GNAS encoding for the protein Gs are responsible for few cases of hyperplasia; (6) expression of illegitimate receptors leads to a specific activation of the PKA pathway depending on the receptor and its ligand. (C) In adrenocortical adenoma, mutations of (1) PRKAR1A and (2) GNAS are observed in a subset of cortisol-secreting adenomas. (3) Mutations of the catalytic subunit alpha leads to an activation of PKA by dissociation from the regulatory subunits. CREB, cAMP-response element-binding protein; pCREB, phospho-CREB.

Catalytic subunits of the protein kinase A

Recently, a comparative genomic hybridization (CGH) study on 35 patients with cortisol-secreting bilateral adrenal hyperplasia demonstrated that 5 patients harbored germline duplications of a region in chromosome 19p that included catalytic alpha subunit of PKA (*PRKACA*).[33] Three patients were young boys with severe disease and micronodular or macronodular bilateral adrenal hyperplasia. The 2 other patients were a mother and her son with mild insidious Cushing syndrome diagnosed after the third decade and caused by bilateral macronodular hyperplasia. Thus, germline duplication of *PRKACA* seems to also be a cause of bilateral adrenal hyperplasia, associated preferentially with early severe Cushing syndrome (see **Fig. 1B**). Increased expression of the catalytic subunit alpha mRNA and protein, higher basal, and stimulated PKA activity were confirmed in tumor samples from these patients.[33] A germline triplication of chromosome 1p31.1, including *PRKACB*, has been recently described in a 19-year-old woman presenting with CNC complex without signs of PPNAD at the time of the publication. Young mice carrying a transgene *PRKACB* exhibited pituitary abnormalities but no adrenal disease.[34]

Primary Bilateral Macronodular Adrenal Hyperplasia

PBMAH is characterized by bilateral adrenal hyperplasia associated with multiple nodules greater than 1 cm. Hypercortisolism is often associated, occurring generally late and insidiously. However, cortisol secretion can vary widely, as many forms diagnosed after the investigation of adrenal incidentaloma present with subclinical Cushing syndrome and a moderate level of cortisol excess. This disease was previously referred to as ACTH-independent macronodular adrenal hyperplasia or massive macro-nodular adrenal dysplasia; but with the recent discovery that local, intra-adrenal secretion of ACTH is responsible for paracrine cortisol hypersecretion,[9] the term *PBMAH* is now preferred.[7] The bilateral nature of the disease and the description of familial forms have suggested a genetic origin.[35–39] PBMAH has served as a model to describe and establish the concept of illegitimate receptors in adrenal Cushing syndrome. Aberrant expression of G protein–coupled receptors (vasopressin V1, serotonin [HT4], catecholamines, angiotensin, gastric inhibitory polypeptide, luteinizing hormone, human chorionic gonadotropin, adrenergic receptors) is observed in most patients with PBMAH (see **Fig. 1B**).[8,40,41] These receptors usually stimulate the cAMP/PKA signaling pathway, as does ACTH. However, no mutations of these receptors have been found; the explanation of this abnormal expression has not yet been elucidated. Variants in *PDE11A* are found in more than one-quarter of patients with PBMAH.[28,29] These variants lead to an activation of the cAMP/PKA pathway in vitro, suggesting that *PDE11A* variants with reduced enzymatic activity might play a role in the genetic predisposition to PBMAH.[29] Rare mutations of the *MC2R* gene, encoding for the ACTH-receptor, have been reported in isolated cases of bilateral hyperplasia (see **Fig. 1B**).[42] In addition, bilateral hyperplasia has been described in other genetic diseases, including the McCune-Albright syndrome (*GNAS1*) (see **Fig. 1B**),[43,44] the multiple endocrine neoplasia type 1 (*MEN1*),[45] the familial adenomatous polyposis (mutations of APC gene),[46,47] and the hereditary leiomyomatosis and renal cell cancer (*fumarate hydratase [FH]*).[48,49] However, McCune-Albright is observed exclusively in rare cases of very young children; somatic GNAS1 mutations are very rare in adults with PBMAH.[43] Mutations of *MEN1*, *APC*, or *FH* do not explain most of the cases of PBMAH in adult patients.

Recently, by a pan-genomic approach using SNP DNA chips to compare tumor and germline DNA in order to identify the region of chromosomal alterations in PBMAH, a copy neutral LOH has been demonstrated at 16p in surgically resected adrenal nodules from patients with PBMAH.[50] By whole-genome sequencing, inactivating mutations of armadillo repeat containing 5 (ARMC5) located at 16p have been identified. Assié and colleagues[50] demonstrated mutations of ARMC5 in 55% of the 33 patients who underwent surgery for clinical Cushing syndrome. The mechanism of ARMC5 inactivation in patients with BMAH follows the Knudson 2-hit model of a tumor suppressor gene: at the germline DNA, one allele presents a mutation (or a large deletion); at the somatic level, the other allele is inactivated by another mutation or by a LOH at 16p.[50] Patients in the cohort from the National Institutes of Health presented a germline ARMC5 mutation in 21% of the 33 index cases.[51] Ten large PBMAH families have been screened by 3 different teams and 8 harbored an ARMC5 mutation.[52–54] To date, 12 stops codons, 17 missenses, 21 frame-shifts, 2 deletions of one or more nucleotide acids, and 2 mutations in splicing sites have been described at the germline or the somatic level.[50–54] Besides, further studies are needed to determinate the implication in PBMAH of common variants described in the general population.[51] All these mutations seemed unique, but the variants p.R898W[50,51] and p.R267X[50,54] have been found in 3 and 5 unrelated index cases (**Fig. 2**). The first preliminary genotype-phenotype correlation analysis suggests that ARMC5 is associated with larger hyperplasia, more nodules, and more severe hypercortisolism.[50,51] The function of ARMC5 and its signaling pathway are unknown. It contains 7 armadillo domains and a BTB domain. Such domains have been demonstrated in other proteins that are known to participate in protein-protein interactions. β-catenin, the most-known armadillo protein, is also involved in adrenal tumors. The first functional studies have shown a role of ARMC5 in apoptosis. Wild-type protein stimulates apoptosis in vitro, whereas this effect is lost with missense mutants.[50]

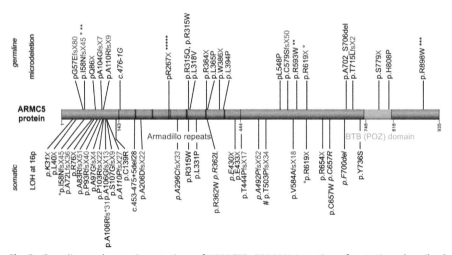

Fig. 2. Germline and somatic mutations of ARMC5 in PBMAH. Location of mutations described to date[50–54] on the ARMC5 protein according to the variant ENSP00000268314 (http://www.ensembl.org/). The location of domains is according to UniProtKB (Uniprot Q96C12-1, http://www.uniprot.org/). Above: germline mutations. Below: somatic mutations and the mutations found on somatic DNA for which the germline or somatic level was not determinate (*italic font*). The open circle indicates mutations described in germline and somatic DNA. The asterisk indicates mutations described for several patients; each star represents one PBMAH index case. The number sign indicates that the mutation p.T503PfsX34 has been described in a meningioma in a patient presenting with a germline mutation of ARMC5.[53]

Finally, new candidate genes have been suggested by whole-exome sequencing (WES). *DOT1L* was mutated in 2 of 7 patients with PBMAH. This gene codes for a histone H3 lysine methyl-transferase that regulates gene transcription and cellular proliferation. A variant in *HDAC9*, a histone deacetylase was found in another tumor of this cohort.[55] The gene endothelin receptor type A was identified as a putative gene of PBMAH by another WES study.[56] Functional studies will be important to confirm the involvement of these newly described gene alterations in the pathophysiology of PBMAH.

CORTISOL-SECRETING ADENOMAS
Activation of the Protein Kinase A Pathway

Alpha subunit of protein G
Beyond McCune-Albright in patients with pediatric PBMAH and rare adults, the gene coding for the alpha subunit of the protein Gs (*GNAS1*) can harbor somatic mutations in rare cortisol secreting tumors (see **Fig. 1**C).[55,57–60] Whole-genome expression profiling (transcriptome) demonstrates activation of different oncogenic pathways such as Wnt/β-catenin pathways for *PRKAR1A*-mutated tumors and MAPK pathways for *GNAS*-mutated tumors.[61]

Catalytic alpha subunit of protein kinase A
Felix Beuschlein and colleagues[33] followed quickly by 3 other teams recently identified somatic-activating mutations of the catalytic alpha subunit of PKA (*PRKACA*) in a subset of cortisol-producing adenomas (CPA) using WES (see **Fig. 1**C).[55,58,62] The c.617A>G/p.L206R hot spot mutation was found in heterozygote state in more than 40% of the CPA considering these 4 cohorts.[63] A unique mutation, the c.595_596insCAC/L199_Cys200insTrp, was found in one patient with a CPA.[33] Mutations of *PRKACA* were mainly found in patients with clinically overt Cushing syndrome. Indeed, patients harboring a mutation are significantly younger at the time of the diagnosis and present with Cushing's syndrome and smaller tumors.[33,55,58,62] The hot spot p.L206R is located in a highly conserved active-site cleft of the catalytic subunits to which the regulatory subunits binds. In vitro experiments demonstrated that the 2 mutants are constitutively hyperactive and are resistant to inhibition by the regulatory subunits R1alpha[58,62] and R2beta.[33] The resistance to regulatory subunits R1alpha inhibition is explained by a loss of interaction between the regulatory subunits and the L206RCα mutant. In adrenal tissue, this mutation leads to activation of the cAMP/PKA pathway and high expression of steroidogenic enzymes.[33,58] The constitutive activation of PKA can be suppressed in vitro by PRKACA inhibitors,[55,62] opening a possible therapeutic opportunity.

Protein kinase A regulatory subunit 1-alpha
Somatic mutations of *PRKAR1A* have been described in CPA both by a candidate gene approach and more recently by WES.[2,55] These mutations are inactivating mutations similar to the one observed in the germline DNA from patients with CNC. CPA with *PRKAR1A* mutations tend to be smaller and exhibit a paradoxic increase in urinary cortisol levels after dexamethasone suppression as often observed in patients with CNC.[2]

Activation of the Wnt/β-Catenin Pathway

The canonical Wnt/β-catenin pathway regulates many cellular processes, including proliferation, differentiation, and apoptosis. In the absence of a Wnt ligand, β-catenin is located in the cytoplasm, phosphorylated by a destruction complex of scaffolding proteins, including Axin and APC and then targeted by E3 ubiquitin ligase for proteosomal degradation. Binding of Wnt ligands to the receptor complex serpentine/low-density lipoprotein receptor leads to recruitment of the disheveled protein and disruption of the destruction complex. Active β-catenin accumulates in the cytoplasm and translocates into the nucleus where it acts as a transcriptional coregulator.[64] Tissier and colleagues[65] first demonstrated the role of activation of the Wnt/β-catenin pathway in the pathogenesis of ACT. They showed by immunohistochemistry that β-catenin was accumulated in the cytoplasm and the nucleus of ACT in 27% of the benign and 31% of the malignant tumors. This particular pattern reflects the activation of this pathway.

The Wnt/β-catenin pathway is activated in 25% to 50% of ACA according to ß-catenin immunohistochemistry analysis.[24,65,66] This activation is explained in 70% of the cases by CTNNB1 mutations (**Fig. 3**).[66] CTNNB1 mutations are more frequent in nonsecreting ACA than cortisol-secreting ACA.[66]

ADRENOCORTICAL CANCER

Cancer of the adrenal cortex is a rare tumor with an overall poor prognosis.[67] It can be responsible for steroid excess, typically cortisol and androgens; but mineralocorticoids and steroid precursors can be also oversecreted. Despite an overall poor outcome there is a certain heterogeneity, and some tumors do not recur after removal or progress slowly when metastatic. Molecular genetics can now give some clue as to the cause of this clinical heterogeneity.

Genes and Pathways Involved in Adrenocortical Cancer

Tumor protein p53
Li-Fraumeni syndrome and germline mutation of TP53 Li-Fraumeni syndrome (LFS) (OMIM No. 151623) is an autosomal disorder characterized by predisposition and early onset of several cancers, including sarcoma, breast carcinoma, brain tumors, leukemia, and ACC.[68,69] Germline mutations of the tumor protein p53 gene (TP53) located at 17p13.1 have been reported in 29% to 90% of cases.[68–71] Pediatric ACCs are related to TP53 germline mutations in more than 70% of cases in Europe and North America.[72] The incidence of pediatric ACC is remarkably high in southern Brazil, where more than 90% of patients carry the germline TP53 mutation p.R337H. In the state of Paraná in Brazil, a systematic screening of newborns found the hot spot in 0.27% of the 171,649 newborns screened. Around 50% of the carriers' children were followed during 3.0 to 6.7 years; the penetrance of ACT was 2.39%.[73] In sporadic ACC in adult patients, germline mutations of TP53 are found in between 3.9% and 5.8% of cases. Several patients did not fulfill the diagnostic criteria for LFS.[74,75] Twenty-five percent of TP53 mutations appear de novo.[76] Beyond these mutations, it has been shown recently that TP53 polymorphisms in adult patients seem to influence overall survival.[77]

TP53 signaling pathway in sporadic adrenocortical cancer The protein p53, named as the guardian of the genome has a fundamental role in the cellular response to stress, oncogene activation, or DNA damage by regulating the cell cycle and apoptosis. It is the most altered gene in sporadic cancers.[76] At the somatic DNA level, mutation of TP53 is a frequent event occurring in between 16% and 70% of ACC if the whole gene is sequenced.[78,79] TP53 is considered a tumor suppressor gene, and both alleles are supposed to be inactivated in the tumor tissue. LOH at 17p13 is observed in 85% of ACCs.[80] However, other mechanisms may lead to TP53 inactivation because LOH and mutation are not associated in every case.[79] The presence of an abnormal nuclear staining of TP53 by immunohistochemistry correlates well with TP53 mutations and

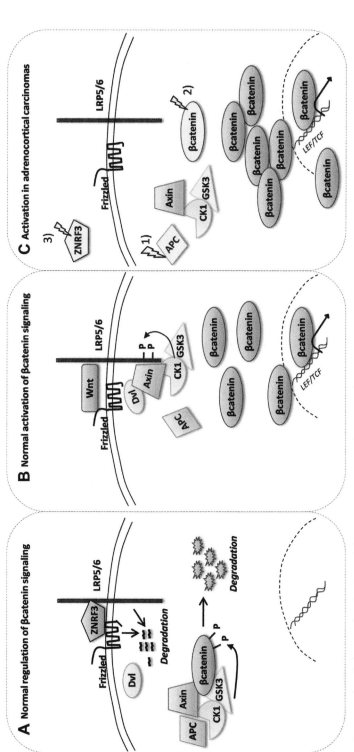

Fig. 3. Normal and abnormal activation of the Wnt-β-catenin pathway in adrenocortical cells. (*A*) In the absence of Wnt ligand, β-catenin is located in the cytoplasm, phosphorylated by a destruction complex of scaffolding proteins, including Axin, APC, CK1, and GSK3, and subsequently targeted by E3 ubiquitin ligase for proteosomal degradation. ZNRF3 leads the Wnt-LRP6 receptors complex to degradation. ZNRF3 regulates the pathway by inhibiting the receptor complex Frizzled/low-density lipoprotein receptor (LRP5/6). (*B*) Binding of Wnt ligands on the receptor complex leads to recruitment of disheveled (Dvl) and disruption of the destruction complex. Active β-catenin accumulates in the cytoplasm, translocates in the nucleus, and acts as a transcriptional coregulator at LEF/TCF (Lymphoid-enhancing factor/T-cell factor) response elements. (*C*) In adrenocortical carcinomas, (1) mutations of *APC* disrupt the destruction complex and set free β-catenin, which accumulates in the cytoplasm and the nucleus; (2) mutated β-catenin escapes degradation and accumulates in the cytoplasm and nucleus; (3) inactivating mutations of *ZNFR3* dissipate the inhibition of the receptor complex.

could be used as a diagnostic tool.[79] Somatic mutations of *TP53* are associated with aggressive tumors and poor outcomes.[79,81]

Other actors of the p53 pathways have been recently shown to play a role in the pathogenesis of ACCs. Overexpression of PTTG1, which encodes securin, a negative regulator of p53, was identified as a marker of poor survival.[82] Loss of retinoblastoma (Rb) protein has been found by immunohistochemistry in 27% of aggressive ACCs. This defect is related in most cases to mutations of the *RB1* gene or its allelic loss.[83] Recently, Assié and colleagues[78] have studied by several genomic approaches a large European cohort of more than 120 ACCs. Mutations of *RB1* were found in 7% of tumors. Eleven percent of the tumors of this cohort harbored mutations of *CDKN2A*, and 2% exhibited high-level amplification of *CDK4*. Thus, overall, 33% of the tumors had alterations of the p53 pathway (**Fig. 4**). Similar findings have been reported in a small series by WES.[58]

The Wnt/β-catenin signaling pathway

Familial adenomatous polyposis Patients with familial adenomatous polyposis (FAP) (OMIM No. 175100) or Gardner syndrome present multiple colonic polyps and an

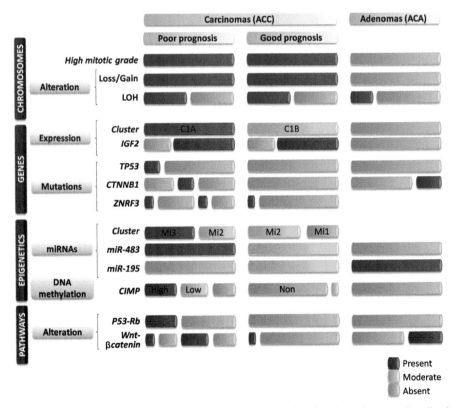

Fig. 4. Molecular defects in adrenocortical carcinomas. Molecular alterations are described at the chromosomal, genetic, and epigenetics levels that help to discriminate malignant from benign tumors as well as to predict prognosis. Cluster associated to different prognoses as described in transcriptome (C1A, C1B), mi-RNAs expression analysis (Mi3, Mi2, Mi1), and methylation study (CIMP-high, -low, -non).[78] Red boxes: the feature is present; green boxes: if quantitative data, the feature is moderately present; blue boxes: the feature is absent. miRNAs, microRNAs.

increased risk of early colon carcinomas. Pigmented retinal lesions, desmoids tumors, osteomas, thyroid adenoma/carcinomas, and other different malignant tumors have also been described.[84] Adrenocortical tumors, especially nonfunctional nodular hyperplasia, CPA, and ACC affects 7% to 13% of patients.[64,85] FAP is caused by germline inactivating mutation of APC, a tumor suppressor gene that inhibits Wnt/β-catenin signaling (see **Fig. 3**). According to the Knudson's model, ACC in patients with FAP exhibits somatic APC mutations as a second hit.[86]

Activation of the Wnt/β-catenin pathway in sporadic adrenocortical cancer Activation of the Wnt/β-catenin signaling pathway is observed according to β-catenin immunohistochemistry in a third of ACC.[46,65] Activation of β-catenin is mainly related to mutation of its gene CTNNB1.[46,65] Sequencing of other actors of the pathway, such as AXIN1, AXIN2, and WTX, failed to show frequent somatic mutations in sporadic ACC.[86–88] However, mutations of APC were recently found in 2% of cases from a large cohort of ACC.[78] Consistently, transcriptome studies have shown an overexpression of Wnt/β-catenin target genes in ACC.[89] Mutations of CTNNB1 or a histologic pattern of its activation are associated with poor outcomes.[46,81] In addition to the observation of a late occurrence of malignancy features in the hyperplastic adrenals from mice with constitutive activation of β-catenin,[90,91] this suggests that Wnt/β-catenin activation is a late driver of tumorigenesis.[64,89] In childhood ACTs, a histologic pattern of β-catenin activation is found in 70% of ACT; but CTNNB1 mutations are not a common event (6%), and it can be associated with TP53 mutations. A decreased expression of Wnt inhibitor genes is observed. Nevertheless, an association with poor prognosis is also found.[92]

Zinc and ring finger 3 (ZNRF3)
ZNRF3 is a cell-surface transmembrane E3 ubiquitin ligase that is a negative regulator of the Wnt/β-catenin pathways (see **Fig. 3**). ZNRF3 leads the Wnt-LRP6 receptors complex to degradation. ZNRF3 is regulated by the R-Spondin protein that regulates the association of ZNRF3 with the related leucine-rich repeat-containing G protein–coupled receptors LGR4. This association results in membrane clearance of ZNFR3 and activation of the Wnt/β-catenin pathway.[93] Recently, ZNRF3 appeared as the most frequently altered gene (21%) in ACCs. In the cohort of 122 ACCs studied by Assié and colleagues,[78] homozygous deletion of the gene was found for 19 tumors, and heterozygous mutations for 7 tumors including 5 with a LOH of the wild type allele. ZNRF3 and CTNNB1 mutations were mutually exclusive (see **Fig. 4**). Transcriptome of tumors with alterations of ZNFR3 shows activation of β-catenin targets but milder than the level observed in CTNNB1-mutated ACC. ZNFR3 also constitutes a new tumor suppressor gene. By the sum of the CTNNB1- and ZNRF3-altered ACC, activation of the Wnt/β-catenin pathway could be present in 39% of ACC.[78]

Insulin-like growth factor 2 (IGF2)
Beckwith-Wiedemann syndrome Beckwith-Wiedemann syndrome (BWS) (OMIM No. 130650) is a pediatric disease leading to visceromegaly (macroglossia, hemihyperplasia), malformations (wall defect, umbilical hernia), and predisposition to embryonal malignancies. Fetal adrenocortical cytomegaly is a specific feature. ACCs are one of the several malignant tumors to which patients are predisposed.[94] Dysregulation of the locus 11p15.5 by genetic and epigenetic alterations is responsible for the disease. This locus includes the genes H19, IGF2, and CDKN1C (p57kip2). H19, a 2,3 kb-long noncoding RNA linked with several cancers, is expressed from the maternal allele, IGF2, from the paternal. Both are regulated by an imprinting center (IC1) usually methylated on the paternal chromosome and unmethylated on the maternal. The

maternal expression of CDKN1C is under the control of another imprinting center (IC2). In BWS, gain of methylation at IC1 (5% of patients) or loss of methylation of IC2 (50% of patients) leads to overexpression of IGF2 by biallelic expression of the gene and reduced expression of CDKN1C and H19. These methylation changes occur with different genomic alterations as DNA methylation changes, uniparental disomy, copy numbers variations, and mutation of *CDKN1C*.[94,95] Beyond these genetic/epigenetic alterations, the physiopathology of BWS is not yet well understood. BWS related to *CDKN1C* mutations or loss of maternal methylation have a lower risk of tumors in comparison with the gain of methylation of IC1,[94] suggesting that overexpression of IGF2 or downregulation of H19 participates in the process of tumorigenesis.

Alteration of the 11p15 locus and insulin-like growth factor 2 overexpression in sporadic adrenocortical cancer IGF2 is a growth factor that stimulates proliferation and inhibits apoptosis in several cell types through the MAPK and PI3K signaling pathways. Overexpression of IGF2 was one of the first molecular events characterized in about 90% of ACCs. Like in BWS, Gicquel and colleagues[4] described a loss of maternal allele methylation, or duplication of the paternal allele, leading to overexpression of IGF2. Several transcriptome studies have confirmed that IGF2 overexpression is observed in more than 85% of ACC and that this gene is the top upregulated gene in ACC as compared with normal adrenal or ACA.[96–99] Overexpression of the IGF-I receptor (IGF1-R), upregulation of IGFBP2, and downregulation of the IGF2 receptors have also been described.[100] An early clinical trial with an inhibitor of the IGF1-R demonstrated partial responses in some patients.[101] In pediatric cases, an overexpression of IGF2 is also found in adenomas; but expression of IGF1-R is higher in ACC and associated with a worse prognosis.[102] However, in adult ACC, overexpression of IGF2 is not associated with a worse prognosis.[103] Furthermore inhibition of the IGF receptors to treat adrenal cancer has not yet proved to be very efficient. A transcriptome study did not show a different profile of gene expression between ACC with or without IGF2 overexpression.[89] Surprisingly, mice models with overexpression of IGF2 fail to show a strong oncogenic potential even in association with β-catenin activation.[100,104] The tumorigenic potential of IGF2 is also misunderstood. Because of the genetic alterations at the 11p15 locus, a possible involvement of H19 or the microRNA miR-483 (see later discussion) located at 11p15 is suggested. Mutations of *CDKN1C* are not commonly found in ACC.[105] H19 is a 2,3 kb-long noncoding RNA linked with several cancers. However, it seems to play a dual role independent of the tumor, either tumor suppressor or oncogene. For example, it could be upregulated by the cMyc transcription factor or downregulated by p53 in function of the tumor models.[106] In ACC, H19 expression is low,[98,107] suggesting a potential tumor suppressor role.

The other genetic alterations
Others syndromes The MEN1 is an autosomal dominant syndrome caused by a germline mutation of the *MEN1* gene (11q13) (OMIM No. 131100). It includes primary hyperparathyroidism (95%), endocrine pancreatic tumors (50%), pituitary adenomas (40%), and thymic carcinoid.[108] ACT and/or hyperplasia are reported in 9% to 55% of the patients. These tumors are mainly benign and nonfunctional tumors, although some malignant lesions and CPA have been described.[45,108] Somatic mutations of *MEN1* were not clearly reported initially in sporadic ACC.[109,110] However, a recent WES revealed somatic *MEN1* mutations in 7% of screened ACC.[78]

The Lynch syndrome or hereditary nonpolyposis colorectal cancer syndrome (OMIM No. 120435) is an autosomal dominant disease secondary to mutations in

DNA mismatch-repair genes. Several other malignant tumors are associated with the disease, including ACC.[111,112] In a recent retrospective cohort of ACC, 3.2% of patients had a Lynch syndrome.[112]

The occurrence of ACC has been reported in patients presenting other syndromes as the CNC but the contribution of the molecular defects to the malignancy is unclear.[113–115]

Other somatic alterations Mutations in *TERT*, *DAXX*, and *ATRX* have been recently found in a European cohort of ACC by WES and SNP analysis.[78] These genes are involved in telomere length maintenance. *TERT* codes for telomerase, and its mutations are involved in several cancers. *DAXX* and *ATRX* mutations have been associated with the maintenance of telomere length by a telomerase-independent mechanism.[78] The specific role of these genes in adrenocortical tumorigenesis warrants further investigation.

Chromosomal Alterations

Some chromosomal alterations can be found by the histologic examination of the tumor. ACC presents with a high mitotic grade associated with abnormal mitotic figures, aneuploidy, or polyploidy.[116] Chromosomal alterations in ACC have been well characterized by different approaches: by conventional CGH,[117–119] by CGH array,[120–122] and, recently, by SNP array.[78,123] Alterations in copy numbers in ACCs are considerably higher in comparison with benign tumors.[120] If the alteration of certain loci is inconstant, copy number gains involving chromosomes 5, 7, 12, and 20 and losses in chromosome 22 were more often reported (see **Fig. 4**). Copy-neutral LOH detected by SNP array occurs in 30% to 90% of ACC.[78,123] SNP array allows the identification of gene amplification or deletion. In the European cohort of ACC, these alterations have been found in the locus of *TERT*, *CD4*, *CDKN2A*, *RB1*, and *ZNFR3* (see earlier discussion) and in the locus 3q13.1 and 4q34.3 where the long noncoding RNA LOC285194 and LINC00290 are respectively located. An implication of the involvement of these 2 noncoding RNA has been suggested.[78] The diagnostic and prognostic potentials of these chromosomal alterations need to be confirmed.[6,120,123] Indeed, ACA presents with LOH in about 25% of cases[123] and can have a gain of material, especially in larger adenomas.[117,118,120]

Epigenetics Alterations in Adrenocortical Cancer

Methylation

DNA methylation is the most characterized epigenetic mechanism of regulation of transcription. This methylation occurs in the cytosine of CpG dinucleotides that are particularly enriched in specific regions of the promoter called *CpG islands*.[124] Beyond the abnormalities described at the IGF2 locus, a global alteration of methylation pattern has been described in ACC by 3 studies done at the genome-wide level.[125–127] In these studies, the ACC presented a hypomethylation of intergenic regions[127] and a global hypermethylation of promoter regions.[125–127] The profile of methylation of ACT could discriminate ACC from ACA.[127] Additionally, the levels of methylation of CpG islands distinguish 2 groups of ACC: one, named non-CIMP (CpG island methylator phenotype), is slightly hypermethylated compared with ACA and another hypermethylated named CIMP. Within the CIMP group, 2 further subgroups were delineated: CIMP-low and CIMP-high, referring to the levels of hypermethylation (see **Fig. 4**). The prognosis was worse for the CIMP carcinomas than the non-CIMP and worse for the CIMP-high than the CIMP-low.[125] The CIMP-high corresponded to the group C1Ax (poor prognosis without mutations) and C1A-p53 (poor prognosis with *TP53* mutations) and the non-CIMP corresponded to the C1A/β-catenin and the C1B group (good prognosis) as determined by transcriptome analysis (see **Fig. 4**).[78,81,125] The hypermethylated genes included genes involved in cell cycle and apoptosis regulation[126] or in cell proliferation and immune response.[125] Their levels of expression are inversely correlated to the level of methylation as expected.[124,126]

microRNAs

MicroRNAs (miRNAs) are small RNAs (approximately 22 nucleotides). They play an important role in the posttranslational regulation of gene expression by targeting mRNAs for cleavage or translational repression. A deregulation of the expression of the miRNAs is involved in several cancers through activation of oncogenes or silencing of suppressor gene tumors. Their profile of expression has been proposed as diagnostic or prognostic markers, achievable in practice because they can be detected in blood.[128] In ACC, a deregulation of several miRNAs has been observed. The determination of their expression profiles in adrenocortical tumors was the aim of several recent studies. The expression of miRNAs seems to differ significantly between ACAs and ACCs. Several miRNAs were particularly highlighted. The difference between the delta cycle threshold of the high-expressed miR-503 and low-expressed miR-511 was proposed to distinguish benign tumor from malignant tumors.[129] A high expression of the miR-483-5p in ACC[130–133] and a low expression of miR-195 and miR-335[130–134] have been well demonstrated. The level of circulating miR-483-5p allows for the distinction between ACC and benign tumors.[133,135] In childhood adrenocortical tumors, a set of miRNAs harbors a differential expression in comparison with normal adrenal tissue. These miRNAs are mainly downregulated (miR-99a, miR-100); however, an upregulation of miR-483 is found in childhood ACC similar to that observed in adult ACC. The profile of miRNA expression shows 3 clusters in ACC associated with different prognoses.[132] In a European cohort of ACC,[78] 3 clusters of miRNA have been differentiated: Mi1, Mi2, and Mi3. Mi1 presents the largest difference of miRNA expression in comparison with normal adrenal samples and is associated to the poor prognosis group C1A (see **Fig. 4**). High levels of miR-483-5p and low levels of miR-195 in tumor tissue[130] or in the blood[133] are associated with a worse prognosis. The miRNA expression pattern could differ for certain specific ACC variants, such as oncocytic ACC.[136] In vitro studies have shown that the level of miR-483-5p and miR-195 affects cell proliferation and death.[132] In particular, the miR-483-3p is inversely correlated with the expression of the proapoptotic protein PUMA (p53 upregulated modulator of apoptosis) suggesting a role for this miR in apoptosis regulation.[132] The gene encoding miR-483-5p is located in the IGF2 locus, and the level of IGF2 expression is directly correlated with this miRNA.[131,135] The miR-99a and miR-100 participate in the regulation of mTOR signaling, a pathway involved in cellular proliferation in ACC.[137]

SUMMARY

Recent advances in the discovery of the genetic alterations of adrenocortical tumors have been possible with genomics methods. However, the genetic defects associated with some adrenocortical tumors, including non-*PRKACA* CPA or non-*ARMC5* PBMAH, are still unknown and represent the new challenge for these whole-genome studies. Large-scale clinical studies are now needed to determine the precise role of the molecular tools derived from these pan-genomic studies in the diagnosis and the prognostication of adrenocortical tumors. The elucidation of the molecular genetics underlying the pathogenesis of adrenocortical tumors paves the way toward personalized medicine. The identification of new genes involved in adrenal cortical tumorigenesis, such as *ARMC5* and *ZNRF3*, opens new questions about their physiologic and pathologic functions. A greater understanding of the role of these new genes is essential in order to develop innovative, targeted therapies for tumors of the adrenal cortex.

REFERENCES

1. Libé R, Bertherat J. Molecular genetics of adrenocortical tumours, from familial to sporadic diseases. Eur J Endocrinol 2005;153:477–87.
2. Bertherat J, Groussin L, Sandrini F, et al. Molecular and functional analysis of PRKAR1A and its locus (17q22-24) in sporadic adrenocortical tumors: 17q losses, somatic mutations, and protein kinase A expression and activity. Cancer Res 2003;63:5308–19.
3. Gicquel C, Raffin-Sanson ML, Gaston V, et al. Structural and functional abnormalities at 11p15 are associated with the malignant phenotype in sporadic adrenocortical tumors: study on a series of 82 tumors. J Clin Endocrinol Metab 1997; 82:2559–65.
4. Gicquel C, Bertagna X, Schneid H, et al. Rearrangements at the 11p15 locus and overexpression of insulin-like growth factor-II gene in sporadic adrenocortical tumors. J Clin Endocrinol Metab 1994;78:1444–53.
5. Reincke M, Karl M, Travis WH, et al. p53 mutations in human adrenocortical neoplasms: immunohistochemical and molecular studies. J Clin Endocrinol Metab 1994;78:790–4.
6. Assié G, Jouinot A, Bertherat J. The 'omics' of adrenocortical tumours for personalized medicine. Nat Rev Endocrinol 2014;10:215–28.
7. Lacroix A. Heredity and cortisol regulation in bilateral macronodular adrenal hyperplasia. N Engl J Med 2013;369:2147–9.
8. Lacroix A. ACTH-independent macronodular adrenal hyperplasia. Best Pract Res Clin Endocrinol Metab 2009;23:245–59.
9. Louiset E, Duparc C, Young J, et al. Intraadrenal corticotropin in bilateral macronodular adrenal hyperplasia. N Engl J Med 2013;369:2115–25.
10. Bertherat J, Horvath A, Groussin L, et al. Mutations in regulatory subunit type 1A of cyclic adenosine 5'-monophosphate-dependent protein kinase (PRKAR1A): phenotype analysis in 353 patients and 80 different genotypes. J Clin Endocrinol Metab 2009;94:2085–91.
11. Stratakis CA, Kirschner LS, Carney JA. Clinical and molecular features of the Carney complex: diagnostic criteria and recommendations for patient evaluation. J Clin Endocrinol Metab 2001;86:4041–6.
12. Bertherat J. Carney complex (CNC). Orphanet J Rare Dis 2006;1:21.
13. Espiard S, Bertherat J. Carney complex. Front Horm Res 2013;41:50–62.
14. Matyakhina L, Pack S, Kirschner LS, et al. Chromosome 2 (2p16) abnormalities in Carney complex tumours. J Med Genet 2003;40:268–77.
15. Casey M, Vaughan CJ, He J, et al. Mutations in the protein kinase A R1alpha regulatory subunit cause familial cardiac myxomas and Carney complex. J Clin Invest 2000;106:R31–8.
16. Kirschner LS, Carney JA, Pack SD, et al. Mutations of the gene encoding the protein kinase A type I-alpha regulatory subunit in patients with the Carney complex. Nat Genet 2000;26:89–92.
17. Horvath A, Bertherat J, Groussin L, et al. Mutations and polymorphisms in the gene encoding regulatory subunit type 1-alpha of protein kinase A (PRKAR1A): an update. Hum Mutat 2010;31:369–79.

18. Groussin L, Kirschner LS, Vincent-Dejean C, et al. Molecular analysis of the cyclic AMP-dependent protein kinase A (PKA) regulatory subunit 1A (PRKAR1A) gene in patients with Carney complex and primary pigmented nodular adrenocortical disease (PPNAD) reveals novel mutations and clues for pathophysiology: augmented PKA signaling is associated with adrenal tumorigenesis in PPNAD. Am J Hum Genet 2002;71:1433–42.

19. Patronas Y, Horvath A, Greene E, et al. In vitro studies of novel PRKAR1A mutants that extend the predicted RIα protein sequence into the 3'-untranslated open reading frame: proteasomal degradation leads to RIα haploinsufficiency and Carney complex. J Clin Endocrinol Metab 2012;97: E496–502.

20. Groussin L, Horvath A, Jullian E, et al. A PRKAR1A mutation associated with primary pigmented nodular adrenocortical disease in 12 kindreds. J Clin Endocrinol Metab 2006;91:1943–9.

21. Sahut-Barnola I, de Joussineau C, Val P, et al. Cushing's syndrome and fetal features resurgence in adrenal cortex-specific Prkar1a knockout mice. PLoS Genet 2010;6:e1000980.

22. Yu B, Ragazzon B, Rizk-Rabin M, et al. Protein kinase A alterations in endocrine tumors. Horm Metab Res 2012;44:741–8.

23. Gaujoux S, Tissier F, Groussin L, et al. Wnt/beta-catenin and 3',5'-cyclic adenosine 5'-monophosphate/protein kinase A signaling pathways alterations and somatic beta-catenin gene mutations in the progression of adrenocortical tumors. J Clin Endocrinol Metab 2008;93:4135–40.

24. Tadjine M, Lampron A, Ouadi L, et al. Detection of somatic beta-catenin mutations in primary pigmented nodular adrenocortical disease (PPNAD). Clin Endocrinol (Oxf) 2008;69:367–73.

25. Horvath A, Mathyakina L, Vong Q, et al. Serial analysis of gene expression in adrenocortical hyperplasia caused by a germline PRKAR1A mutation. J Clin Endocrinol Metab 2006;91:584–96.

26. Horvath A, Boikos S, Giatzakis C, et al. A genome-wide scan identifies mutations in the gene encoding phosphodiesterase 11A4 (PDE11A) in individuals with adrenocortical hyperplasia. Nat Genet 2006;38:794–800.

27. Libé R, Horvath A, Vezzosi D, et al. Frequent phosphodiesterase 11A gene (PDE11A) defects in patients with Carney complex (CNC) caused by PRKAR1A mutations: PDE11A may contribute to adrenal and testicular tumors in CNC as a modifier of the phenotype. J Clin Endocrinol Metab 2011;96:E208–14.

28. Libé R, Fratticci A, Coste J, et al. Phosphodiesterase 11A (PDE11A) and genetic predisposition to adrenocortical tumors. Clin Cancer Res 2008;14:4016–24.

29. Vezzosi D, Libé R, Baudry C, et al. Phosphodiesterase 11A (PDE11A) gene defects in patients with acth-independent macronodular adrenal hyperplasia (AIMAH): functional variants may contribute to genetic susceptibility of bilateral adrenal tumors. J Clin Endocrinol Metab 2012;97:E2063–9.

30. Horvath A, Mericq V, Stratakis CA. Mutation in PDE8B, a cyclic AMP-specific phosphodiesterase in adrenal hyperplasia. N Engl J Med 2008;358:750–2.

31. Rothenbuhler A, Horvath A, Libé R, et al. Identification of novel genetic variants in phosphodiesterase 8B (PDE8B), a cAMP-specific phosphodiesterase highly expressed in the adrenal cortex, in a cohort of patients with adrenal tumours. Clin Endocrinol (Oxf) 2012;77:195–9.

32. Tsai LC, Shimizu-Albergine M, Beavo JA. The high-affinity cAMP-specific phosphodiesterase 8B controls steroidogenesis in the mouse adrenal gland. Mol Pharmacol 2011;79:639–48.

33. Beuschlein F, Fassnacht M, Assié G, et al. Constitutive activation of PKA catalytic subunit in adrenal Cushing's syndrome. N Engl J Med 2014;370:1019–28.
34. Forlino A, Vetro A, Garavelli L, et al. PRKACB and Carney complex. N Engl J Med 2014;370:1065–7.
35. Gagliardi L, Hotu C, Casey G, et al. Familial vasopressin-sensitive ACTH-independent macronodular adrenal hyperplasia (VPs-AIMAH): clinical studies of three kindreds. Clin Endocrinol (Oxf) 2009;70:883–91.
36. Imöhl M, Köditz R, Stachon A, et al. Catecholamine-dependent hereditary Cushing's syndrome - follow-up after unilateral adrenalectomy. Med Klin (Munich) 1983;2002(97):747–53 [in Germany].
37. Lee S, Hwang R, Lee J, et al. Ectopic expression of vasopressin V1b and V2 receptors in the adrenal glands of familial ACTH-independent macronodular adrenal hyperplasia. Clin Endocrinol (Oxf) 2005;63:625–30.
38. Miyamura N, Taguchi T, Murata Y, et al. Inherited adrenocorticotropin-independent macronodular adrenal hyperplasia with abnormal cortisol secretion by vasopressin and catecholamines: detection of the aberrant hormone receptors on adrenal gland. Endocrine 2002;19:319–26.
39. Vezzosi D, Cartier D, Régnier C, et al. Familial adrenocorticotropin-independent macronodular adrenal hyperplasia with aberrant serotonin and vasopressin adrenal receptors. Eur J Endocrinol 2007;156:21–31.
40. Hofland J, Hofland LJ, van Koetsveld PM, et al. ACTH-independent macronodular adrenocortical hyperplasia reveals prevalent aberrant in vivo and in vitro responses to hormonal stimuli and coupling of arginine-vasopressin type 1a receptor to 11β-hydroxylase. Orphanet J Rare Dis 2013;8:142.
41. Libé R, Coste J, Guignat L, et al. Aberrant cortisol regulations in bilateral macronodular adrenal hyperplasia: a frequent finding in a prospective study of 32 patients with overt or subclinical Cushing's syndrome. Eur J Endocrinol 2010;163: 129–38.
42. Swords FM, Noon LA, King PJ, et al. Constitutive activation of the human ACTH receptor resulting from a synergistic interaction between two naturally occurring missense mutations in the MC2R gene. Mol Cell Endocrinol 2004;213:149–54.
43. Fragoso MC, Domenice S, Latronico AC, et al. Cushing's syndrome secondary to adrenocorticotropin-independent macronodular adrenocortical hyperplasia due to activating mutations of GNAS1 gene. J Clin Endocrinol Metab 2003;88: 2147–51.
44. Weinstein LS, Shenker A, Gejman PV, et al. Activating mutations of the stimulatory G protein in the McCune-Albright syndrome. N Engl J Med 1991;325: 1688–95.
45. Gatta-Cherifi B, Chabre O, Murat A, et al. Adrenal involvement in MEN1. Analysis of 715 cases from the Groupe d'etude des Tumeurs Endocrines database. Eur J Endocrinol 2012;166:269–79.
46. Gaujoux S, Grabar S, Fassnacht M, et al. β-catenin activation is associated with specific clinical and pathologic characteristics and a poor outcome in adrenocortical carcinoma. Clin Cancer Res 2011;17:328–36.
47. Hsiao HP, Kirschner LS, Bourdeau I, et al. Clinical and genetic heterogeneity, overlap with other tumor syndromes, and atypical glucocorticoid hormone secretion in adrenocorticotropin-independent macronodular adrenal hyperplasia compared with other adrenocortical tumors. J Clin Endocrinol Metab 2009; 94:2930–7.
48. Matyakhina L, Freedman RJ, Bourdeau I, et al. Hereditary leiomyomatosis associated with bilateral, massive, macronodular adrenocortical disease and

atypical Cushing syndrome: a clinical and molecular genetic investigation. J Clin Endocrinol Metab 2005;90:3773–9.

49. Shuch B, Ricketts CJ, Vocke CD, et al. Adrenal nodular hyperplasia in hereditary leiomyomatosis and renal cell cancer. J Urol 2013;189:430–5.

50. Assié G, Libé R, Espiard S, et al. ARMC5 mutations in macronodular adrenal hyperplasia with Cushing's syndrome. N Engl J Med 2013;369:2105–14.

51. Faucz FR, Zilbermint M, Lodish MB, et al. Macronodular adrenal hyperplasia due to mutations in an armadillo repeat containing 5 (ARMC5) gene: a clinical and genetic investigation. J Clin Endocrinol Metab 2014;99:E1113–9.

52. Alencar GA, Lerario AM, Nishi MY, et al. ARMC5 mutations are a frequent cause of primary macronodular adrenal hyperplasia. J Clin Endocrinol Metab 2014;99:E1501–9.

53. Elbelt U, Trovato A, Kloth M, et al. Molecular and clinical evidence for an ARMC5 tumor syndrome: concurrent inactivating germline and somatic mutations are associated with both primary macronodular adrenal hyperplasia and meningioma. J Clin Endocrinol Metab 2015;100(1):E119–28.

54. Gagliardi L, Schreiber AW, Hahn CN, et al. ARMC5 mutations are common in familial bilateral macronodular adrenal hyperplasia. J Clin Endocrinol Metab 2014;99:E1784–92.

55. Cao Y, He M, Gao Z, et al. Activating hotspot L205R mutation in PRKACA and adrenal Cushing's syndrome. Science 2014;344:913–7.

56. Zhu J, Cui L, Wang W, et al. Whole exome sequencing identifies mutation of EDNRA involved in ACTH-independent macronodular adrenal hyperplasia. Fam Cancer 2013;12:657–67.

57. Dall'Asta C, Ballarè E, Mantovani G, et al. Assessing the presence of abnormal regulation of cortisol secretion by membrane hormone receptors: in vivo and in vitro studies in patients with functioning and non-functioning adrenal adenoma. Horm Metab Res 2004;36:578–83.

58. Goh G, Scholl UI, Healy JM, et al. Recurrent activating mutation in PRKACA in cortisol-producing adrenal tumors. Nat Genet 2014;46(6):613–7.

59. Kobayashi H, Usui T, Fukata J, et al. Mutation analysis of Gsalpha, adrenocorticotropin receptor and p53 genes in Japanese patients with adrenocortical neoplasms: including a case of Gsalpha mutation. Endocr J 2000;47:461–6.

60. Libé R, Mantovani G, Bondioni S, et al. Mutational analysis of PRKAR1A and Gs(alpha) in sporadic adrenocortical tumors. Exp Clin Endocrinol Diabetes 2005;113:248–51.

61. Almeida MQ, Azevedo MF, Xekouki P, et al. Activation of cyclic AMP signaling leads to different pathway alterations in lesions of the adrenal cortex caused by germline PRKAR1A defects versus those due to somatic GNAS mutations. J Clin Endocrinol Metab 2012;97:E687–93.

62. Sato Y, Maekawa S, Ishii R, et al. Recurrent somatic mutations underlie corticotropin-independent Cushing's syndrome. Science 2014;344:917–20.

63. Espiard S, Ragazzon B, Bertherat J. Protein kinase A alterations in adrenocortical tumors. Horm Metab Res 2014;46(12):869–75.

64. Berthon A, Martinez A, Bertherat J, et al. Wnt/β-catenin signalling in adrenal physiology and tumour development. Mol Cell Endocrinol 2012;351:87–95.

65. Tissier F, Cavard C, Groussin L, et al. Mutations of beta-catenin in adrenocortical tumors: activation of the Wnt signaling pathway is a frequent event in both benign and malignant adrenocortical tumors. Cancer Res 2005;65:7622–7.

66. Bonnet S, Gaujoux S, Launay P, et al. Wnt/β-catenin pathway activation in adrenocortical adenomas is frequently due to somatic CTNNB1-activating mutations,

which are associated with larger and nonsecreting tumors: a study in cortisol-secreting and -nonsecreting tumors. J Clin Endocrinol Metab 2011;96:E419–26.

67. Libè R, Fratticci A, Bertherat J. Adrenocortical cancer: pathophysiology and clinical management. Endocr Relat Cancer 2007;14:13–28.

68. Bougeard G, Sesboüé R, Baert-Desurmont S, et al. Molecular basis of the Li-Fraumeni syndrome: an update from the French LFS families. J Med Genet 2008;45:535–8.

69. Malkin D, Li FP, Strong LC, et al. Germ line p53 mutations in a familial syndrome of breast cancer, sarcomas, and other neoplasms. Science 1990;250:1233–8.

70. Ruijs MW, Verhoef S, Rookus MA, et al. TP53 germline mutation testing in 180 families suspected of Li-Fraumeni syndrome: mutation detection rate and relative frequency of cancers in different familial phenotypes. J Med Genet 2010; 47:421–8.

71. Srivastava S, Zou ZQ, Pirollo K, et al. Germ-line transmission of a mutated p53 gene in a cancer-prone family with Li-Fraumeni syndrome. Nature 1990;348:747–9.

72. Faria AM, Almeida MQ. Differences in the molecular mechanisms of adrenocortical tumorigenesis between children and adults. Mol Cell Endocrinol 2012;351: 52–7.

73. Custódio G, Parise GA, Kiesel Filho N, et al. Impact of neonatal screening and surveillance for the TP53 R337H mutation on early detection of childhood adrenocortical tumors. J Clin Oncol 2013;31:2619–26.

74. Herrmann LJ, Heinze B, Fassnacht M, et al. TP53 germline mutations in adult patients with adrenocortical carcinoma. J Clin Endocrinol Metab 2012;97: E476–85.

75. Raymond VM, Else T, Everett JN, et al. Prevalence of germline TP53 mutations in a prospective series of unselected patients with adrenocortical carcinoma. J Clin Endocrinol Metab 2013;98:E119–25.

76. Wasserman JD, Zambetti GP, Malkin D. Towards an understanding of the role of p53 in adrenocortical carcinogenesis. Mol Cell Endocrinol 2012;351:101–10.

77. Heinze B, Herrmann LJ, Fassnacht M, et al. Less common genotype variants of TP53 polymorphisms are associated with poor outcome in adult patients with adrenocortical carcinoma. Eur J Endocrinol 2014;170:707–17.

78. Assié G, Letouzé E, Fassnacht M, et al. Integrated genomic characterization of adrenocortical carcinoma. Nat Genet 2014;46:607–12.

79. Libè R, Groussin L, Tissier F, et al. Somatic TP53 mutations are relatively rare among adrenocortical cancers with the frequent 17p13 loss of heterozygosity. Clin Cancer Res 2007;13:844–50.

80. Gicquel C, Bertagna X, Gaston V, et al. Molecular markers and long-term recurrences in a large cohort of patients with sporadic adrenocortical tumors. Cancer Res 2001;61:6762–7.

81. Ragazzon B, Libé R, Gaujoux S, et al. Transcriptome analysis reveals that p53 and {beta}-catenin alterations occur in a group of aggressive adrenocortical cancers. Cancer Res 2010;70:8276–81.

82. Demeure MJ, Coan KE, Grant CS, et al. PTTG1 overexpression in adrenocortical cancer is associated with poor survival and represents a potential therapeutic target. Surgery 2013;154:1405–16 [discussion: 1416].

83. Ragazzon B, Libé R, Assié G, et al. Mass-array screening of frequent mutations in cancers reveals RB1 alterations in aggressive adrenocortical carcinomas. Eur J Endocrinol 2014;170:385–91.

84. Half E, Bercovich D, Rozen P. Familial adenomatous polyposis. Orphanet J Rare Dis 2009;4:22.

85. Beuschlein F, Reincke M, Königer M, et al. Cortisol producing adrenal adenoma–a new manifestation of Gardner's syndrome. Endocr Res 2000;26: 783–90.

86. Gaujoux S, Pinson S, Gimenez-Roqueplo A-P, et al. Inactivation of the APC gene is constant in adrenocortical tumors from patients with familial adenomatous polyposis but not frequent in sporadic adrenocortical cancers. Clin Cancer Res 2010;16:5133–41.

87. Chapman A, Durand J, Ouadi L, et al. Identification of genetic alterations of AXIN2 gene in adrenocortical tumors. J Clin Endocrinol Metab 2011;96: E1477–81.

88. Guimier A, Ragazzon B, Assié G, et al. AXIN genetic analysis in adrenocortical carcinomas updated. J Endocrinol Invest 2013;36:1000–3.

89. Assie G, Giordano TJ, Bertherat J. Gene expression profiling in adrenocortical neoplasia. Mol Cell Endocrinol 2012;351:111–7.

90. Berthon A, Sahut-Barnola I, Lambert-Langlais S, et al. Constitutive beta-catenin activation induces adrenal hyperplasia and promotes adrenal cancer development. Hum Mol Genet 2010;19:1561–76.

91. Heaton JH, Wood MA, Kim AC, et al. Progression to adrenocortical tumorigenesis in mice and humans through insulin-like growth factor 2 and β-catenin. Am J Pathol 2012;181:1017–33.

92. Leal LF, Mermejo LM, Ramalho LZ, et al. Wnt/beta-catenin pathway deregulation in childhood adrenocortical tumors. J Clin Endocrinol Metab 2011;96:3106–14.

93. Hao HX, Xie Y, Zhang Y, et al. ZNRF3 promotes Wnt receptor turnover in an R-spondin-sensitive manner. Nature 2012;485:195–200.

94. Weksberg R, Shuman C, Beckwith JB. Beckwith-Wiedemann syndrome. Eur J Hum Genet 2010;18:8–14.

95. Baskin B, Choufani S, Chen YA, et al. High frequency of copy number variations (CNVs) in the chromosome 11p15 region in patients with Beckwith-Wiedemann syndrome. Hum Genet 2014;133:321–30.

96. De Fraipont F, El Atifi M, Cherradi N, et al. Gene expression profiling of human adrenocortical tumors using complementary deoxyribonucleic Acid microarrays identifies several candidate genes as markers of malignancy. J Clin Endocrinol Metab 2005;90:1819–29.

97. De Reyniès A, Assié G, Rickman DS, et al. Gene expression profiling reveals a new classification of adrenocortical tumors and identifies molecular predictors of malignancy and survival. J Clin Oncol 2009;27:1108–15.

98. Giordano TJ, Kuick R, Else T, et al. Molecular classification and prognostication of adrenocortical tumors by transcriptome profiling. Clin Cancer Res 2009;15: 668–76.

99. Giordano TJ, Thomas DG, Kuick R, et al. Distinct transcriptional profiles of adrenocortical tumors uncovered by DNA microarray analysis. Am J Pathol 2003; 162:521–31.

100. Ribeiro TC, Latronico AC. Insulin-like growth factor system on adrenocortical tumorigenesis. Mol Cell Endocrinol 2012;351:96–100.

101. Haluska P, Worden F, Olmos D, et al. Safety, tolerability, and pharmacokinetics of the anti-IGF-1R monoclonal antibody figitumumab in patients with refractory adrenocortical carcinoma. Cancer Chemother Pharmacol 2010;65: 765–73.

102. Almeida MQ, Fragoso MC, Lotfi CF, et al. Expression of insulin-like growth factor-II and its receptor in pediatric and adult adrenocortical tumors. J Clin Endocrinol Metab 2008;93:3524–31.

103. Guillaud-Bataille M, Ragazzon B, de Reyniès A, et al. IGF2 promotes growth of adrenocortical carcinoma cells, but its overexpression does not modify phenotypic and molecular features of adrenocortical carcinoma. PloS One 2014;9: e103744.

104. Drelon C, Berthon A, Val P. Adrenocortical cancer and IGF2: is the game over or our experimental models limited? J Clin Endocrinol Metab 2013;98:505–7.

105. Barzon L, Chilosi M, Fallo F, et al. Molecular analysis of CDKN1C and TP53 in sporadic adrenal tumors. Eur J Endocrinol 2001;145:207–12.

106. Guo G, Kang Q, Chen Q, et al. High expression of long non-coding RNA H19 is required for efficient tumorigenesis induced by Bcr-Abl oncogene. FEBS Lett 2014;588:1780–6.

107. Gao ZH, Suppola S, Liu J, et al. Association of H19 promoter methylation with the expression of H19 and IGF-II genes in adrenocortical tumors. J Clin Endocrinol Metab 2002;87:1170–6.

108. Agarwal SK. Multiple endocrine neoplasia type 1. Front Horm Res 2013;41: 1–15.

109. Heppner C, Reincke M, Agarwal SK, et al. MEN1 gene analysis in sporadic adrenocortical neoplasms. J Clin Endocrinol Metab 1999;84:216–9.

110. Kjellman M, Roshani L, Teh BT, et al. Genotyping of adrenocortical tumors: very frequent deletions of the MEN1 locus in 11q13 and of a 1-centimorgan region in 2p16. J Clin Endocrinol Metab 1999;84:730–5.

111. Karamurzin Y, Zeng Z, Stadler ZK, et al. Unusual DNA mismatch repair-deficient tumors in Lynch syndrome: a report of new cases and review of the literature. Hum Pathol 2012;43:1677–87.

112. Raymond VM, Everett JN, Furtado LV, et al. Adrenocortical carcinoma is a lynch syndrome-associated cancer. J Clin Oncol 2013;31:3012–8.

113. Anselmo J, Medeiros S, Carneiro V, et al. A large family with Carney complex caused by the S147G PRKAR1A mutation shows a unique spectrum of disease including adrenocortical cancer. J Clin Endocrinol Metab 2012;97:351–9.

114. Bertherat J. Adrenocortical cancer in Carney complex: a paradigm of endocrine tumor progression or an association of genetic predisposing factors? J Clin Endocrinol Metab 2012;97:387–90.

115. Morin E, Mete O, Wasserman JD, et al. Carney complex with adrenal cortical carcinoma. J Clin Endocrinol Metab 2012;97:E202–6.

116. Cibas ES, Medeiros LJ, Weinberg DS, et al. Cellular DNA profiles of benign and malignant adrenocortical tumors. Am J Surg Pathol 1990;14:948–55.

117. Dohna M, Reincke M, Mincheva A, et al. Adrenocortical carcinoma is characterized by a high frequency of chromosomal gains and high-level amplifications. Genes Chromosomes Cancer 2000;28:145–52.

118. Kjellman M, Kallioniemi OP, Karhu R, et al. Genetic aberrations in adrenocortical tumors detected using comparative genomic hybridization correlate with tumor size and malignancy. Cancer Res 1996;56:4219–23.

119. Zhao J, Speel EJ, Muletta-Feurer S, et al. Analysis of genomic alterations in sporadic adrenocortical lesions. Gain of chromosome 17 is an early event in adrenocortical tumorigenesis. Am J Pathol 1999;155:1039–45.

120. Barreau O, de Reynies A, Wilmot-Roussel H, et al. Clinical and pathophysiological implications of chromosomal alterations in adrenocortical tumors: an integrated genomic approach. J Clin Endocrinol Metab 2012;97:E301–11.

121. Stephan EA, Chung TH, Grant CS, et al. Adrenocortical carcinoma survival rates correlated to genomic copy number variants. Mol Cancer Ther 2008; 7:425–31.

122. Szabó PM, Tamási V, Molnár V, et al. Meta-analysis of adrenocortical tumour genomics data: novel pathogenic pathways revealed. Oncogene 2010;29: 3163–72.
123. Ronchi CL, Sbiera S, Leich E, et al. Single nucleotide polymorphism array profiling of adrenocortical tumors–evidence for an adenoma carcinoma sequence? PloS One 2013;8:e73959.
124. Kulis M, Esteller M. DNA methylation and cancer. Adv Genet 2010;70:27–56.
125. Barreau O, Assié G, Wilmot-Roussel H, et al. Identification of a CpG island methylator phenotype in adrenocortical carcinomas. J Clin Endocrinol Metab 2013; 98:E174–84.
126. Fonseca AL, Kugelberg J, Starker LF, et al. Comprehensive DNA methylation analysis of benign and malignant adrenocortical tumors. Genes Chromosomes Cancer 2012;51:949–60.
127. Rechache NS, Wang Y, Stevenson HS, et al. DNA methylation profiling identifies global methylation differences and markers of adrenocortical tumors. J Clin Endocrinol Metab 2012;97:E1004–13.
128. Lujambio A, Lowe SW. The microcosmos of cancer. Nature 2012;482:347–55.
129. Tömböl Z, Szabó PM, Molnár V, et al. Integrative molecular bioinformatics study of human adrenocortical tumors: microRNA, tissue-specific target prediction, and pathway analysis. Endocr Relat Cancer 2009;16:895–906.
130. Soon PS, Tacon LJ, Gill AJ, et al. miR-195 and miR-483-5p identified as predictors of poor prognosis in adrenocortical cancer. Clin Cancer Res 2009;15: 7684–92.
131. Patterson EE, Holloway AK, Weng J, et al. MicroRNA profiling of adrenocortical tumors reveals miR-483 as a marker of malignancy. Cancer 2011;117:1630–9.
132. Özata DM, Caramuta S, Velázquez-Fernández D, et al. The role of microRNA deregulation in the pathogenesis of adrenocortical carcinoma. Endocr Relat Cancer 2011;18:643–55.
133. Chabre O, Libé R, Assie G, et al. Serum miR-483-5p and miR-195 are predictive of recurrence risk in adrenocortical cancer patients. Endocr Relat Cancer 2013; 20:579–94.
134. Schmitz KJ, Helwig J, Bertram S, et al. Differential expression of microRNA-675, microRNA-139-3p and microRNA-335 in benign and malignant adrenocortical tumours. J Clin Pathol 2011;64:529–35.
135. Patel D, Boufraqech M, Jain M, et al. MiR-34a and miR-483-5p are candidate serum biomarkers for adrenocortical tumors. Surgery 2013;154:1224–8 [discussion: 1229].
136. Duregon E, Rapa I, Votta A, et al. MicroRNA expression patterns in adrenocortical carcinoma variants and clinical pathologic correlations. Hum Pathol 2014; 45:1555–62.
137. Doghman M, El Wakil A, Cardinaud B, et al. Regulation of insulin-like growth factor-mammalian target of rapamycin signaling by microRNA in childhood adrenocortical tumors. Cancer Res 2010;70:4666–75.

Adrenal Incidentalomas

A Disease of Modern Technology
Offering Opportunities for Improved Patient Care

Adriana G. Ioachimescu, MD, PhD[a], Erick M. Remer, MD[b],
Amir H. Hamrahian, MD[c],*

KEYWORDS

- Adrenal incidentaloma • Noncontrast CT attenuation • Percentage washout
- Tumor size • Pheochromocytoma

KEY POINTS

- Noncontrast computed tomography attenuation is superior to adrenal tumor size in differentiating benign adenomas from malignant tumors.
- Absolute and relative percentage washout may be used to further characterize lipid-poor adrenal tumors.
- Pheochromocytoma is extremely unlikely in patients with lipid-rich adrenal tumors.
- Any degree of increase of plasma or urinary metanephrine fraction in a patient with adrenal incidentaloma should prompt a careful evaluation for an underlying pheochromocytoma.

Since the initial report of an adrenal incidentaloma (AI) in 1941, the diagnosis of AI has become increasingly prevalent contemporaneously with advances in imaging techniques.[1,2] The two main questions that should be answered are the secretory and malignant potential of the mass. A practical approach in the investigation and follow-up of adrenal incidentalomas incorporating authors' experience is presented in this review.

DEFINITION

Adrenal incidentalomas (AIs) are adrenal masses discovered serendipitously by radiological evaluation in the absence of clinical features suggestive of adrenal disease. The definition usually encompasses lesions larger than 1 cm that are detected outside the work-up for staging of known cancers. Adrenal diseases inadvertently missed on clinical evaluation are not under the strict definition of AIs.

Disclosure: The authors have nothing to disclose.
[a] Emory University School of Medicine, 1365 B Clifton Road, Northeast, B6209, Atlanta, GA 30322, USA; [b] Imaging Institute, Cleveland Clinic, 9500 Euclid Avenue, A21, Cleveland, OH 44195, USA; [c] Endocrinology, Cleveland Clinic Abu Dhabi, Abu Dhabi, UAE
* Corresponding author.
E-mail address: hamraha@clevelandclinicabudhabi.ae

Endocrinol Metab Clin N Am 44 (2015) 335–354
http://dx.doi.org/10.1016/j.ecl.2015.02.005
0889-8529/15/$ – see front matter © 2015 Elsevier Inc. All rights reserved.

endo.theclinics.com

EPIDEMIOLOGY
Autopsy Studies

Autopsy studies have shown a wide range of prevalence of 1.1% to 32% for adrenal nodules, which reflects the heterogeneity of published data, especially with regard to age at death and inclusion of metastatic lesions.[3–5] A summary of 25 autopsy studies indicates a prevalence of 6%. AIs are detected with increased prevalence at older ages. One study identified AIs in 7% of those who died after the age of 70 years. In contrast, only 1% of those younger than 30 years had AIs.[6] Other investigators confirmed the age-dependent occurrence of adrenal cortical adenomas.[2] No gender difference was observed in autopsy studies.

Computed Tomography Studies

Earlier computed tomography (CT) studies from 1980s reported a prevalence of 0.9%.[2] However, as CT resolution improved over time, the prevalence of AIs also increased. Further, the increasing use of CT imaging for nonspecific symptoms has likely contributed to the increased identification of AIs. AIs were detected in 4.4% of chest CT scans performed as part of a high-resolution lung cancer screening program in Italy in 2006.[7] Because only 1 metastasis of lung cancer was identified in this study of 520 subjects, it is unlikely that the prevalence of AIs was overestimated. In contrast, a 2011 study conducted in a routine clinical practice setting indicated a prevalence of only 0.98% for abdominal CT and 0.81% for chest CT scans.[8] However, the prevalence may have been underestimated, because only radiology reports and not the films were reviewed in this study.

The diagnosis of AI identified on CT peaks in the sixth and seventh decades of life. However, based on autopsy studies, it is expected that the prevalence of AIs continues to increase after age 70 years. Some studies showed a higher prevalence of AIs in women, which may be the result of referral bias caused by higher frequency of abdominal complaints in women than in men.[9] An equal prevalence between the genders is supported by autopsy studies.

Differential diagnosis of adrenal incidentaloma

At least 38 different diagnoses have been identified in patients with incidentally detected adrenal masses.[2] The main categories are nonfunctioning cortical adenomas (70%–80%), pheochromocytomas (PHEOs) (1.1%–11%), subclinical Cushing syndrome (5%–20%), primary aldosteronism (1%–2%), primary adrenocortical carcinomas (ACCs) (<5%), and metastases (2.5%).[2,4,10–14] A list of disorders that may present as AIs is shown in **Box 1**. AIs are bilateral in about 10% to 15% of cases.[15,16] Nonadrenal lesions may also present as AIs (**Fig. 1**).[17]

CLINICAL EVALUATION

A thorough clinical evaluation is of paramount importance in patients with AIs, because identification of an AI may provide an opportunity for clinicians to detect an underlying secretory tumor. History should assess manifestations of hypercortisolemia, primary aldosteronism, catecholamine excess, hyperandrogenism, and abdominal complaints. New-onset or worsened hypertension, impaired glucose metabolism, and bone loss may suggest excess cortisol secretion. A history of new-onset sustained or paroxysmal hypertension, blood pressure fluctuations during general anesthesia, syncopal events, and orthostatic blood pressure changes may suggest an underlying PHEO.

Several cancers, including lung, breast, renal, and melanoma, have potential to metastasize to the adrenal glands, so history of malignancy and weight loss should

---

Box 1
Adrenal abnormalities that can present as AIs

1. Adrenal cortical masses.

    Benign: adenoma, nodular hyperplasia,[a] congenital adrenal hyperplasia.[a]

    Malignant: primary ACC.

2. Adrenal medullary tumors: PHEO,[a] ganglioneuroma, neuroblastoma.

3. Other adrenal tumors.

    Benign: myelolipoma,[a] teratoma, hamartoma, lipoma, hemangioma, lymphangioma, adrenal adenomatoid tumor.

    Malignant: metastases,[a] primary adrenal lymphoma,[a] primary adrenal melanoma.

4. Infections[a]: fungal (Histoplasma, coccidioidomycosis, blastomycosis), viral (cytomegalovirus), parasitic (echinococcosis), bacterial (tuberculosis, syphilis).

5. Infiltration[a]: sarcoidosis, amyloidosis.

6. Cysts and pseudocysts.

7. Hemorrhage,[a] hematoma.

8. Nonadrenal disorders such as schwannoma, leiomyosarcoma, retroperitoneal lipoma.

    [a]May present as bilateral adrenal masses.

---

be obtained (**Figs. 2** and **3**). A combination of features reflecting cortisol and androgen excess in the setting of an adrenal mass should alert for the possibility of underlying primary ACC. A history of smoking and medication use including anticoagulants needs to be established.

Family history should be ascertained for components of multiple endocrine neoplasia type 2, von Hippel-Lindau syndromes, neurofibromatosis type 1, Carney complex, and Carney triad. Although genetic syndromes are usually rare in patients with AI, their detection has important implications in patients with bilateral adrenal lesions and silent PHEOs. Unilateral or bilateral adrenal masses may be seen in patients with homozygous or heterozygous congenital adrenal hyperplasia.[18] However, such an association may be related to the increased volume of adrenal tissue or intratumoral functional impairment of enzyme activity, rather than a true enzymatic defect.[19]

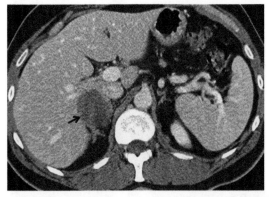

Fig. 1. Well-circumscribed schwannoma (*arrow*) next to the right adrenal gland with mild heterogeneous enhancement. Larger schwannomas are more likely to undergo degenerative changes, including cyst formation (up to 66%), calcification, hemorrhage, and hyalinization.

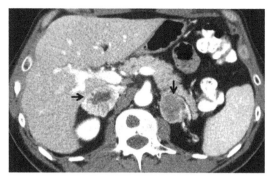

Fig. 2. Bilateral metastases (*arrows*). Contrast-enhanced CT shows brisk enhancement of bilateral adrenal masses (right>left) from renal cell carcinoma metastases.

RADIOLOGICAL CHARACTERISTICS

After the detection of an AI, a decision must be made about whether further dedicated adrenal studies are necessary. For example, postcontrast CT studies may not provide sufficient information about the risk of malignancy and may need to be repeated by doing a noncontrast CT study with or without contrast (adrenal protocol). In addition, AIs detected by abdominal ultrasonography or nuclear medicine studies have to be further investigated.

Choice of Adrenal Imaging Studies

Adrenal CT is the cornerstone of imaging for AIs, establishing the size, lipid content, and imaging phenotype, including heterogeneity, calcifications, irregular borders, local invasion, and areas of necrosis. All of these imaging characteristics can help

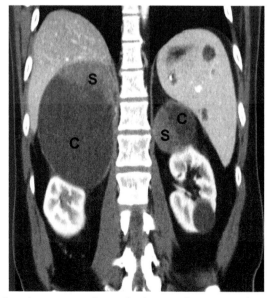

Fig. 3. Bilateral adrenal metastases. Coronal reformat of contrast-enhanced CT shows bilateral, large cystic (C) and solid (S) adrenal metastases from melanoma.

to assess the risk of malignancy. MRI scans can also be used to establish the risk of malignancy, but they are more expensive and are generally reserved for selected cases in which CT imaging is contraindicated or equivocal to delineate the malignancy risk. Functional imaging studies of the adrenal glands have a limited role in evaluation of selected patients with AIs.

Size of the Adrenal Incidentalomas

The risk of malignancy traditionally relied heavily on the size of the adrenal masses. In a retrospective study by Musella and colleagues,[20] the proportion of ACCs among 282 surgically resected AIs was 25% in adrenal masses with a maximal diameter greater than 6 cm, 1.2% for tumors measuring 4 to 6 cm, and 0% in lesions smaller than 4 cm. The likelihood ratios derived from a large cohort of ACCs yielded probabilities of 10%, 19%, and 47% for malignancy in adrenal cortical tumors greater than or equal to 4 cm, greater than or equal to 6 cm, and greater than or equal to 8 cm, respectively.[21] Note that there is no safe absolute tumor size cutoff to rule out malignancy because there are reports of ACCs less than 4 cm in size.[22]

The tumor size should be evaluated in the context of other radiological features because the risk of malignancy for a homogeneous mass greater than 4 cm with no areas of necrosis or calcification and a noncontrast CT less than 10 Hounsfield units (HU) is close to 0% (**Fig. 4**).[23–25] In addition, myelolipoma, a benign fat-containing tumor, can reach sizable dimensions with negative HU typically in a range −40 HU or less (**Fig. 5**).

Metastatic lesions to the adrenal glands are usually smaller than ACCs. However, in most cases a history of prior malignancy is present, which can direct further work-up and management.[23]

Computed Tomography Scan

The CT scan is the primary tool for evaluation of adrenal masses. It provides information on the adrenal tumor size and density, as well as calcification, areas of necrosis, and local invasion (**Figs. 6 and 7**).

Noncontrast computed tomography attenuation coefficient

A low attenuation value measurement of an adrenal nodule is secondary to high fat concentration in the sterol-producing adrenal cortical tissue and has a specificity close to 100% for diagnosing adenoma and, thus, in differentiating benign from

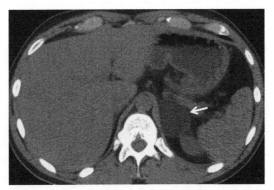

Fig. 4. Large left adrenal adenoma (*arrow*) shows typical features of well-defined margins, homogeneous attenuation, and attenuation measurement of less than 10 HU on unenhanced CT despite its size of 4.7 cm.

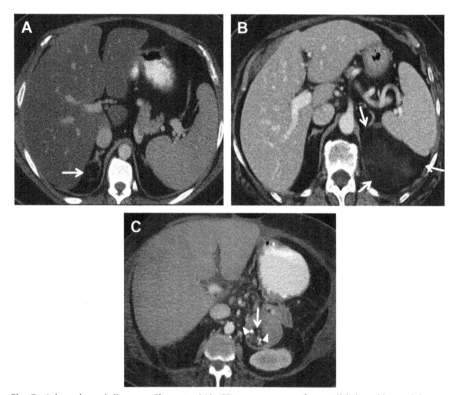

Fig. 5. Adrenal myelolipoma. Characteristic CT appearances of a small (*A*) and large (*B*) myelolipomas that include bulk fat of varying degrees (*arrows*) without (*A, B*) or with calcifications (*arrowhead*) (*C*). Note that fat in myelolipoma has the same attenuation as subcutaneous or retroperitoneal fat.

potentially malignant lesions (**Fig. 8**).[18,23–29] In addition, a combination of adrenal mass size less than 4 cm and an attenuation value less than or equal to 20 HU had 100% specificity to predict a benign lesion.[23] The unenhanced CT attenuation value is a better predictor of benign tumors than adrenal tumor size.[23,24]

ACCs and PHEOs typically have attenuation values greater than 30 HU. In our experience the lowest attenuation value for adrenal PHEO has been 17 HU.[30] There has

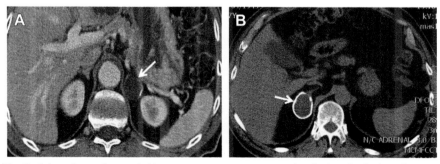

Fig. 6. Adrenal cysts (*arrows*). Homogeneous water attenuation (~0 HU) of adrenal masses without (*A*) and with (*B*) circumferential dense calcification.

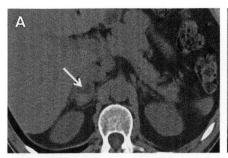
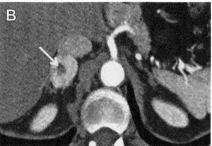

Fig. 7. PHEO. (*A*) Right adrenal soft tissue attenuation mass with central low attenuation (*arrow*). (*B*) Mass shows marked enhancement after intravenous contrast administration except for the central area of necrosis (*arrow*), which is a common finding in PHEO.

been a report of unenhanced CT attenuation values less than 10 HU in 2 patients with symptomatic adrenal PHEO.[31] However, these tumors were very small, less than 1.5 cm, and one of the reported patients had adrenal medullary hyperplasia on pathology. In other cases in which a low attenuation value for PHEO has been reported, the measurement technique has been questioned.[32] The region of interest during measurement of attenuation value should encompass two-thirds of the largest axial diameter of the mass and should avoid boundaries to prevent volume averaging with tissue outside the nodule. Only homogeneous regions of the tumor should be selected, avoiding areas with cystic and necrotic changes. The highest CT attenuation values in mixed tumors should be used for clinical decision making (**Fig. 9**) with the exception of myelolipomas in which a small fat-containing area (<−40 HU) would establish the diagnosis. Based on the accumulating data in the literature and our own experience, we only perform biochemical investigation for PHEO in patients with AIs in whom the CT attenuation value is greater than 10 HU.[30,32,33]

Computed tomography washout and enhancement patterns

Although an unenhanced CT attenuation value less than or equal to 10 HU is an excellent predictor of benign histology, 20% to 30% of adrenal adenomas are lipid poor (**Fig. 10**).[34] That is, there is insufficient sterol content to diminish the overall attenuation of the adrenal nodule below the diagnostic threshold. In such cases additional imaging is needed diagnose an adenoma and to avoid unnecessary surgery. If unenhanced CT shows an attenuation value greater than 10 HU, postcontrast images should be

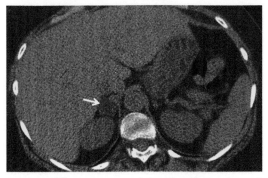

Fig. 8. Typical adenoma. Small homogeneous right adrenal mass (*arrow*) measures less than 10 HU on unenhanced CT.

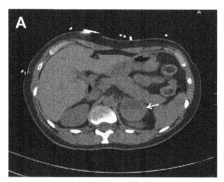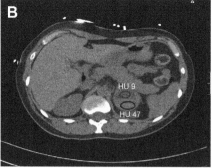

Fig. 9. (*A, B*) Patient with a heterogeneous left adrenal mass (*arrow*) on noncontrast CT scan (*A*). The CT attenuation is 9 HU in the upper part of the mass and 47 HU in the lower part (*B*). The final pathology was consistent with PHEO.

obtained at 1 and 15 minutes in order to calculate the washout percentage (**Fig. 11**). An absolute percentage washout greater than 60% and/or a relative percentage washout greater than 40% at 15 minutes suggests an adenoma.[35–37]

Studies with shorter postcontrast time delays have been done; however, a 15-minute delayed scan seems to have the best sensitivity (87%) and specificity (94%) in distinguishing between adenomas and nonadenomas.[35–39] Note that PHEOs may display washout characteristics similar to adenomas.[33,40]

The enhancement pattern of an adrenal lesion after contrast administration may also be used as a clue to differentiate adenomas from nonadenomatous lesions. In a recent study by Northcutt and colleagues,[41] comparing 41 adenomas with 12 PHEOs, none of the adenomas had an enhancement attenuation greater than 85 HU within 60 seconds after contrast administration compared with more than 50% of PHEOs that enhanced more than 110 HU.

Chemical shift T1-weighted MRI can reliably identify lipid-rich lesions by a reduction in signal intensity during out-of-phase compared with in-phase images (**Fig. 12**).[42] Chemical shift MRI may further characterize adrenal tumors with borderline

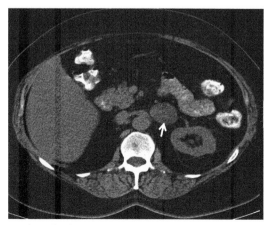

Fig. 10. A lipid-poor adrenal adenoma measuring 3 cm with a noncontrast CT attenuation value of 29 HU (*arrow*). Measurement of washout characteristics is indicated in patients with lipid-poor adrenal masses.

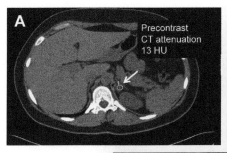
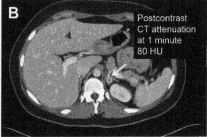
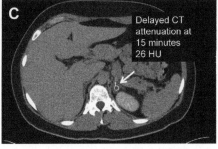

Fig. 11. (*A–C*). Left adrenal adenoma diagnosed by CT washout. Small left adrenal nodule measures greater than 10 HU on unenhanced scan (13 HU) (*A*). One-minute portal venous phase (*B*) and 15-minute delayed (*C*) scans were performed. Absolute washout = (enhanced−delayed)/(enhanced−unenhanced) = (80−26)/(80−13) × 100 = 81%, which is highly suggestive of adenoma.

unenhanced CT attenuation values or washout characteristics.[43,44] However, there are rare reports of ACC, PHEO, and clear cell renal and hepatocellular carcinoma metastases showing a signal loss on out-of-phase images.[22] Very high signal intensity on T2-weighted MRI is characteristic but not pathognomonic for PHEO. However, it may be absent in up to 35% of cases (**Fig. 13**).[45,46] The criteria used for defining hyperintensity may have an impact on its prevalence in patients with PHEO.[47]

Quantitative analysis of chemical shift MRI and diffusion-weighted imaging may help to characterize the hyperattenuating adrenal lesions, especially differentiating lipid-poor adenomas and benign PHEOs from malignant tumors.[48]

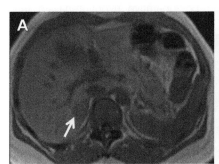
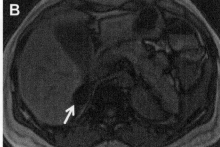

Fig. 12. Incidental right adrenal adenoma (*arrows*) on MRI performed for evaluation of the pancreas. In-phase (*A*) and opposed-phase (*B*) T1-weighted gradient echo images show homogeneous, marked signal intensity loss on opposed-phase image compared with in-phase image, which is diagnostic of adenoma.

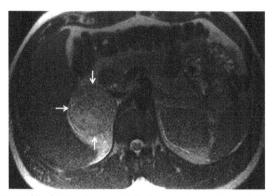

Fig. 13. PHEO. T2-weighted MRI shows mildly hyperintense 4-cm right adrenal mass (*arrows*). Mass signal intensity is visually slightly less than that of retroperitoneal fat and cerebrospinal fluid. Up to 35% of PHEOs are not light-bulb bright on T2-weighted MRI.

Functional Imaging

There is a limited role for functional imaging in the diagnostic work-up of patients with AIs. Scintigraphic studies with iodine-meta-iodobenzylguanidine (^{123}I-MIBG), and PET studies using ^{18}F-fluoro-2-deoxy-D-glucose (^{18}F-FDG), ^{18}F-3,4-dihydroxyphenylalanine (^{18}F-DOPA), and ^{18}F-fluorodopamine (^{18}F-FDA) may be used if an underlying multifocal or metastatic PHEO is suspected.[49] ^{18}F-FDA and ^{18}F-FDG have higher sensitivity than MIBG.[50,51]

^{18}F-FDG–PET and PET-CT scans may be useful to detect extra-adrenal disease in patients suspected to have an underlying malignancy. The study relies on trapping of ^{18}F-FDG by metabolically active malignant cells. In a study of 165 adrenal lesions in 150 patients, all 139 benign lesions had a quantitative standardized uptake value of 0.54 to 3.34 SUV. A 2.31 SUV threshold provided 100% sensitivity to detect all 29 malignant lesions and was associated with an approximately 5% false-positive rate for benign lesions (**Fig. 14**).[52] There is small false-negative result in patients with small, hemorrhagic, or necrotic metastatic lesions.

Adrenal scintigraphy with radioiodinated [131]I-6b-iodomethyl-19-norcholesterol (NP-59) highlights the adrenocortical hyperfunctioning lesions, but has limited clinical availability. We do not recommend it for routine evaluation of AIs. A recent small study showed that positive 19-iodocholesterol scintigraphy in patients with AI had better predictability for development of prolonged postoperative hypoadrenalism than

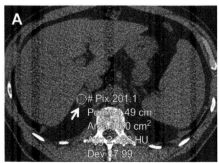
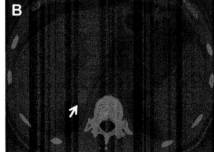

Fig. 14. False-positive PET/CT. (*A*) Unenhanced CT shows right adrenal adenoma that measures 3 HU (*arrow*). (*B*) Up to 5% of adenomas may be hypermetabolic on PET/CT (*arrow*).

hormonal work-up for subclinical Cushing syndrome. It was able to predict the metabolic outcome, identifying the patients who could benefit from adrenalectomy irrespective of hormonal diagnosis.[53]

Imaging phenotypes of the most frequent types of AIs are summarized in **Table 1**. An unenhanced adrenal CT scan reliably identifies benign tumors based on noncontrast attenuation values less than or equal to 10 HU. For lipid-poor adrenal masses, we suggest delayed contrast-enhanced CT studies for washout calculation. MRI should be considered when CT is inconclusive or iodinated CT contrast cannot safely be administered. Functional scans should be considered for selected cases to detect extra-adrenal PHEOs or malignant lesions.

BIOCHEMICAL EVALUATION AND MANAGEMENT IMPLICATIONS

Up to 30% of patients with AIs harbor excess cortisol, catecholamine, or aldosterone secretion depending on the criteria used to define excess hormone secretion. Screening for subclinical excess is indicated in all patients with AIs. Patients with lipid-poor adrenal masses need to be evaluated for PHEO. Primary aldosteronism should be ruled out in patients with hypertension and/or hypokalemia. Measurement of testosterone and dehydroepiandrosterone sulfate (DHEAS) should be considered in women with virilization, new-onset symptoms suggestive of hyperandrogenism, or adrenal masses suspicious for ACCs. Although several guidelines have been released over the years,[13,54,55] only 50% to 82% of patients diagnosed with AI undergo hormonal evaluations in clinical practice.[8,56,57]

Subclinical Cushing Syndrome

The first reports on subclinical Cushing syndrome (SCS) were published by Beier-waltes and colleagues[58] in 1972 and subsequently by Chabonnel and colleagues[59] in 1981. SCS is best defined as the subtle autonomous production of cortisol from an adrenal mass, which is usually associated with suppression of cortisol production from the contralateral gland, but no overt clinical features of Cushing syndrome.[6,55] Based on the criteria used, prevalence of up to 20% in patients with AIs has been reported.[2,60]

At present, there is a large body of literature linking SCS to comorbidities including hypertension, abnormal glucose metabolism, obesity, dyslipidemia, vertebral fractures, and osteoporosis.[61–65] There are emerging data on the long-term consequences of SCS, including a higher rate of cardiovascular events and all-cause

Table 1
Imaging phenotypes of the most common types of AIs. Necrosis, hemorrhage, calcifications, irregular borders, and local invasion are seen more frequently in patients with ACC and PHEO

Type	Size (cm)	Nonenhanced Attenuation	CT Washout >60% (Absolute)	Loss of Signal Intensity on T1-weighted Out-of-phase MRI
Cortical adenoma	Small (<4)	Low in 70% (<10 HU)	Yes	Yes
Primary cortical carcinoma	Large (>4)	High (>30 HU)	No	No
Metastasis	Variable	High (>10 HU)	No, except RCC, HCC	No, except RCC, HCC
PHEO	Large (>3)	High (>17 HU)	variable	No

Abbreviations: HCC, hepatocellular carcinoma; RCC, renal cell carcinoma.

mortality compared with patients with normal cortisol levels.[66] A full review of biochemical evaluation and management of SCS is discussed in Adrenal Mild Hypercortisolism by Goddard and colleagues.

Primary Aldosteronism

The estimated prevalence of primary aldosteronism among patients with AI is up to 2%.[2,12–14,19,67] Evaluation for primary aldosteronism is recommended in patients with AIs in the presence of hypertension regardless of their potassium levels.[55,68–70] A few patients with well-documented primary aldosteronism had hypokalemia in the absence of hypertension, therefore evaluation for primary aldosteronism in such patients is also indicated.[71] A detailed review of biochemical evaluation and management of patients with primary aldosteronism is discussed in another article in this issue.

Pheochromocytoma

Patients with AIs should be evaluated for PHEO regardless of their blood pressure status, because up to 50% of patients with incidentally discovered PHEO are normotensive.[67,72–74] The prevalence of PHEO in patients with AIs is about 3%, but a prevalence ranging from 1.1% to 11% has been reported.[4,11,12,60] There are accumulating data in the literature that evaluation for PHEO in AIs with a noncontrast CT attenuation less than or equal to 10 HU is not needed.[23,30,32] Accordingly the authors only evaluate for PHEO in patients with lipid-poor AIs.

Biochemical evaluation

Both plasma and 24-hour urine metanephrine levels are reasonable initial screening tests in patients with AIs. Normal plasma metanephrine level rules out a diagnosis of PHEO in almost all patients except very rare dopamine-secreting tumors, which are usually extra-adrenal.[75] When normotensive reference ranges are used for plasma and urine metanephrines, the diagnostic specificity of plasma metanephrines is similar to or better than that of urine metanephrines.[30] Accordingly, the authors prefer plasma metanephrines as the first-line diagnostic test because of its excellent diagnostic sensitivity and convenience.[55,75,76]

Modest plasma and urine normetanephrine level increases (<4-fold above upper normal limit) in adrenal masses greater than 5 cm are almost always false-positive.[30] However, any degree of increase in plasma or urinary metanephrine fraction in patients with AIs should be carefully evaluated for an underlying adrenal PHEO.[30]

Management

PHEOs should be surgically removed after medical preparation to reduce the risk of a cardiovascular event during the surgery. All patients with PHEO should be treated with an alpha adrenoceptor blocker for at least 7 to14 days preoperatively.[77–79] Calcium channel blockers may be used for better control of hypertension or in those patients who cannot tolerate adequate alpha-blockade. β-Blockers are often required to control the tachycardia that may occur during alpha-blocking receptor treatment. Preoperative volume repletion by increased salt intake is recommended before surgery. Patients who continue to be symptomatic on alpha-blockade and beta-blockade may require a brief preoperative course of metyrosine to block catecholamine synthesis.[80]

Patient should be monitored for hypotension or hypoglycemia postoperatively. Because there are no definitive pathologic diagnostic criteria for malignancy, patients with apparently benign PHEO should be followed annually for at least 5 years and then intermittently afterward.[81,82]

Primary Adrenocortical Carcinoma

ACC is a rare malignancy that usually carries a grave prognosis unless complete surgical resection can be achieved early in the course of the disease. A large series of patients with ACC identified cortisol overproduction and advanced tumor stage and tumor grade as negative prognostic factors.[83] ACC comprised less than 5% of all AIs in a pooled analysis from 26 international studies.[19] Most ACCs have noncontrast CT HU values greater than 30.[23] Concerning features for malignancy include microcalcification, irregular shape and border, necrosis, and a heterogeneous enhancement pattern (**Fig. 15**).

Close follow-up by a multidisciplinary team consisting of an endocrinologist, oncologist, and surgeon is recommended. Postoperative treatment with mitotane is associated with longer recurrence-free survival.[83]

Adrenal Metastases

Adrenal metastases are common in patients with carcinoma of lung, breast, renal cell, and ovary, and in patients with melanoma, but have been described in many other malignant diseases (see **Figs. 2** and **3**). In cases of bilateral metastases, adrenal function needs to be evaluated. Adrenal biopsy may be of value in selected patients in whom the diagnosis of a metastatic lesion to the adrenal gland would change the treatment plan or prognosis. Any biopsy attempt should be preceded by biochemical exclusion of PHEO. Surgical treatment may improve survival in cases of solitary metastases, but the management should be decided after a thorough oncologic evaluation.[84]

Follow-up of Patients with Adrenal Incidentalomas

The management of patients with AIs is summarized in **Fig. 16**.

In a recent large Italian prospective study, 8.2% of patients developed new SCS after greater than or equal to 5 years of follow-up.[85] Autonomous cortisol secretion usually correlates with adenoma size; adenomas larger than 2.4 cm are more likely to be associated with worsening of hypercortisolemia.[85] Accordingly, patients managed conservatively should have clinical and biochemical evaluation for up to 5 years until further studies define the optimal follow-up period in such patients. A through initial diagnostic approach can be the basis of a subsequent tailored approach.[86]

Repeat imaging of adrenal masses with borderline characteristics in 3 to 6 months and then annually for 2 years is reasonable. There is no good evidence supporting continued radiological surveillance in patients with AIs, which is associated with increased radiation exposure, higher health care expenditures, and potentially significant emotional impact.[60]

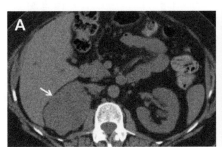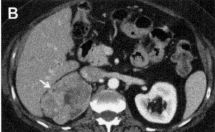

Fig. 15. Adrenal cortical carcinoma. Right adrenal mass measuring 6 cm with a soft tissue attenuation greater than 30 HU (*arrows*) on unenhanced CT (*A*) shows heterogeneous enhancement (*B*) after intravenous contrast administration.

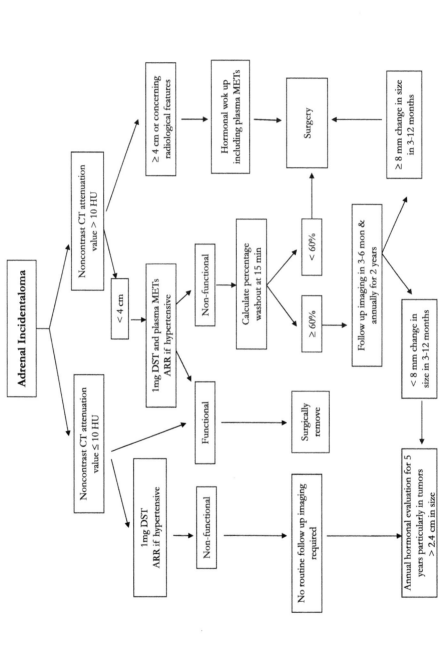

Fig. 16. Algorithm for investigating patients with AIs. ARR, aldosterone/renin ratio; DST, dexamethasone suppression test; METs, metanephrines.

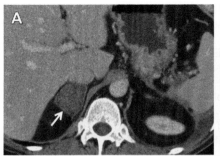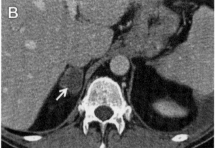

Fig. 17. Adrenal hematoma (*arrows*). Right adrenal hematoma (*A*) with an interval decrease in size on follow-up CT (*B*).

Changes in adrenal mass size

AIs can increase (up to 10%), decrease (up to 5%), or remain unchanged in size over the years.[87] A decrease in the size and the attenuation value of an adrenal mass on noncontrast CT studies may be a clue to the presence of an adrenal hematoma (**Fig. 17**). An adrenal mass growth cutoff that can reliably confirm or exclude malignancy has not been identified. Surgical resection may be considered for an increase greater than or equal to 0.8 cm in maximal diameter of an adrenal mass, if corroborated by other imaging and clinical findings.[88]

SUMMARY

The incidence of AI is expected to increase because of improved resolution of CT imaging and its use for nonspecific symptoms. Increased awareness among practitioners is necessary for the best cost-effective approach to AIs. We recommend dedicated adrenal imaging to assess the potential for malignancy. Noncontrast CT attenuation characteristics of AIs is the most important radiological characteristic to differentiate between benign adenomas, hyperplasia, or cysts and malignant adrenal tumors. Screening for subclinical excess is indicated in all patients with AIs. Patients with lipid-poor tumors need to be evaluated for PHEO regardless of their blood pressure status. Primary aldosteronism should be ruled out in patients with hypertension and/or hypokalemia. Adrenal androgens are measured in patients with clinical signs of androgen excess. Identification of AIs should be considered as an opportunity because there is growing literature linking AIs to several cardiovascular risk factors, and may be associated with increased mortality. Surgery is indicated for most secretory tumors and those with radiological features concerning for malignancy.

REFERENCES

1. Korobkin M, White EA, Kressel HY, et al. Computed tomography in the diagnosis of adrenal disease. AJR Am J Roentgenol 1979;132(2):231–8.
2. Young WF Jr. Management approaches to adrenal incidentalomas. A view from Rochester, Minnesota. Endocrinol Metab Clin North Am 2000;29(1):159–85, x.
3. Kloos RT, Gross MD, Francis IR, et al. Incidentally discovered adrenal masses. Endocr Rev 1995;16(4):460–84.
4. Young WF Jr. Clinical practice. The incidentally discovered adrenal mass. N Engl J Med 2007;356(6):601–10.

5. Kawano M, Kodama T, Ito Y, et al. Adrenal incidentaloma–report of 14 operated cases and analysis of 4-year autopsy series of Japan. Nihon Geka Gakkai Zasshi 1989;90(12):2031–6 [in Japanese].

6. Kannan S, Remer EM, Hamrahian AH. Evaluation of patients with adrenal incidentalomas. Curr Opin Endocrinol Diabetes Obes 2013;20(3):161–9.

7. Bovio S, Cataldi A, Reimondo G, et al. Prevalence of adrenal incidentaloma in a contemporary computerized tomography series. J Endocrinol Invest 2006;29(4): 298–302.

8. Davenport C, Liew A, Doherty B, et al. The prevalence of adrenal incidentaloma in routine clinical practice. Endocrine 2011;40(1):80–3.

9. Mantero F, Terzolo M, Arnaldi G, et al. A survey on adrenal incidentaloma in Italy. Study group on adrenal tumors of the Italian Society of Endocrinology. J Clin Endocrinol Metab 2000;85(2):637–44.

10. Kim J, Bae KH, Choi YK, et al. Clinical characteristics for 348 patients with adrenal incidentaloma. Endocrinol Metab (Seoul) 2013;28(1):20–5.

11. Kasperlik-Zaluska AA, Otto M, Cichocki A, et al. Incidentally discovered adrenal tumors: a lesson from observation of 1,444 patients. Horm Metab Res 2008;40(5): 338–41.

12. Bulow B, Jansson S, Juhlin C, et al. Adrenal incidentaloma - follow-up results from a Swedish prospective study. Eur J Endocrinol 2006;154(3):419–23.

13. Terzolo M, Stigliano A, Chiodini I, et al. AME position statement on adrenal incidentaloma. Eur J Endocrinol 2011;164(6):851–70.

14. Kim HY, Kim SG, Lee KW, et al. Clinical study of adrenal incidentaloma in Korea. Korean J Intern Med 2005;20(4):303–9.

15. Barzon L, Fallo F, Sonino N, et al. Development of overt Cushing's syndrome in patients with adrenal incidentaloma. Eur J Endocrinol 2002; 146(1):61–6.

16. Angeli A, Osella G, Ali A, et al. Adrenal incidentaloma: an overview of clinical and epidemiological data from the National Italian Study Group. Horm Res 1997; 47(4–6):279–83.

17. Alguraan Z, Agcaoglu O, El-Hayek K, et al. Retroperitoneal masses mimicking adrenal tumors. Endocr Pract 2012;18(3):335–41.

18. Jaresch S, Kornely E, Kley HK, et al. Adrenal incidentaloma and patients with homozygous or heterozygous congenital adrenal hyperplasia. J Clin Endocrinol Metab 1992;74(3):685–9.

19. Barzon L, Sonino N, Fallo F, et al. Prevalence and natural history of adrenal incidentalomas. Eur J Endocrinol 2003;149(4):273–85.

20. Musella M, Conzo G, Milone M, et al. Preoperative workup in the assessment of adrenal incidentalomas: outcome from 282 consecutive laparoscopic adrenalectomies. BMC Surg 2013;13:57.

21. Sturgeon C, Shen WT, Clark OH, et al. Risk assessment in 457 adrenal cortical carcinomas: how much does tumor size predict the likelihood of malignancy? J Am Coll Surg 2006;202(3):423–30.

22. McDermott S, O'Connor OJ, Cronin CG, et al. Radiological evaluation of adrenal incidentalomas: current methods and future prospects. Best Pract Res Clin Endocrinol Metab 2012;26(1):21–33.

23. Hamrahian AH, Ioachimescu AG, Remer EM, et al. Clinical utility of noncontrast computed tomography attenuation value (Hounsfield units) to differentiate adrenal adenomas/hyperplasias from nonadenomas: Cleveland Clinic experience. J Clin Endocrinol Metab 2005;90(2):871–7.

24. Korobkin M, Brodeur FJ, Yutzy GG, et al. Differentiation of adrenal adenomas from nonadenomas using CT attenuation values. AJR Am J Roentgenol 1996; 166(3):531–6.

25. Lee MJ, Hahn PF, Papanicolaou N, et al. Benign and malignant adrenal masses: CT distinction with attenuation coefficients, size, and observer analysis. Radiology 1991;179(2):415–8.

26. Miyake H, Maeda H, Tashiro M, et al. CT of adrenal tumors: frequency and clinical significance of low-attenuation lesions. AJR Am J Roentgenol 1989;152(5): 1005–7.

27. Funahashi H, Imai T, Tanaka Y, et al. Discrepancy between PNMT presence and relative lack of adrenaline production in extra-adrenal pheochromocytoma. J Surg Oncol 1994;57(3):196–200.

28. Boland GW, Lee MJ, Gazelle GS, et al. Characterization of adrenal masses using unenhanced CT: an analysis of the CT literature. AJR Am J Roentgenol 1998; 171(1):201–4.

29. Nwariaku FE, Champine J, Kim LT, et al. Radiologic characterization of adrenal masses: the role of computed tomography–derived attenuation values. Surgery 2001;130(6):1068–71.

30. Kannan S, Purysko A, Faiman C, et al. Biochemical and radiological relationships in patients with pheochromocytoma: lessons from a case control study. Clin Endocrinol (Oxf) 2014;80(6):790–6.

31. Blake MA, Krishnamoorthy SK, Boland GW, et al. Low-density pheochromocytoma on CT: a mimicker of adrenal adenoma. AJR Am J Roentgenol 2003; 181(6):1663–8.

32. Sane T, Schalin-Jantti C, Raade M. Is biochemical screening for pheochromocytoma in adrenal incidentalomas expressing low unenhanced attenuation on computed tomography necessary? J Clin Endocrinol Metab 2012;97(6):2077–83.

33. Park BK, Kim CK, Kwon GY, et al. Re-evaluation of pheochromocytomas on delayed contrast-enhanced CT: washout enhancement and other imaging features. Eur Radiol 2007;17(11):2804–9.

34. Mayo-Smith WW, Boland GW, Noto RB, et al. State-of-the-art adrenal imaging. Radiographics 2001;21(4):995–1012.

35. Caoili EM, Korobkin M, Francis IR, et al. Adrenal masses: characterization with combined unenhanced and delayed enhanced CT. Radiology 2002;222(3): 629–33.

36. Kamiyama T, Fukukura Y, Yoneyama T, et al. Distinguishing adrenal adenomas from nonadenomas: combined use of diagnostic parameters of unenhanced and short 5-minute dynamic enhanced CT protocol. Radiology 2009;250(2): 474–81.

37. Korobkin M, Brodeur FJ, Francis IR, et al. Delayed enhanced CT for differentiation of benign from malignant adrenal masses. Radiology 1996;200(3):737–42.

38. Foti G, Faccioli N, Mantovani W, et al. Incidental adrenal lesions: accuracy of quadriphasic contrast enhanced computed tomography in distinguishing adenomas from nonadenomas. Eur J Radiol 2012;81(8):1742–50.

39. Korobkin M, Brodeur FJ, Francis IR, et al. CT time-attenuation washout curves of adrenal adenomas and nonadenomas. AJR Am J Roentgenol 1998;170(3): 747–52.

40. Yoon JK, Remer EM, Herts BR. Incidental pheochromocytoma mimicking adrenal adenoma because of rapid contrast enhancement loss. AJR Am J Roentgenol 2006;187(5):1309–11.

41. Northcutt BG, Raman SP, Long C, et al. MDCT of adrenal masses: can dual-phase enhancement patterns be used to differentiate adenoma and pheochromocytoma? AJR Am J Roentgenol 2013;201(4):834–9.

42. Outwater EK, Siegelman ES, Radecki PD, et al. Distinction between benign and malignant adrenal masses: value of T1-weighted chemical-shift MR imaging. AJR Am J Roentgenol 1995;165(3):579–83.

43. Israel GM, Korobkin M, Wang C, et al. Comparison of unenhanced CT and chemical shift MRI in evaluating lipid-rich adrenal adenomas. AJR Am J Roentgenol 2004;183(1):215–9.

44. Haider MA, Ghai S, Jhaveri K, et al. Chemical shift MR imaging of hyperattenuating (>10 HU) adrenal masses: does it still have a role? Radiology 2004;231(3):711–6.

45. Rha SE, Byun JY, Jung SE, et al. Neurogenic tumors in the abdomen: tumor types and imaging characteristics. Radiographics 2003;23(1):29–43.

46. Francis IR, Korobkin M. Pheochromocytoma. Radiol Clin North Am 1996;34(6):1101–12.

47. Jacques AE, Sahdev A, Sandrasagara M, et al. Adrenal phaeochromocytoma: correlation of MRI appearances with histology and function. Eur Radiol 2008;18(12):2885–92.

48. Song J, Zhang C, Liu Q, et al. Utility of chemical shift and diffusion-weighted imaging in characterization of hyperattenuating adrenal lesions at 3.0T. Eur J Radiol 2012;81(9):2137–43.

49. Timmers HJ, Kozupa A, Chen CC, et al. Superiority of fluorodeoxyglucose positron emission tomography to other functional imaging techniques in the evaluation of metastatic SDHB-associated pheochromocytoma and paraganglioma. J Clin Oncol 2007;25(16):2262–9.

50. Timmers HJ, Chen CC, Carrasquillo JA, et al. Staging and functional characterization of pheochromocytoma and paraganglioma by 18F-fluorodeoxyglucose (18F-FDG) positron emission tomography. J Natl Cancer Inst 2012;104(9):700–8.

51. Timmers HJ, Chen CC, Carrasquillo JA, et al. Comparison of 18F-fluoro-L-DOPA, 18F-fluoro-deoxyglucose, and 18F-fluorodopamine PET and 123I-MIBG scintigraphy in the localization of pheochromocytoma and paraganglioma. J Clin Endocrinol Metab 2009;94(12):4757–67.

52. Boland GW, Blake MA, Holalkere NS, et al. PET/CT for the characterization of adrenal masses in patients with cancer: qualitative versus quantitative accuracy in 150 consecutive patients. AJR Am J Roentgenol 2009;192(4):956–62.

53. Ricciato MP, Di Donna V, Perotti G, et al. The role of adrenal scintigraphy in the diagnosis of subclinical Cushing's syndrome and the prediction of postsurgical hypoadrenalism. World J Surg 2014;38(6):1328–35.

54. Mantero F, Masini AM, Opocher G, et al. Adrenal incidentaloma: an overview of hormonal data from the National Italian Study Group. Horm Res 1997;47(4–6):284–9.

55. Zeiger MA, Thompson GB, Duh QY, et al. American Association of Clinical Endocrinologists and American Association of Endocrine Surgeons Medical Guidelines for the Management of Adrenal Incidentalomas: executive summary of recommendations. Endocr Pract 2009;15(5):450–3.

56. Herrera MF, Grant CS, van Heerden JA, et al. Incidentally discovered adrenal tumors: an institutional perspective. Surgery 1991;110(6):1014–21.

57. Eldeiry LS, Garber JR. Adrenal incidentalomas, 2003 to 2005: experience after publication of the National Institutes of Health consensus statement. Endocr Pract 2008;14(3):279–84.

58. Beierwaltes WH, Sturman MF, Ryo U, et al. Imaging functional nodules of the adrenal glands with 131-I-19-iodocholesterol. J Nucl Med 1974;15(4):246–51.
59. Charbonnel B, Chatal JF, Ozanne P. Does the corticoadrenal adenoma with "pre-Cushing's syndrome" exist? J Nucl Med 1981;22(12):1059–61.
60. Cawood TJ, Hunt PJ, O'Shea D, et al. Recommended evaluation of adrenal incidentalomas is costly, has high false-positive rates and confers a risk of fatal cancer that is similar to the risk of the adrenal lesion becoming malignant; time for a rethink? Eur J Endocrinol 2009;161(4):513–27.
61. Akaza I, Yoshimoto T, Iwashima F, et al. Clinical outcome of subclinical Cushing's syndrome after surgical and conservative treatment. Hypertens Res 2011;34(10):1111–5.
62. Chiodini I, Morelli V, Masserini B, et al. Bone mineral density, prevalence of vertebral fractures, and bone quality in patients with adrenal incidentalomas with and without subclinical hypercortisolism: an Italian multicenter study. J Clin Endocrinol Metab 2009;94(9):3207–14.
63. Chiodini I, Morelli V, Salcuni AS, et al. Beneficial metabolic effects of prompt surgical treatment in patients with an adrenal incidentaloma causing biochemical hypercortisolism. J Clin Endocrinol Metab 2010;95(6):2736–45.
64. Morelli V, Eller-Vainicher C, Salcuni AS, et al. Risk of new vertebral fractures in patients with adrenal incidentaloma with and without subclinical hypercortisolism: a multicenter longitudinal study. J Bone Miner Res 2011;26(8):1816–21.
65. Toniato A, Merante-Boschin I, Opocher G, et al. Surgical versus conservative management for subclinical Cushing syndrome in adrenal incidentalomas: a prospective randomized study. Ann Surg 2009;249(3):388–91.
66. Di Dalmazi G, Vicennati V, Garelli S, et al. Cardiovascular events and mortality in patients with adrenal incidentalomas that are either non-secreting or associated with intermediate phenotype or subclinical Cushing's syndrome: a 15-year retrospective study. Lancet Diabetes Endocrinol 2014;2(5):396–405.
67. Mansmann G, Lau J, Balk E, et al. The clinically inapparent adrenal mass: update in diagnosis and management. Endocr Rev 2004;25(2):309–40.
68. Funder JW, Carey RM, Fardella C, et al. Case detection, diagnosis, and treatment of patients with primary aldosteronism: an endocrine society clinical practice guideline. J Clin Endocrinol Metab 2008;93(9):3266–81.
69. Mysliwiec J, Zukowski L, Grodzka A, et al. Diagnostics of primary aldosteronism: is obligatory use of confirmatory tests justified? J Renin Angiotensin Aldosterone Syst 2012;13(3):367–71.
70. Rossi GP, Bernini G, Caliumi C, et al. A prospective study of the prevalence of primary aldosteronism in 1,125 hypertensive patients. J Am Coll Cardiol 2006;48(11):2293–300.
71. Kono T, Ikeda F, Oseko F, et al. Normotensive primary aldosteronism: report of a case. J Clin Endocrinol Metab 1981;52(5):1009–13.
72. Grumbach MM, Biller BM, Braunstein GD, et al. Management of the clinically inapparent adrenal mass ("incidentaloma"). Ann Intern Med 2003;138(5):424–9.
73. Mannelli M, Lenders JW, Pacak K, et al. Subclinical phaeochromocytoma. Best Pract Res Clin Endocrinol Metab 2012;26(4):507–15.
74. Stenstrom G, Svardsudd K. Pheochromocytoma in Sweden 1958–1981. An analysis of the National Cancer Registry Data. Acta Med Scand 1986;220(3):225–32.
75. Lenders JW, Pacak K, Walther MM, et al. Biochemical diagnosis of pheochromocytoma: which test is best? JAMA 2002;287(11):1427–34.

76. Sawka AM, Jaeschke R, Singh RJ, et al. A comparison of biochemical tests for pheochromocytoma: measurement of fractionated plasma metanephrines compared with the combination of 24-hour urinary metanephrines and catecholamines. J Clin Endocrinol Metab 2003;88(2):553–8.
77. Adler JT, Meyer-Rochow GY, Chen H, et al. Pheochromocytoma: current approaches and future directions. Oncologist 2008;13(7):779–93.
78. Goldstein RE, O'Neill JA Jr, Holcomb GW 3rd, et al. Clinical experience over 48 years with pheochromocytoma. Ann Surg 1999;229(6):755–64 [discussion: 755–64].
79. Pacak K. Preoperative management of the pheochromocytoma patient. J Clin Endocrinol Metab 2007;92(11):4069–79.
80. Lenders JW, Duh QY, Eisenhofer G, et al. Pheochromocytoma and paraganglioma: an Endocrine Society clinical practice guideline. J Clin Endocrinol Metab 2014;99(6):1915–42.
81. Amar L, Servais A, Gimenez-Roqueplo AP, et al. Year of diagnosis, features at presentation, and risk of recurrence in patients with pheochromocytoma or secreting paraganglioma. J Clin Endocrinol Metab 2005;90(4):2110–6.
82. Bravo EL. Evolving concepts in the pathophysiology, diagnosis, and treatment of pheochromocytoma. Endocr Rev 1994;15(3):356–68.
83. Else T, Williams AR, Sabolch A, et al. Adjuvant therapies and patient and tumor characteristics associated with survival of adult patients with adrenocortical carcinoma. J Clin Endocrinol Metab 2014;99(2):455–61.
84. Uberoi J, Munver R. Surgical management of metastases to the adrenal gland: open, laparoscopic, and ablative approaches. Curr Urol Rep 2009;10(1):67–72.
85. Morelli V, Reimondo G, Giordano R, et al. Long-term follow-up in adrenal incidentalomas: an Italian multicenter study. J Clin Endocrinol Metab 2014;99(3):827–34.
86. Arnaldi G, Boscaro M. Adrenal incidentaloma. Best Pract Res Clin Endocrinol Metab 2012;26(4):405–19.
87. Yener S, Ertilav S, Secil M, et al. Prospective evaluation of tumor size and hormonal status in adrenal incidentalomas. J Endocrinol Invest 2010;33(1):32–6.
88. Pantalone KM, Gopan T, Remer EM, et al. Change in adrenal mass size as a predictor of a malignant tumor. Endocr Pract 2010;16(4):577–87.

Primary Aldosteronism
Challenges in Diagnosis and Management

Sandi-Jo Galati, MD

KEYWORDS

- Primary aldosteronism • Aldosterone-producing adenoma
- Bilateral adrenal hyperplasia • Endocrine hypertension

KEY POINTS

- Primary aldosteronism (PA) imparts significant cardiovascular, cerebrovascular, and renal morbidity, which is disproportionate to the degree of hypertension.
- Recent prevalence studies suggest PA is common, perhaps accounting for 10% of patients with hypertension, and most cases are not accompanied by hypokalemia.
- Recent advances in understanding the underlying molecular pathophysiology of the rare causes of hereditary PA have provided further insight into to mechanisms leading to sporadic disease.
- The preferred screening test for PA is the aldosterone/renin ratio (ARR), which must be interpreted in the context of the antihypertensive agents in use.
- Elevated ARRs are suspicious for true disease but require confirmatory testing. The choice of confirmatory test depends on patient and institution preference and capabilities.
- Surgery or targeted medical therapy is available and effective both for hypertension management and reversal of the end-organ damage effects of aldosterone excess.

INTRODUCTION AND DISEASE PREVALENCE

In 1954, Jerome Conn described the index patient with an aldosterone-producing adenoma (APA), a young woman hospitalized with uncontrolled hypertension and hypokalemia with tetany. Bilateral adrenalectomy was planned in hopes of achieving control of her symptoms. An adrenal mass was identified and resected in the operating room, sparing her from lifelong steroid dependence while resolving her hypokalemia, tetany, and hypertension.[1,2] Throughout his career, Conn continued to seek out and treat patients with primary aldosteronism (PA), ultimately postulating that it was common among hypertensive patients; potentially present in up to one-fifth of cases; and, unlike in his index patient, hypokalemia was not synonymous with the disease.[3,4] This

The author has nothing to disclose.
Trumbull, CT 06611, USA
E-mail address: sandijo.galati@gmail.com

Endocrinol Metab Clin N Am 44 (2015) 355–369
http://dx.doi.org/10.1016/j.ecl.2015.02.010
0889-8529/15/$ – see front matter © 2015 Elsevier Inc. All rights reserved.

endo.theclinics.com

estimate was subsequently questioned and debunked by Fishman and colleagues[5] who suggested the disease was rare and present in less than 1% of all hypertensive patients, an estimate that persisted for nearly 30 years along with the indoctrination that hypertension due to PA was invariably accompanied by hypokalemia.[6]

Worldwide prevalence studies conducted over the last 20 years in subjects with hypertension have suggested a much higher prevalence, ranging from 5% to 12%.[7–9] In 1994, Gordon and colleagues[7] reported a prospective study of 199 Australian subjects with hypertension and normokalemia identifying PA as the underlying cause in 8.5% to 12% of subjects. A subsequent study of 380 Chinese subjects living in Singapore identified PA as the underlying cause of hypertension in 5%.[8] The largest study to date, the PA Prevalence in Hypertensives (PAPY) study, reported an 11.2% prevalence of PA in 1125 hypertensive subjects recruited from 14 Italian centers.[9] Further, increased prevalence rates have been described in specific patient populations, including those with resistant hypertension (20%), diabetes with hypertension (13%–14%), and hypertension with obstructive sleep apnea (34%).[10–16]

Recent increased screening and diagnosis of PA is also related to the recognition that hypokalemia is not a requisite finding in the disease. There is an 11-fold increased incidence of disease in patients with concomitant hypertension and potassium less than 3.2 mEq/L compared with normokalemic (potassium >3.5 mEq/L) patients.[17] In practice, however, most patients with PA are not hypokalemic. Recent studies demonstrate a 9% to 37% overall incidence of hypokalemia in patients with documented PA, suggesting that normokalemia should not exclude hypertensive patients from being screened for the disease.[9,18]

It is important to recognize that most of these recent prevalence studies were conducted at referral centers where populations consist mainly of patients with resistant hypertension. Therefore, some experts maintain that PA is a rare finding in the general hypertensive population.[19] In a 2012-2013 study of 296 hypertensive subjects in a New York City general internal medicine clinic population, only 4.7% screened positive for PA. Further, those who screened positive for PA were more likely to have resistant hypertension and required more antihypertensive agents for blood pressure treatment (both statistically significant). The participation of these subjects with subsequent confirmatory testing was poor, with only 6 completing confirmatory testing and, of these, only 2 testing positive for PA, an overall prevalence of only 0.67% (Galati, 2013). This may reflect certain genetic characteristics of the population studied or confirm the suspicions of those who believe PA is a disease of patients with resistant hypertension.

PATHOPHYSIOLOGY AND GENETICS

Aldosterone binds to the mineralocorticoid receptor (MR) on the distal nephron where it promotes gene expression of epithelium sodium channels (ENaCs). ENaC receptors increase sodium and water absorption and promote volume expansion.[20] Aldosterone synthesis and release principally depends on the presence of angiotensin II binding to its receptor on the zona glomerulosa of the adrenal cortex, although adrenocorticotrophic hormone (ACTH) and hyperkalemia can also stimulate its secretion. Angiotensin II is converted from angiotensin I by angiotensin-converting enzyme (ACE). Angiotensin I is converted from angiotensinogen in a reaction catalyzed by renin. Renin is released in response to volume receptors juxtaglomerular apparatus and chemoreceptors in the macula densa of the kidney.[21] Therefore, aldosterone release is normally modulated by renin-sensed alterations in salt and volume status. In PA, however, aldosterone synthesis and release is independent of renin. As a result, there is constitutive promotion of ENaC expression resulting with excess salt and water reabsorption; reflexive vasoconstriction; and, ultimately, hypertension.[20,21]

PA most frequently is the result of excess aldosterone production by both adrenal glands, so-called bilateral adrenal hyperplasia, which accounts for two-thirds of cases. APAs account for only one-third of cases. Rarely, unilateral hyperplasia, adrenocortical carcinoma, or ectopic aldosterone production are diagnosed. Finally, 3 hereditary causes have been recently described: familial hyperaldosteronism 1, 2, and 3 (FH 1, 2, 3).

Although rare, the hereditary causes of PA also have provided further insight into the molecular pathophysiology of PA. FH 1, or glucocorticoid-remediable aldosteronism, results from a recombination of the genes encoding the cytochrome P450 enzymes 11-β hydroxylase and aldosterone synthase, creating a chimeric gene. Affected families present with severe hypertension, hypokalemia, and overproduction of aldosterone and the hybrid steroids 18-hydroxycortisol and 18-oxocortisol. The ACTH-dependent promoter region from 11-β hydroxylase is coupled to aldosterone synthase; therefore, aldosterone synthase gene expression is controlled by ACTH (rather than angiotensin II or potassium). Thus, the disease is effectively managed by suppressing ACTH with dexamethasone treatment.[22]

FH 3 was described in a family with severe hypertension, hypokalemia, and elevated aldosterone and hybrid steroids that, unlike in FH 1, were unsuppressed after administration of dexamethasone.[23] A mutation in the gene KCNJ5 encoding the selectivity component of the Kir 3.4 potassium channel was identified, ultimately resulting in loss of channel selectivity to potassium, constitutive depolarization of the cell, and uncontrolled aldosterone synthesis and release (**Fig. 1**).[24] Subsequently, somatic KCNJ5 mutations were identified in high frequency ranging from 34% to 65% of sporadic APAs.[25–29] Several other germline mutation genotypes affecting the KCNJ5 potassium selectivity region of the channel have been identified resulting in variable disease severity.[30] Interestingly, germline mutations outside of this potassium channel selectivity region have also been described and may account for a small percentage of presumed sporadic PA.[31]

Recent research has focused on elucidating other molecular pathways that lead to the development of sporadic PA, either from neoplasia in unilateral disease or hyperplasia in unilateral or bilateral disease. These mechanisms include enhanced aldosterone synthesis from increased expression of steroidogenic enzymes,[32–34] increased Wnt/β-catenin activity leading to APA development,[34] and presence of agonistic autoantibodies against the angiotensin II receptor.[35]

In addition to the distal nephron, MR has been identified in the colon, salivary glands, vasculature, heart, adipose tissue, and hippocampus,[36] where both genomic and nongenomic effects occur.[37] Specifically, aldosterone-mediated oxidative stress has been demonstrated in the vasculature by inducing endothelial dysfunction[38] and increasing arterial stiffness and intima to media thickness by promoting deposition of collagen within arterial walls.[39–42]

These cellular changes are translated clinically by the mounting evidence that continues to support the multisystem sequelae of aldosterone excess that are both independent of blood pressure control as well as out of proportion to the degree of hypertension.

Cardiovascular effects are the most well studied and include left ventricular remodeling and hypertrophy, increased risk of coronary artery disease, nonfatal myocardial infarctions, strokes, atrial fibrillation, and heart failure.[43–50] There is also mounting evidence for development of type 2 diabetes, insulin resistance and the metabolic syndrome,[51–54] obstructive sleep apnea,[55] renal disease,[56–58] psychiatric disease,[59] and bone loss[60] in patients with untreated aldosterone excess.

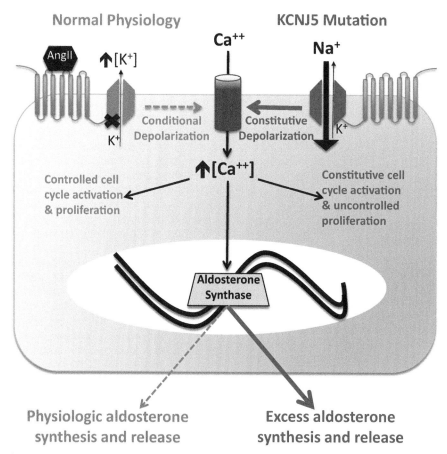

Fig. 1. Molecular pathophysiology of KCNJ5 mutation. In normal physiologic circumstances, angiotensin II (Ang II) binds to its receptor on the zona glomerulosa cells, decreases potassium efflux, and depolarizes the cell allowing calcium entry. Rising calcium concentrations ultimately stimulate aldosterone synthesis and secretion, as well as cell proliferation. KCNJ5 gene mutations result in unselective potassium Kir 3.4 channels. The loss of selectivity results in constitutive cell depolarization with aldosterone synthesis and secretion in the absence of Ang II and uncontrolled cellular proliferation. (*From* Galati SJ, Hopkins SM, Cheesman KC, et al. Primary aldosteronism: emerging trends. Trends Endocrinol Metab 2013;24(9):424; with permission.)

SCREENING AND CONFIRMATION OF DISEASE

Published guidelines have identified high-prevalence subgroups of patients for whom screening is recommended. These include patients with moderate-to-severe hypertension, resistant hypertension, spontaneous or diuretic-induced hypokalemia, hypertension with a family history of early-onset disease, hypertension with an adrenal incidentaloma, a history of cerebrovascular accident occurring before age 40, or with a first-degree relative with PA.[61] However, with the mounting evidence of the prevalence of PA in hypertensive patients regardless of serum potassium levels,[7–9] as well as the increased cardiovascular and renal sequelae, which is present regardless of blood pressure control, an argument exists for screening all patients with hypertension[62–65] although this remains highly controversial.[19]

The aldosterone/renin ratio (ARR) is the screening test for PA, having the highest sensitivity and specificity for disease detection. The ARR is calculated by dividing the plasma aldosterone concentration (PAC) in ng/dL or pmol/L by the plasma renin activity (PRA) measured in ng per mL per hour.

Again, in normal physiology, aldosterone synthesis and secretion depends on renin-stimulated angiotensin II production in low-volume states. Conversely, PA is a renin-independent state in which aldosterone synthesis and secretion occurs independent of volume status. The ARR reflects this pathophysiology of PA, in which values suggestive of underlying disease are characterized by high aldosterone with low renin levels. Threshold values vary by institution but, in general, an ARR greater than 20 ng/dL per ng/mL/h and PAC greater than 10 ng/dL with a suppressed renin are accepted values for a positive screening test[18] and minimize false-negative screens.[66]

The challenge in using the ARR as a screening test for PA is that many factors confound the interpretation of the results. Volume status, age, posture, time of day, potassium, dietary sodium, renal disease, and antihypertensive agent use must be considered and the ARR must be interpreted in the context of these factors.[66,67] For instance, ACE inhibitors (ACEis) and angiotensin-receptor blockers (ARBs) are commonly used antihypertensive agents that exert their action on the renin-angiotensin-aldosterone pathway. Use of an ACEi or ARB would be expected to increase PRA levels; lower PAC levels; and therefore, result in a low ARR. An elevated PAC, suppressed PRA, and elevated ARR in patients taking these drugs would, therefore, prompt suspicion for disease.

With the exception of the mineralocorticoid-receptor antagonists, spironolactone and eplerenone, the ARR can be interpreted with the use of any antihypertensive agent or clinical circumstance as long as the impact on PAC and PRA is understood (**Table 1**). Patients who are on a mineralocorticoid-receptor blocker require a 6-week medication withdrawal before screening, during which agents that do not

Table 1
The effects of antihypertensive drug classes on aldosterone, renin, and the aldosterone/renin ratio

	Aldosterone	Renin	ARR
β-blockers	↓	↓	↑
Central α-blockers	↓	↓	↑
ACEi, ARBs	↓	↑	↓
K+ sparing diuretics	↑	↑	↓
K+ wasting diuretics	↕	↑	↓
CCBs (DHP only)	↕	↑	↓
Renin inhibitors	↓	↓↑ *	*

*The effect of renin inhibitors depends on the methodology used to measure renin.
Abbreviations: ACEi, angiotensin-converting enzyme inhibitor; ARBs, angiotensin-receptor blockers; CCBs, calcium-channel blockers; DHP, dihydropyridine.
Data from Funder JW, Carey RM, Fardella C, et al. Case detection, diagnosis, and treatment of patients with primary aldosteronism: an endocrine society clinical practice guideline. J Clin Endocrinol Metab 2008;93:3266–81.

Table 2
Confirmatory testing in primary aldosteronism

	Protocol	Interpretation	Clinical Pearls	Reference
Intravenous saline load	• Infusion of 2 L of 0.9% normal saline over 2 h[a] • Infusion should begin in the morning • Renin, PAC, cortisol, and potassium levels are drawn preinfusion and postinfusion of saline	• PAC >10 ng/dL postinfusion is highly suggestive of PA • PAC <5 ng/dL is less likely consistent with PA • PAC between 5–10 ng/dL is indeterminate and may represent PA or low-renin hypertension	• Potassium supplementation is required for patients with hypokalemia • During the test potassium tends to remain stable • Caution in patients with uncontrolled HTN, congestive heart failure, or arrhythmias	60,94,95
Oral salt load	• Goal sodium intake is >6 g/d for 3 d (combination of dietary intake and sodium chloride tabs) • 24-h urine collection for sodium, creatinine, and aldosterone starting on day 3 of salt load	• 24-h urinary aldosterone excretion >12 mcg/24 h is consistent with PA • 24-h urinary sodium exceeding 200 mEq/24 h indicates adequate sodium intake	• Potassium supplementation and daily potassium measurements required for patients with hypokalemia • Caution in patients with uncontrolled HTN, congestive heart failure, or arrhythmias • False negatives may occur in renal insufficiency	60,94
Captopril challenge test	• Patient is administered 25–50 mg of oral captopril after sitting or standing for 1 h • PAC, renin, and cortisol levels are measured before captopril administration and 1–2 h after	• PAC is suppressed by 30% or more if PA is not present • ARR is >30–50, PAC remains elevated (>8.5 ng/dL or greater) and renin remains suppressed in PA	• High false-positive or false-negative rate • Results may be variable, particularly in BAH, where there are reports of PAC suppression • Poor test performance also seen with high ARR • Safer in patients at risk of volume overload	94,95

| Fludrocortisone suppression test | • Patients receive 0.1 mg of fludrocortisones every 6 h for 4 d
• Potassium supplements are also administered 4 times daily and serum potassium is measured 4 times daily to maintain values of >4.0 mmol/L
• High sodium diet + sodium chloride tabs are administered
• On the morning of day 4, plasma cortisol is measured at 7 or 8 AM and 10 AM and PAC and renin are measured at 10 AM with the patient in the seated position | • PAC >6 ng/dL confirms PA provided
  ○ Renin is suppressed to <1 ng/mL/h (<8.4 mU/L)
  ○ Plasma potassium is normal
  ○ 10 AM cortisol is lower than 7–8 AM cortisol to exclude ACTH effect[b] | • Considered by some to be the most reliable test
• Requires inpatient admission for monitoring
• Potassium supplementation and daily potassium measurements required for patients with hypokalemia
• Caution in patients with uncontrolled HTN, congestive heart failure or arrhythmias
• False-negatives can occur in renal insufficiency | 60,93,96,97 |

Abbreviations: BAH, bilateral adrenal hyperplasia; HTN, hypertension.

[a] A recent study has demonstrated improved sensitivity for disease detection when the intravenous saline load is performed in the seated, rather than recumbent position.[95]

[b] Dexamethasone may be administered on the final day of the fludrocortisones suppression test to eliminate any potential contribution of ACTH-induced aldosterone secretion.[97]

affect the ARR can be substituted. These include peripheral α-adrenergic antagonists (prazosin, doxazosin, or terazosin), hydralazine, or nondihydropyridine calcium channel blockers (verapamil and diltiazem).[67,68]

The ARR is a screening test designed to identify patients who may have disease. A suspicious ARR must be followed with a confirmatory test to distinguish bilateral from potentially surgical unilateral disease. These confirmatory tests include the oral sodium loading test, saline infusion, fludrocortisone suppression, or captopril challenge. There is insufficient evidence to support 1 confirmatory test over another[61] and, similar to the ARR, confounding factors, such as position, may affect test results. Therefore, selection of the appropriate confirmatory test tends to be specific to both patient and institution (**Table 2**).

LOCALIZATION OF DISEASE

Adrenal vein sampling (AVS) is the only method currently available to reliably distinguish aldosterone excess from a unilateral source, typically an APA, from bilateral disease. However, AVS is both technically difficult to perform and lacks procedural standardization, which can make interpretation of the results challenging. Therefore, to ensure diagnostic accuracy, it should be performed only at a center that is skilled in the procedure and interpreted with knowledge of the procedure protocols.

Cannulating the short right adrenal vein that drains directly into the inferior vena cava represents the most significant procedural limitation of AVS. Computed tomography (CT) scan to localize the right adrenal vein, point-of-care cortisol testing, and CT angiography to confirm catheter placement improve cannulation success.[69–72]

Calculating a peripheral cortisol/adrenal cortisol ratio is used to confirm catheter placement with a ratio of 10:1, suggestive of adequate cannulation of the adrenal veins.[73] Sampling then proceeds in either a simultaneous or sequential fashion with continuous, intermittent, or no ACTH stimulation. A ratio of PAC/cortisol from the high side to PAC/cortisol from the low side greater than 4:1 is consistent with an APA,[73] whereas lower ratios are consistent with bilateral disease. Further confirmatory evidence of the presence of an APA is the suppression of secretion from the contralateral side, in which the unaffected adrenal PAC/cortisol quotient is less than peripheral PAC/cortisol quotient in 93% of cases.[73]

The presence of cortisol cosecretion from an APA, which may be present in up to 10% of cases,[74] may further confound AVS by resulting in loss of laterality. In cases in which mild hypercortisolism is suspected, plasma metanephrines[75] or catecholamine levels[76] have been used to confirm cannulization and, in the case of catecholamines, lateralization.[76]

CT is typically used to exclude the presence of adrenocortical carcinoma[61] in addition to providing further information regarding the adrenal anatomy before AVS.[71] In a retrospective study of 263 subjects with unilateral PA, use of CT or MRI in conjunction with AVS with subsequent adrenalectomy resulted in a 95.5% cure rate.[77] CT or MRI alone accurately detected disease in only 58.6% of cases, although CT or MRI accurately localized disease in 100% of patients younger than age 35.1.[77] In general, concordance between CT and AVS has been demonstrated to be as low, although the value of CT localization may be greater among patients younger than age 40.[73,77,78]

Use of clinical data in addition to imaging has also been suggested to correctly localize disease. In a retrospective study of patients with confirmed PA who underwent AVS, CT predicted localization unilateral localization with 100% accuracy if the adrenal adenoma was less than 10 mm and either hypokalemia of 3.5 mEq/dL or glomerular filtration rate (GFR) of 100 mL/min was present.[79] However, subsequent application of this prediction score to other patient registries demonstrated lack of specificity.[80,81] Further prospective data are required before CT can be used to localize disease, even in specific patient subsets. Simply stated, even in patients with proven PA in whom a small adrenal incidentaloma has been identified on imaging, AVS at an experienced center is strongly recommended to avoid improper localization.

SURGICAL VERSUS MEDICAL MANAGEMENT AND TREATMENT OUTCOMES

For most patients with localized APA, unilateral laparoscopic adrenalectomy is the preferred management approach, both improving blood pressure and correcting hypokalemia, as well as being cost-effective.[82]

Cure (defined as blood pressure <140/90) rates range from 30% to 60%[83–85] and depend on: family history of hypertension, preoperative requirement of 2 or fewer antihypertensive medications, age younger than 50 years, less than 5-year duration of hypertension, presence of increased serum creatinine, presence of hypokalemia, high urinary aldosterone secretion, and response to spironolactone.[77,83–86]

Patients who are not surgical candidates or have bilateral disease can be managed medically and achieve blood pressure control with a mineralocorticoid-receptor antagonist, either spironolactone or eplerenone, although typically additional antihypertensive agents are required.[87] Spironolactone has antagonistic properties at the androgen receptor in addition to the MR and agonistic properties at the progesterone receptor, which can result in painful gynecomastia, erectile dysfunction, decreased libido in men, and menstrual irregularity in women. Eplerenone is a selective mineralocorticoid-receptor antagonist and, therefore, lacks these side effects.[88] However, studies comparing the efficacy of eplerenone and spironolactone in patients with PA demonstrated greater blood pressure reduction with spironolactone use.[89] Amiloride, an ENaC channel antagonist, is also effective in controlling blood pressure and improving hypokalemia without the side effects of spironolactone.[90] Finally, aldosterone synthase inhibitors may be a future treatment option; however, studies thus far have demonstrated decreased efficacy compared with MR-antagonists while promoting concern for the possibility of decreasing cortisol synthesis.[91]

In a prospective study of 54 subjects treated for PA, Catena and colleagues[83] reported either medical or surgical treatment reversed the excess risk of myocardial infarctions, sustained arrhythmias, need for revascularization procedures, or cerebrovascular events after 7.4 years of follow-up. However, a subsequent study by Bernini and colleagues[92] demonstrated either medical or surgical management of PA resulted in blood pressure control; however, significant decreases in left-ventricular mass were detected only in the surgically-treated group after 2.5 years of follow-up. This suggests that there is accelerated improvement in cardiometabolic parameters occurring in those patients treated surgically. Prospective data extending beyond 2.5 years in this cohort will be essential to determine if and when medical therapy is efficacious.

Mortality data is limited to 1 retrospective analysis of the German Conn's Registry. There was no difference in all-cause mortality in 337 patients after medical or surgical treatment of PA compared with controls matched for age, sex, body mass index, and blood pressure. This suggests treatment reverses any excess mortality risk associated with aldosterone excess. Interestingly, all-cause mortality was reduced in patients with PA treated with adrenalectomy compared with those who were medically-treated.[93]

SUMMARY

PA is the most common identifiable endocrine cause of hypertension. Recent prevalence studies suggest that PA may be more common in select high-risk populations than historically estimated. Patients on any antihypertensive agents, with the exception of MR antagonists, can be screened with the ARR and all positive screens should be confirmed before subtype differentiation. Again, the risk of cardiovascular, cerebrovascular, and renal disease exceeds what is expected for the degree of blood pressure elevation when aldosterone excess is present. Therefore, any treatment, either medical or surgical, must improve blood pressure, correct metabolic abnormalities that may be present, and reverse the risks of excess cardiovascular and renal morbidity.

REFERENCES

1. Young WF. Primary aldosteronism: renaissance of a syndrome. Clin Endocrinol 2007;669(5):607–18.
2. Conn JW. Presidential address. Part I: painting background. Part II: primary aldosteronism, a new clinical syndrome. J Lab Clin Med 1955;45:3–17.
3. Conn JW, Knopf RF, Nesbit RM, et al. Clinical characteristics of primary aldosteronism from analysis of 145 cases. Am J Surg 1964;107:159–72.
4. Conn JW. Plasma renin activity in primary aldosteronism: importance in differential diagnosis and in research of essential hypertension. JAMA 1964;190:222–5.
5. Fishman LM, Küchel O, Liddle GW, et al. Incidence of primary aldosteronism uncomplicated "essential" hypertension. A prospective study with elevated aldosterone secretion and suppressed plasma renin activity used as diagnostic criteria. JAMA 1968;205:497–502.
6. Kaplan NM. Hypokalemia in the hypertensive patient, with observations on the incidence of primary aldosteronism. Ann Intern Med 1967;66:1079–90.
7. Gordon RD, Stowasser MD, Tunny TJ, et al. High prevalence in primary aldosteronism in 199 patients referred with hypertension. Clin Exp Pharmacol Physiol 1994;21(4):315–8.
8. Loh KC, Koay ES, Khaw MC, et al. Prevalence of primary aldosteronism among Asian hypertensive patients in Singapore. J Clin Endocrinol Metab 2000;85:2854–9.
9. Rossi GP, Bernini G, Caliumi C, et al. PAPY Study Investigators. A prospective study of the prevalence of primary aldosteronism in 1,125 hypertensive patients. J Am Coll Cardiol 2006;48(11):2293–300.
10. Calhoun DA, Nishizaka MK, Zaman MA, et al. Hyperaldosteronism among black and white subjects with resistant hypertension. Hypertension 2002;40(6):892–6.
11. Gallay BJ, Ahmad S, Xu L, et al. Screening for primary aldosteronism without discontinuing hypertensive medications: plasma aldosterone-renin ratio. Am J Kidney Dis 2001;37(4):699–705.
12. Strauch B, Zelinka T, Hampf M, et al. Prevalence of primary aldosteronism in moderate to severe hypertension in the Central Europe region. J Hum Hypertens 2003;17(5):349–52.
13. Mukherjee JJ, Khoo CM, Thai AC, et al. Type 2 diabetic patients with resistant hypertension should be screened for primary aldosteronism. Diab Vasc Dis Res 2010;7(1):6–13.
14. Umpierrez GE, Cantey P, Smiley D, et al. Primary aldosteronism in diabetic subjects with resistant hypertension. Diabetes Care 2007;30(7):1699–703.

15. Li N, Wang M, Wang H, et al. Prevalence of primary aldosteronism in hypertensive subjects with hyperglycemia. Clin Exp Hypertens 2013;35(3):175–82.
16. Di Murro A, Petramala L, Cotesta D, et al. Renin-angiotensin-aldosterone system in patients with sleep apnoea: prevalence of primary aldosteronism. J Renin Angiotensin Aldosterone Syst 2010;11(3):165–72.
17. Goldenberg K, Snyder DK. Screening for primary aldosteronism: hypokalemia in hypertensive patients. J Gen Intern Med 1986;1(6):368–72.
18. Mulatero P, Stowasser M, Loh KC, et al. Increased diagnosis of primary aldosteronism, including surgically correctable forms, in centers from five continents. J Clin Endocrinol Metab 2004;89(3):1045–50.
19. Kaplan NM. Primary aldosteronism: A contrarian view. Rev Endocr Metab Disord 2011;12:49–52.
20. Funder JW. Aldosterone and mineralocorticoid receptors in the cardiovascular system. Prog Cardiovasc Dis 2010;53:393–400.
21. Young WF Jr. Endocrine hypertension. In: Melmed S, Polonsky KS, Larsen PR, et al, editors. Williams textbook of endocrinology. 12th edition. Philadelphia: Elsevier; 2012. p. 545–77.
22. Lenzini L, Caroccia B, Campos AG, et al. Lower expression of TWIK-related acid-sensitive K+ channel 2 (TASK-2) gene is a hallmark of aldosterone-producing adenoma causing human primary aldosteronism. J Clin Endocrinol Metab 2014;99:E674–82.
23. Robertson S, MacKenzie SM, Alvarez-Madrazo S, et al. MicroRNA-24 is a novel regulator of aldosterone and cortisol production in the human adrenal cortex. Hypertension 2013;62:572–8.
24. Berthon A, Drelon C, Ragazzon B, et al. WNT/β-catenin signaling is activated in aldosterone-producing adenomas and controls aldosterone production. Hum Mol Genet 2014;23:889–905.
25. Rossiotto G, Regolisti G, Rossi F, et al. Elevation of angiotensin-II type-1-receptor autoantibodies titer in primary aldosteronism as a result of an aldosterone-producing adenoma. Hypertension 2013;61:526–33.
26. Lifton RP, Dluly RG, Powers M, et al. A chimaeric 11b–hydroxylase/aldosterone synthase gene causes glucocorticoid-remediable aldosteronism in human hypertension. Nature 2002;355:262–5.
27. Geller DS, Zhang J, Wisgerhof MV, et al. A novel form of mendelian hypertension featuring nonglucocorticoid-remediable aldosteronism. J Clin Endocrinol Metab 2008;93:3117–23.
28. Choi M, Scholl UI, Yue P, et al. K+ channel mutations in adrenal aldosterone-producing adenomas and hereditary hypertension. Science 2011;331:768–72.
29. Boulkroun S, Beuschlein F, Rossi GP, et al. Prevalence, clinical and molecular correlates of KCNJ5 mutations in primary aldosteronism. Hypertension 2012;52:592–8.
30. Azizan EA, Murthy M, Stowasser M, et al. Somatic mutations affecting the selectivity filter of KCNJ5 are frequent in 2 large unselected collections of adrenal aldosteronomas. Hypertension 2012;59:587–91.
31. Taguchi R, Yamada M, Nakajima Y, et al. Expression and mutations of KCNJ5 mRNA in Japanese patients with aldosterone-producing adenomas. J Clin Endocrinol Metab 2012;97:1311–9.
32. Azizan EA, Lam BY, Newhouse SJ, et al. Microarray, qPCR, and KCNJ5 sequencing of aldosterone-producing adenomas reveal differences in genotype and phenotype between zona glomerulosa- and zona fasciculate-like tumors. J Clin Endocrinol Metab 2012;97:E819–29.

33. Monticone S, Hattangady NG, Nishimoto K, et al. Effect of KCNJ5 mutations on gene expression in aldosterone-producing adenomas and adrenocortical cells. J Clin Endocrinol Metab 2012;97:E1567–72.
34. Scholl U, Nelson-Williams C, Yue P, et al. Hypertension with or without adrenal hyperplasia due to different inherited mutations in the potassium channel KCNJ5. Proc Natl Acad Sci U S A 2012;109:2533–8.
35. Murthy M, Xu S, Massimo G, et al. Role for germline mutations and a rare coding single nucleotide polymorphism within the KCNJ5 potassium channel in a large cohort of sporadic cases of primary aldosteronism. Hypertension 2014;63:783–9.
36. Hawkins UA, Gomez-Sanchez EP, Gomez-Sanchez CM, et al. The ubiquitous mineralocorticoid receptor: clinical implications. Curr Hypertens Rep 2012;14: 573–80.
37. Gros R, Ding Q, Sklar LA, et al. GPR30 expression is required for the mineralocorticoid receptor-independent rapid vascular effects of aldosterone. Hypertension 2011;57:442–51.
38. Stehr CB, Mellado R, Ocaranza MP, et al. Increased oxidative stress, subclinical inflammation, and myocardial fibrosis markers in primary aldosteronism patients. J Hypertens 2010;28:2120–6.
39. Wu VC, Lo SC, Chen YL, et al. Endothelial progenitor cells in primary aldosteronism: a biomarker of severity for aldosterone vasculopathy and prognosis. J Clin Endocrinol Metab 2011;96:3175–83.
40. Rizzoni D, Paiardi S, Rodella L, et al. Changes in extracellular matrix in subcutaneous small resistance arteries of patients with primary aldosteronism. J Clin Endocrinol Metab 2006;91:2638–42.
41. Holaj R, Zelinka T, Wichterle D, et al. Increased intima-media thickness and carotid artery fibrosis in patients with primary aldosteronism. J Hypertens 2007; 25:1451–7.
42. Bernini G, Galetta F, Franzoni F, et al. Arterial stiffness, intima-media thickness and carotid artery fibrosis in patients with primary aldosteronism. J Hypertens 2008;26:2399–405.
43. Rossi GP, Sacchetto A, Pavan E, et al. Remodeling of the left ventricle in primary aldosteronism due to Conn's adenoma. Circulation 1997;95:1471–8.
44. Matsumura K, Fujii K, Oniki H, et al. Role of aldosterone in left ventricular hypertrophy in hypertension. Am J Hypertens 2006;19:13–8.
45. Milliez P, Girerd X, Plouin PF, et al. Evidence for an increased rate of cardiovascular events in patients with primary aldosteronism. J Am Coll Cardiol 2005;45: 1243–8.
46. Muiesan ML, Salvetti M, Paini A, et al. Inappropriate left ventricular mass in patients with primary aldosteronism. Hypertension 2008;52:529–34.
47. Born-Frontsberg E, Reincke M, Rump LC, et al. Cardiovascular and cerebrovascular comorbidities of hypokalemic and normokalemic primary aldosteronism: results of the German Conn's registry. J Clin Endocrinol Metab 2009;94:1125–30.
48. Mulatero P, Monticone S, Bertello C, et al. Long-term cardio- and cerebrovascular events in patients with primary aldosteronism. J Clin Endocrinol Metab 2013;98: 4826–33.
49. Savard S, Amar L, Plouin PF, et al. Cardiovascular complications associated with primary aldosteronism: a controlled cross-sectional study. Hypertension 2013;62: 331–6.
50. Fallo F, Pilon C, Urbanet R. Aldosterone and metabolic syndrome. Horm Metab Res 2012;44:208–14.

51. Fischer E, Adolf C, Pallouf A, et al. Aldosterone excess impairs first phase insulin secretion in primary aldosteronism. J Clin Endocrinol Metab 2013;98:2513–20.
52. Rossi GP, Belfiore A, Bernini G, et al. Body mass index predicts plasma aldosterone concentrations in overweight-obese primary hypertensive patients. J Clin Endocrinol Metab 2008;93:2566–71.
53. Reincke M, Meisinger C, Holle R, et al. Is primary aldosteronism associated with diabetes mellitus? Results of the German Conn's registry. Horm Metab Res 2010; 42:435–9.
54. Sim JJ, Yan EH, Liu IL, et al. Positive relationship of sleep apnea to hyperaldosteronism in an ethnically diverse population. J Hypertens 2011;29:1553–9.
55. Rossi GP, Bernini G, Desideri G, et al. Renal damage in primary aldosteronism: results of the PAPY study. Hypertension 2006;48:232–8.
56. Novello M, Catena C, Nadalini E, et al. Renal cysts and hypokalemia in primary aldosteronism: results of long-term follow-up after treatment. J Hypertens 2007; 25:1443–50.
57. Reincke M, Rump LC, Quinkler M, et al. Participants of German Conn's Registry. Risk factors associated with a low glomerular filtration rate in primary aldosteronism. J Clin Endocrinol Metab 2009;94:869–75.
58. Fourkiotis VG, Hanslik G, Hanusch F, et al. Aldosterone and the kidney. Horm Metab Res 2012;44(3):194–201.
59. Apostolopoulou K, Kunzel HE, Gerum S, et al. Gender differences in anxiety and depressive symptoms in patients with primary aldosteronism: a cross-sectional study. World J Biol Psychiatry 2012;15(1):26–35.
60. Salcuni AS, Palmieri S, Carnevale V, et al. Bone involvement in aldosteronism. J Bone Miner Res 2012;27:2217–22.
61. Funder JW, Carey RM, Fardella C, et al. Case detection, diagnosis, and treatment of patients with primary aldosteronism: an endocrine society clinical practice guideline. J Clin Endocrinol Metab 2008;93:3266–81.
62. Stowasser M. Primary aldosteronism: revival of a syndrome. J Hypertens 2000; 19:363–6.
63. Gordon RD, Stowasser M, Rutherford JC. Primary aldosteronism: are we diagnosing and operating on too few patients? World J Surg 2001;25:941–7.
64. Stowasser M, Gordon RD, Gunasekera TG, et al. High rate of detection of primary aldosteronism, including surgically treatable forms, after 'non-selective' screening of hypertensive patients. J Hypertens 2003;21:2149–57.
65. Gordon RD. The challenge of a more robust and reproducible methodology in screening for primary aldosteronism. J Hypertens 2004;22:251–5.
66. Stowasser M, Ahmed AH, Pimenta E, et al. Factors affecting the aldosterone/renin ratio. Horm Metab Res 2012;44:170–6.
67. Doi SA, Abalkhail S, Al-Qudhaiby MM, et al. Optimal use and interpretation of the aldosterone renin ratio to detect aldosterone excess in hypertension. J Hum Hypertens 2006;20:482–9.
68. Mulatero P, Rabbia F, Milan A, et al. Drug effects on aldosterone/plasma renin activity ratio in primary aldosteronism. Hypertension 2002;4:597–907.
69. Betz MJ, Degenhart C, Fischer E, et al. Adrenal vein sampling using rapid cortisol assays in primary aldosteronism is useful in centers with low success rates. Eur J Endocrinol 2011;165:301–6.
70. Rossi E, Regolisti G, Perazzoli F, et al. Intraprocedural cortisol measurement increased adrenal vein sampling success rate in primary aldosteronism. Am J Hypertens 2011;24:1280–5.

71. Stowasser M, Gordon RD, Rutherford JC, et al. Diagnosis and management of primary aldosteronism. J Renin Angiotensin Aldosterone Syst 2001;2:156–69.

72. Onozawa S, Murata S, Tajima H, et al. Evaluation of right adrenal vein cannulation by computed tomography angiography in 140 consecutive patients undergoing adrenal venous sampling. Eur J Endocrinol 2014;170:601–8.

73. Young WF, Stanson AW, Thompson GB, et al. Role for adrenal venous sampling in primary aldosteronism. Surgery 2004;136:1227–35.

74. Fujimoto K, Honjo S, Tatsuoka H, et al. Primary aldosteronism associated with subclinical Cushing syndrome. J Endocrinol Invest 2013;36:564–7.

75. Dekkers T, Deinum J, Schultzekool LJ, et al. Plasma metanephrine for assessing the selectivity of adrenal venous sampling. Hypertension 2013;62:1152–7.

76. Baba Y, Hayashi S, Nakajo M. Are catecholamine-derived indexes in adrenal venous sampling useful for judging selectivity and laterality in patients with primary aldosteronism? Endocrine 2013;43:611–7.

77. Lim V, Guo Q, Grant CS, et al. Accuracy of adrenal imaging and adrenal venous sampling in predicting surgical cure of primary aldosteronism. J Clin Endocrinol Metab 2014;99:2712.

78. Nwariaku FE, Miller BS, Auchus R, et al. Primary hyperaldosteronism: effect of adrenal vein sampling on surgical outcome. Arch Surg 2006;141:497–503.

79. Küpers EM, Amar L, Raynaud A, et al. A clinical prediction score to diagnose unilateral primary aldosteronism. J Clin Endocrinol Metab 2012;97:3530–7.

80. Reister A, Fischer E, Degenhart C, et al. Age below 40 or a recently proposed clinical prediction score cannot bypass adrenal vein sampling in primary aldosteronism. J Clin Endocrinol Metab 2014;90(6):E1035–9.

81. Candy SW, Soh LM, Lau JH, et al. Diagnosing unilateral primary aldosteronism - comparison of a clinical prediction score, computed tomography and adrenal venous sampling. Clin Endocrinol (Oxf) 2013;81:25–30.

82. Sywak M, Pasieka JL. Long-term follow-up and cost benefit of adrenalectomy in patients with primary aldosteronism. Br J Surg 2002;89:1587–93.

83. Letavernier E, Peyrard S, Amar L, et al. Blood pressure outcome of adrenalectomy in patients with primary hyperaldosteronism with or without unilateral adenoma. J Hypertens 2008;26:1816–23.

84. Meyer A, Brabant G, Behrend M. Long-term follow-up after adrenalectomy for primary aldosteronism. World J Surg 2005;29:155–9.

85. Catena C, Colussi G, Di Fabio A, et al. Mineralocorticoid antagonists treatment versus surgery in primary aldosteronism. Horm Metab Res 2010;42:440–5.

86. Wang W, Hu W, Zhang X, et al. Predictors of successful outcome after adrenalectomy for primary aldosteronism. Int Surg 2012;97:104–11.

87. Ghose RP, Hall PM, Bravo EL. Medical management of aldosterone-producing adenomas. Ann Intern Med 1999;131:105–8.

88. De Gasparo M, Joss U, Ramjoué HP, et al. Three new epoxy-spirolactone derivatives: characterization in vivo and in vitro. J Pharmacol Exp Ther 1987;240:650–6.

89. Parthasarathy HK, Ménard J, White WB, et al. A double-blind, randomized study comparing the antihypertensive effect of eplerenone and spironolactone in patients with hypertension and evidence of primary aldosteronism. J Hypertens 2011;29:980–90.

90. Lim PO, Young WF, MacDonald TM. A review of the medical treatment of primary aldosteronism. J Hypertens 2001;19:353–61.

91. Amar L, Azizi M, Menard J, et al. Sequential comparison of aldosterone synthase inhibition and mineralocorticoid blockade in patients with primary aldosteronism. J Hypertens 2013;31:624–9.

92. Bernini G, Bacca A, Carli V, et al. Cardiovascular changes in patients with primary aldosteronism after surgical or medical treatment. J Endocrinol Invest 2012;35: 274–80.
93. Reincke M, Fischer E, Gerum S, et al. Observational study mortality in treated primary aldosteronism: the German Conn's registry. Hypertension 2012;60:618–24.
94. Mulatero P, Monticone S, Bertello C, et al. Confirmatory tests in the diagnosis of primary aldosteronism. Horm Metab Res 2010;42:406–10.
95. Ahmed AH, Cowley D, Wolley M, et al. Seated saline suppression testing for the diagnosis of primary aldosteronism: a preliminary study. J Clin Endocrinol Metab 2014;99:2745–53.
96. Westerdahl C, Bergenfelz A, Isaksson A, et al. Captopril suppression: limitations for confirmation of primary aldosteronism. J Renin Angiotensin Aldosterone Syst 2001;2:156–69.
97. Gouli A, Kaltsas G, Tzonou A, et al. High prevalence of autonomous aldosterone secretion among patients with essential hypertension. Eur J Clin Invest 2011;41: 1227–36.

Adrenal Mild Hypercortisolism

Gillian M. Goddard, MD[a,b], Aarti Ravikumar, MD[a], Alice C. Levine, MD[a,*]

KEYWORDS

- Adrenal • Adrenal incidentaloma • Mild hypercortisolism
- Subclinical Cushing syndrome • Cushing syndrome • Cortisol

KEY POINTS

- Mild hypercortisolism is also known as subclinical Cushing syndrome, and is usually caused by benign adrenal adenomas.
- The definition of mild hypercortisolism is debatable, but the most sensitive diagnostic test is failure of suppression of AM cortisol after low-dose dexamethasone suppression test (LDDST).
- Using an AM cortisol level of less than 1.8 µg/dL after LDDST gives high sensitivity but low specificity compared with using an AM cortisol level of less than 5 µg/dL after LDDST, which gives a lower sensitivity but a higher specificity.
- Mild hypercortisolism has been associated with the same comorbidities as overt Cushing syndrome: metabolic syndrome, osteoporosis, increased risk of cardiovascular events, and increased mortality. However, causality has not been demonstrated.
- Treatment options include surgical resection of the affected adrenal gland and medical therapies.

INTRODUCTION

Adrenal incidentalomas (AIs) are becoming increasingly common as more abdominal imaging is performed. Most of these lesions are benign and cortical in origin. The most common secretory syndrome associated with these adrenal adenomas is that of mild hypercortisolism, also known as subclinical Cushing syndrome (SCS). This syndrome is a rapidly changing and controversial subject with no consensus regarding the diagnostic criteria and management recommendations. However, recent reports are beginning to shed light on the prevalence, associated comorbidities, and newer treatment options for adrenal hypercortisolism.

Disclosure: The authors have nothing to disclose.
[a] The Hilda and J. Lester Gabrilove Division of Endocrinology, Diabetes and Bone Diseases, Department of Internal Medicine, Icahn School of Medicine at Mount Sinai, One Gustave L. Levy Place, Box 1055, New York, NY 10029-6574, USA; [b] Lennox Hill Hospital, North Shore-LIJ Health System, New York, NY 10075, USA
* Corresponding author.
E-mail address: alice.levine@mountsinai.org

IS SUBCLINICAL CUSHING SYNDROME REALLY SUBCLINICAL?

Since its conceptualization, mild hypercortisolism has been referred to as SCS because classic signs and symptoms of Cushing syndrome, including moon facies, striae, increased dorsocervical and supraclavicular fat pads, and proximal muscle wasting, are absent. In addition, although there may be mild derangements in cortisol production, urinary free cortisol levels 2 to 3 times the upper limit of normal and grossly abnormal midnight salivary cortisol levels are typically absent. The traditional thinking was that these low levels of excess cortisol were not associated with any comorbidities.[1,2]

However, SCS has been shown to be associated with increased insulin resistance and changes in body composition in women.[3] Most recently, 3 studies found an increased risk of cardiovascular disease and mortality in patients with SCS.[4–6]

Given the clinical implications of having even modest increases of cortisol level, we argue this is not a subclinical disease, and that it would best be termed mild hypercortisolism.

FREQUENCY OF INCIDENTALOMAS AND MILD HYPERCORTISOLISM

AIs are estimated to be present in approximately 7% of the population.[7] With an increase in abdominal imaging, the reported prevalence is higher and the incidence increases with advancing age. The probability of detecting an AI in patients between the ages of 20 and 29 years is approximately 0.2%, as opposed to approximately 7% in a patient more than 70 years of age.[8,9] Previously Cushing syndrome was estimated to be present in 4% to 5% of patients with AIs.[7] However, in studies that also include patients with mild hypercortisolism, the incidence is reported to be closer to 30%.[5]

DEFINING MILD HYPERCORTISOLISM

Laboratory testing should be performed in patients with known adrenal disorders with or without evidence of clinical signs and symptoms of excess cortisol.[1,7] Particular attention should be paid to those patients with associated comorbidities, including resistant hypertension, obesity, impaired glucose tolerance, and lipid derangements.[1]

Much of the variability in the reported frequency of mild hypercortisolism among patients with adrenal adenomas can be attributed to differences in the biochemical definition of this disease. There is controversy over which laboratory cutoffs should be used. As with classic Cushing syndrome, a combination of simple laboratory testing and dynamic testing is helpful.

The most sensitive test for the detection of mild hypercortisolism from adrenal nodules is the 1-mg overnight, low-dose dexamethasone suppression test (LDDST).[10] Historically, a morning serum cortisol of more than 5 µg/dL (>138 nmol/L) after 1 mg of dexamethasone was considered diagnostic of the disorder,[1] which is not intuitive given that in classic Cushing syndrome a morning serum cortisol level of greater than 1.8 µg/dL (>50 nmol/L) after LDDST is considered diagnostic. The discrepancy arises because, in the case of symptomatic Cushing syndrome, the clinician's index of suspicion is high and there is a high pretest probability of disease so therefore the likelihood of a false-positive test is reduced. In contrast, in patients with mild hypercortisolism, symptoms are subtle so the clinician's index of suspicion is lower and therefore a test with greater specificity is preferable, despite the loss of sensitivity. In addition, until recently, there were few treatment options other than surgical adrenalectomy for hypercortisolism caused by adrenal adenomas.

At present, the definition of a positive LDDST to confirm mild hypercortisolism is not consistent in the literature. Many investigators use a morning serum cortisol level of greater than 5 μg/dL after LDDST, which has a low sensitivity (44%–58%) but a high specificity (83%–100%). In contrast, some reports use a lower AM cortisol value after LDDST (cortisol level >1.8 μg/dL). This definition results in a higher sensitivity (75%–100%) but a lower specificity (67%–72%) (**Fig. 1**).[1] There is a risk of having false-positive values when using the cutoff of 1.8 μg/dL and the potential for overdiagnosis.[11] Other values, including a morning cortisol level of greater than 2.2 μg/dL or greater than 3.0 μg/dL after LDDST, have been advocated as offering the best balance of sensitivity and specificity when evaluating patients with AI for mild hypercortisolism.[1]

Increased urinary free cortisol (UFC) level from a 24-hour urine collection may support the diagnosis. Mild increases of up to 2 times the upper limit of normal are often seen. However, patients with mild hypercortisolism often have normal UFC levels.[2]

The use of midnight salivary cortisol (MSC) has been explored in the diagnosis of mild hypercortisolism, but its utility seems limited. One study compared the MSC concentrations of patients with adrenal adenomas and known mild hypercortisolism with MSC concentrations from patients with adrenal adenomas and no evidence of excess cortisol secretion. MSC concentrations in the two groups were identical.[12] Other similar studies have replicated this outcome.[13] As with UFC, mild increases of MSC level support the diagnosis of mild hypercortisolism, but a normal MSC level does not rule out the disease.

Most published reports define mild hypercortisolism as a disease of the adrenal glands resulting from benign-appearing incidentalomas.[1] However, it is important to confirm this cause biochemically. Once hypercortisolism is established, a morning adrenocorticotropic hormone (ACTH) level that is suppressed (<10 ng/mL) confirms ACTH-independent hypercortisolism caused by an adrenal disorder. However, in mild hypercortisolism the degree of excess cortisol production may not be sufficient to entirely suppress the hypothalamus-pituitary-adrenal (HPA) axis and a low-normal morning ACTH level may be seen. In those cases, it is important to check the morning ACTH level after LDDST. If the ACTH level is not suppressed in the setting of an increased dexamethasone level, other causes, such as pituitary or ectopic ACTH overproduction, should be considered.[14]

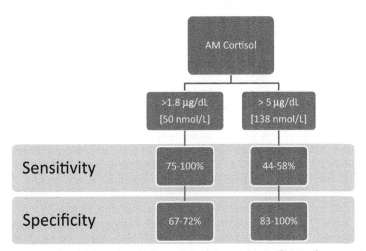

Fig. 1. Diagnosis of mild hypercortisolism. Sensitivity and specificity of AM cortisol after LDDST for diagnosing mild hypercortisolism. (*Data from* Chiodini I. Diagnosis and treatment of subclinical hypercortisolism. J Clin Endocrinol Metab 2011;96(5):1223–36.)

Other supportive laboratory testing may include dehydroepiandrosterone (DHEA)/sulfated DHEA (DHEAS) levels, which are often low in the setting of autonomous adrenal cortisol secretion; however, in older patients, nonspecific decreases in DHEA/DHEAS levels are also detected.[15]

MILD HYPERCORTISOLISM: ASSOCIATED COMORBIDITIES

Recent reports have established that the comorbidities associated with mild hypercortisolism are similar to those reported in patients with overt Cushing syndrome: the metabolic syndrome, osteoporosis, increased cardiovascular disease, and increased mortality.

METABOLIC SYNDROME

In 2002, Terzolo and colleagues[16] studied patients with AIs and SCS, defined as at least 2 of following criteria: increased UFC level, cortisol level greater than 5 μg/dL after LDDST, suppressed ACTH level, or disturbed cortisol circadian rhythm. Twelve patients met these criteria and were compared with controls (euthyroid patients with multinodular goiter). The controls were age, sex, and body mass index (BMI) matched. A 120-minute, 75-g oral glucose tolerance test was done for both groups. The fasting plasma glucose and insulin levels were similar in the two groups. However, glucose levels were higher and insulin sensitivity lower in the patients with SCS at 60, 90, and 120 minutes after ingestion of 75 g of glucose. Fasting triglyceride levels were higher in the SCS group, which is an indirect measure of insulin resistance. Given that the two groups were BMI matched, the investigators concluded that the observed insulin resistance in the SCS group was likely caused by excess cortisol.[16]

OSTEOPOROSIS

The risk of osteoporosis caused by mild hypercortisolism has also been reported. Chiodini and colleagues[17] published an article in 2009 that concerned a multicenter, retrospective study done in Italy evaluating the bone mineral density (BMD), prevalence of vertebral fractures, and bone quality in patients with AIs with and without subclinical hypercortisolism (SH). SH was defined as 2 out of 3 of UFC level greater than 70 μg/24 h, cortisol level greater than 3 μg/dL after LDDST, and ACTH level less than 10 pg/mL. The primary end point measured was the spinal deformity index (SDI), in which the number and severity of vertebral fractures are integrated; the SDI has been suggested to be associated with vertebral fracture risk over time. Of the 287 patients with AIs, SH was present (SH+) in 85 patients and absent (SH−) in 202 patients. All of the patients with AI (287) were age, BMI, and gender matched to 194 controls without AI. The study showed that the patients with AIs (SH+) had lower BMD at the lumbar spine (trabecular bone) and femoral neck (cortical bone), more metabolic syndrome, and increased SDI compared with both those with AI (SH-) and controls. The odds radio (OR) for vertebral fractures was 7.27 (P = .0001; confidence interval, 3.94 to >13.41) for patients who were SH+ regardless of age, BMD, menopause, and gender.[17]

In 2011, the same group conducted a multicenter, prospective, longitudinal study evaluating SDI and vertebral fractures at baseline and after 12 and 24 months in patients who were SH+ and SH− with AIs.[18] The definition was the same as in the retrospective analysis. In the prospective study, Morelli and colleagues reported that the prevalences of fractures and SDI were higher in the SH+ group regardless of age, sex, BMI, BMD, and menopausal status. Also, those who were SH+ had a higher risk of vertebral fractures than those who were SH− (OR, 12.264; P = .001).

CARDIOVASCULAR DISEASE

SH has long been reported to be associated with an increased risk of cardiovascular disease. Recently, several studies reaffirmed this association and further implied that even mild degrees of hypercortisolism are deleterious to overall cardiovascular health. Di Dalmazi and colleagues[5] performed a retrospective analysis of 198 outpatients with AIs over 15 years. They categorized the patients with AI as stable nonsecreting (cortisol level <1.8 μg/dL after LDDST; n = 114), stable intermediate (cortisol level 1.8–5 μg/dL after LDDST), or subclinical Cushing (cortisol level >5 μg/dL after LDDST; n = 61). In addition, 23 patients had a demonstrated worsening of their hypercortisolism during the course of the study, and moved from the nonsecreting to intermediate or intermediate to subclinical Cushing groups. The reported incidence of cardiovascular events was higher in patients with the stable intermediate or subclinical Cushing patterns (16.7%; $P = .04$) and also in those patients with worsened secreting patterns (28.4%; $P = .02$) compared with those with stable nonsecreting adenomas (6.7%). Survival rates for all-cause mortality were lower in adenomas with stable intermediate and subclinical Cushing secreting patterns compared with nonsecreting patterns (57% vs 91.2%; $P = .005$).

More recently, Androulakis and colleagues[6] published a case-control study evaluating cardiovascular risk in patients with apparently nonfunctioning AIs and no known cardiovascular risk factors (ie, hypertension, hyperlipidemia, or diabetes). Sixty patients were subdivided into those with cortisol-secreting AIs (CSAIs) and nonfunctioning AIs (NFAIs). Both groups were compared with 32 healthy controls with normal adrenal imaging. The definition of CSAIAI was an AM cortisol level +2 standard deviations greater than the control group after LDDST, which translated to a cortisol level greater than 1.09 μg/dL; a value that is lower than previously suggested cutoffs even in patients with overt Cushing syndrome. Twenty-four patients had CSAI and 34 had NFAI using this definition. The study measured intimal media thickness (IMT) and flow-mediated vasodilatation (FMD); 2 measures that are associated with atherosclerosis and cardiovascular risk. The IMT was greater and FMD less in the subjects with cortisol-secreting adenomas compared with the subjects with NFAIs. In a previous report, even patients with nonfunctioning AIs (defined as cortisol level <1.8 μg/dL after LDDST) also had less FMD compared with age-matched, sex-matched, BMI-matched subjects and cardiometabolic controls.[19]

A very recent study by Debono and colleagues[20] also confirmed this association. In a retrospective study of 206 patients, all with adrenal adenomas, patients were categorized as having cortisol concentrations greater than 1.8 μg/dL after 1-mg LDDST or having cortisol concentrations less than 1.8 μg/dL after 1-mg LDDST. Increase in cortisol concentration after LDDST was associated with decreased survival. Fifty percent of the deaths in the group were from cardiovascular causes.

TREATMENT OF MILD HYPERCORTISOLISM
Surgery

The usual treatment of adrenal Cushing syndrome is unilateral adrenalectomy to remove the gland that contains the hyperfunctioning adrenal nodule. There have been several studies assessing the effectiveness of unilateral adrenalectomy in patients with mild hypercortisolism. One such retrospective, longitudinal study evaluated 108 subjects, all with AIs, of whom 55 underwent unilateral adrenalectomy and 53 did not undergo surgery. Metabolic improvements after surgery were seen in those patients with 2 or more of the following preoperatively: UFC level greater than

70 μg/24 hours, ACTH level less than 10 pg/mL, or cortisol level greater than 3.0 μg/dL (83 nmol/L) after LDDST (sensitivity, 65%; specificity, 69%).[21]

However, the patients who did not meet criteria for mild hypercortisolism but who had surgery for other indications (eg, suspicious appearance of adenoma on imaging) also had evidence of improvement in metabolic parameters. These data imply that the so-called nonsecretory adenomas may have had very mild hypercortisolism that might have been detected using a more sensitive cutoff, such as cortisol level greater than 1.8 μg/dL after LDDST. Alternatively, there may be other, as-yet undetermined factors secreted by adrenal cortical adenomas that contribute to features of the metabolic syndrome.

A review of the surgical literature assessed 10 studies with a total of 101 patients meeting the criteria for mild hypercortisolism. The definition of mild hypercortisolism varied between studies, ranging from cortisol levels greater than 1 μg/dL to cortisol levels greater than 5 μg/dL after LDDST. Outcomes, including improvements in blood pressure, body weight, and fasting glucose level, were mixed. Only 1 of the 10 studies assessed possible improvements in bone health and showed no significant improvement in bone density after unilateral adrenalectomy.[1]

A prospective randomized controlled trial was performed over 15 years assigning patients with AIs to either conservative management or surgical resection with laparoscopic adrenalectomy.[22] Conservative management was performed by 2 experienced endocrinologists who monitored and treated the patients for diabetes mellitus, hypertension, hyperlipidemia, obesity, and osteoporosis if necessary. No medical therapy was given that specifically targeted the hypercortisolism in either group. Forty-five patients enrolled: 23 underwent surgery and 22 were treated conservatively. The diagnosis of SCS was made by 2 HPA axis alterations, of which 1 had to be failure to suppress on LDDST, with cutoff of morning serum cortisol level greater than 2.5 μg/dL and no signs of Cushing syndrome on physical examination. Mean follow-up was 7.7 years (2–17 years). Surgery proved beneficial for patients with mild hypercortisolism that was accompanied by any of the following: diabetes (5 of 8 normalized or improved; 62.5%), arterial hypertension (12 of 18 normalized or improved; 67%), and central obesity (3 of 6 normalized; 50%). However, the only statistically significant improvement in metabolic parameters was improvement in blood pressure ($P = .046$).

Medical Treatment of Mild Hypercortisolism

Historically, medical treatment options for Cushing syndrome have been limited, both in the number of options available and in their efficacy. Ketoconazole has been used for many years, although it does not have an US Food and Drug Administration (FDA)–approved indication for the treatment of Cushing syndrome. More recently, mifepristone, a glucocorticoid receptor antagonist, was approved for the treatment of hyperglycemia caused by Cushing syndrome. More medical options are under active investigation (**Fig. 2**).

Mifepristone acts as a potent glucocorticoid receptor blocker. It does not lower cortisol levels and may cause an increase in serum cortisol measurements. To determine efficacy, surrogate markers of cortisol action, such as improvement in insulin sensitivity, must be followed. Side effects include nausea, fatigue, and muscle aches.[23] Rarely, adrenal insufficiency can occur because of excessive glucocorticoid receptor blockade. In addition, patients may experience hypertension and hypokalemia caused by cortisol activity at the mineralocorticoid receptor, which is not blocked by mifepristone.

Mifepristone has been used in the only study of medical treatment of mild hypercortisolism. Debono and colleagues[24] conducted a pilot study of mifepristone in

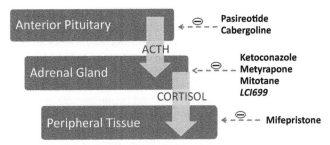

Fig. 2. Medical treatment of Cushing syndrome. The medical therapies that are available and where they inhibit cortisol synthesis or action.

6 patients, all with mild hypercortisolism (defined as a serum cortisol level >1.8 μg/dL after both a 1-mg overnight and 2-mg 48-hour dexamethasone suppression test) and normal glucose parameters. After 4 weeks of treatment with mifepristone, insulin sensitivity measured by HOMA-IR (The homeostatic model assessment [HOMA] is a method used to quantify insulin resistance [IR]), Matsuda index, and insulin area under the curve all improved, as did fasting insulin levels. Fasting glucose levels were not improved but were not noted to be increased at baseline.

Ketoconazole, an antifungal agent, has been the most widely prescribed medication for Cushing syndrome. The medication has not been FDA approved for this indication and the FDA recently issued a safety warning about the use of ketoconazole for the treatment of fungal infection and the risk of liver toxicity. As of this publication, ketoconazole is still available.

Metyrapone, an 11β-hydroxylase inhibitor, has long been used in Europe for the treatment of Cushing syndrome. It is not easily available in the United States. Another, more potent 11β-hydroxylase inhibitor under investigation is LCI699 (Novartis).[25,26] Both of these medications block the conversion of 11-deoxycortisol to cortisol, thus lowering serum concentrations of cortisol. The inhibition of cortisol synthesis leads to a buildup of steroid precursors that are shunted into other steroid synthesis pathways, potentially resulting in undesirable, androgenic side effects such as hirsutism in women. Recent proof-of-concept studies of LCI699 have been promising but the compound is not yet commercially available. Pasireotide, a selective somatostatin analogue, binds and activates somatostatin receptors SSTR2 and SSTR5, and acts at the level of the pituitary to decrease the secretion of ACTH in Cushing disease.[27] However, this is not an effective treatment of adrenal Cushing syndrome.

The chemotherapeutic agent mitotane is cytotoxic to adrenal cortical tissue. It is currently FDA approved for the treatment of adrenal cortical carcinoma. Mitotane often renders patients adrenally insufficient and has neurologic side effects. Therefore, this medication is typically reserved only for patients with adrenocortical carcinoma.

To date there is little evidence for or against the use of medical therapies for the treatment of mild hypercortisolism caused by adrenal adenomas. Future studies may help determine which medications are most effective and which patients may benefit most from surgical intervention.

SUMMARY

AIs are becoming increasingly common and nearly one-third may be producing low levels of excess cortisol. The definition of mild hypercortisolism is much debated. Using a cortisol cutoff of greater than 1.8 μg/dL after LDDST results in a higher sensitivity (90%) but with a trade-off of lower specificity (70%). Recent studies have shown an association between mild hypercortisolism and the metabolic syndrome, cardiovascular disease, osteoporosis, and increased mortality. These association studies make a compelling argument that any degree of hypercortisolism, over time, is deleterious to bone, metabolic health, and cardiovascular health. However, these studies have not established causality. There are surgical and medical options, including mifepristone and ketoconazole, available to treat mild hypercortisolism caused by adrenal adenomas. Additional further medical therapies are being evaluated.

The data regarding the efficacy of various treatments in patients with only mild degrees of hypercortisolism are sparse. In addition, most of the previous reports use varying definitions of the disorder, further complicating the interpretation of the data. Prospective studies are sorely needed in order to better define the disorder and determine whether medical or surgical therapy should be considered in patients with adrenal adenomas and mild hypercortisolism.

REFERENCES

1. Chiodini I. Clinical review: diagnosis and treatment of subclinical hypercortisolism. J Clin Endocrinol Metab 2011;96(5):1223–36.
2. De Leo M, Cozzolino A, Colao A, et al. Subclinical Cushing's syndrome. Best Pract Res Clin Endocrinol Metab 2012;26(4):497–505.
3. Garrapa GG, Pantanetti P, Arnaldi G, et al. Body composition and metabolic features in women with adrenal incidentaloma or Cushing's syndrome. J Clin Endocrinol Metab 2001;86(11):5301–6.
4. Morelli V, Reimondo G, Giordano R, et al. Long-term follow-up in adrenal incidentalomas: an Italian multicenter study. J Clin Endocrinol Metab 2014;99(3):827–34.
5. Di Dalmazi G, Vicennati V, Garelli S, et al. Cardiovascular events and mortality in patients with adrenal incidentalomas that are either non-secreting or associated with intermediate phenotype or subclinical Cushing's syndrome: a 15-year retrospective study. Lancet Diabetes Endocrinol 2014;2(5):396–405.
6. Androulakis II, Kaltsas GA, Kollias GE, et al. Patients with apparently nonfunctioning adrenal incidentalomas may be at increased cardiovascular risk due to excessive cortisol secretion. J Clin Endocrinol Metab 2014;99(8):2754–62.
7. Young WF Jr. Clinical practice. The incidentally discovered adrenal mass. N Engl J Med 2007;356(6):601–10.
8. Young WF Jr. Management approaches to adrenal incidentalomas. A view from Rochester, Minnesota. Endocrinol Metab Clin North Am 2000;29(1):159–85, x.
9. Kloos RT, Gross MD, Francis IR, et al. Incidentally discovered adrenal masses. Endocr Rev 1995;16(4):460–84.
10. Morelli V, Masserini B, Salcuni AS, et al. Subclinical hypercortisolism: correlation between biochemical diagnostic criteria and clinical aspects. Clin Endocrinol (Oxf) 2010;73(2):161–6.
11. Stewart PM. Is subclinical Cushing's syndrome an entity or a statistical fallout from diagnostic testing? Consensus surrounding the diagnosis is required before optimal treatment can be defined. J Clin Endocrinol Metab 2010;95(6):2618–20.
12. Masserini B, Morelli V, Bergamaschi S, et al. The limited role of midnight salivary cortisol levels in the diagnosis of subclinical hypercortisolism in patients with adrenal incidentaloma. Eur J Endocrinol 2009;160(1):87–92.
13. Ceccato F, Barbot M, Zilio M, et al. Performance of salivary cortisol in the diagnosis of Cushing's syndrome, adrenal incidentaloma, and adrenal insufficiency. Eur J Endocrinol 2013;169(1):31–6.

14. Newell-Price J, Trainer P, Besser M, et al. The diagnosis and differential diagnosis of Cushing's syndrome and pseudo-Cushing's states. Endocr Rev 1998;19(5):647–72.
15. Rossi R, Tauchmanova L, Luciano A, et al. Subclinical Cushing's syndrome in patients with adrenal incidentaloma: clinical and biochemical features. J Clin Endocrinol Metab 2000;85(4):1440–8.
16. Terzolo M, Pia A, Ali A, et al. Adrenal incidentaloma: a new cause of the metabolic syndrome? J Clin Endocrinol Metab 2002;87(3):998–1003.
17. Chiodini I, Morelli V, Masserini B, et al. Bone mineral density, prevalence of vertebral fractures, and bone quality in patients with adrenal incidentalomas with and without subclinical hypercortisolism: an Italian multicenter study. J Clin Endocrinol Metab 2009;94(9):3207–14.
18. Morelli V, Eller-Vainicher C, Salcuni AS, et al. Risk of new vertebral fractures in patients with adrenal incidentaloma with and without subclinical hypercortisolism: a multicenter longitudinal study. J Bone Miner Res 2011;26(8):1816–21.
19. Erbil Y, Ozbey N, Barbaros U, et al. Cardiovascular risk in patients with nonfunctional adrenal incidentaloma: myth or reality? World J Surg 2009;33(10):2099–105.
20. Debono M, Bradburn M, Bull M, et al. Cortisol as a marker for increased mortality in patients with incidental adrenocortical adenomas. J Clin Endocrinol Metab 2014;99(12):4462–70.
21. Eller-Vainicher C, Morelli V, Salcuni AS, et al. Accuracy of several parameters of hypothalamic-pituitary-adrenal axis activity in predicting before surgery the metabolic effects of the removal of an adrenal incidentaloma. Eur J Endocrinol 2010;163(6):925–35.
22. Toniato A, Merante-Boschin I, Opocher G, et al. Surgical versus conservative management for subclinical Cushing syndrome in adrenal incidentalomas: a prospective randomized study. Ann Surg 2009;249(3):388–91.
23. Fleseriu M, Biller BM, Findling JW, et al. Mifepristone, a glucocorticoid receptor antagonist, produces clinical and metabolic benefits in patients with Cushing's syndrome. J Clin Endocrinol Metab 2012;97(6):2039–49.
24. Debono M, Chadarevian R, Eastell R, et al. Mifepristone reduces insulin resistance in patient volunteers with adrenal incidentalomas that secrete low levels of cortisol: a pilot study. PLoS One 2013;8(4):e60984.
25. Trainer PJ. Next generation medical therapy for Cushing's syndrome–can we measure a benefit? J Clin Endocrinol Metab 2014;99(4):1157–60.
26. Bertagna X, Pivonello R, Fleseriu M, et al. LCI699, a potent 11beta-hydroxylase inhibitor, normalizes urinary cortisol in patients with Cushing's disease: results from a multicenter, proof-of-concept study. J Clin Endocrinol Metab 2014;99(4):1375–83.
27. Colao A, Petersenn S, Newell-Price J, et al. A 12-month phase 3 study of pasireotide in Cushing's disease. N Engl J Med 2012;366(10):914–24.

Management of Adrenal Tumors in Pregnancy

Deirdre Cocks Eschler, MD[a],*, Nina Kogekar, BA[b], Rachel Pessah-Pollack, MD, FACE[c,d]

KEYWORDS

- Pregnancy • Cushing syndrome • Adrenal cell carcinoma • Adrenal tumor
- Pheochromocytoma • Hyperaldosteronism

KEY POINTS

- Adrenal diseases including Cushing syndrome (CS), primary aldosteronism (PA), pheochromocytoma, and adrenocortical carcinoma are uncommon in pregnancy; a high degree of clinical suspicion must exist.
- Physiologic changes to the hypothalamus-pituitary-adrenal axis in a normal pregnancy result in increased cortisol, renin, and aldosterone levels, thus making the diagnosis of CS and PA in pregnancy challenging. However, catecholamines are not altered in pregnancy and allow a laboratory diagnosis of pheochromocytoma that is similar to that of the nonpregnant state.
- Although adrenal tumors in pregnancy result in significant maternal and fetal morbidity, and sometimes mortality, early diagnosis and appropriate treatment often improve outcomes.

INTRODUCTION

Adrenal diseases, including Cushing syndrome (CS), primary aldosteronism (PA), pheochromocytoma, and adrenocortical carcinoma (ACC), are uncommon in pregnancy. Normal physiologic changes to the hypothalamus-pituitary-adrenal (HPA) axis during pregnancy result in a physiologic hypercortisol state and changes in the renin-aldosterone-angiotensin system (RAAS) result in increased renin and aldosterone production in healthy pregnant women. Normal pregnant women are able to overcome these hormonal changes without adverse consequences, but such changes pose a challenge to the diagnosis of a disease state in pregnancy. Undiagnosed CS,

Disclosure: The authors have nothing to disclose.
[a] Endocrinology Division, Department of Medicine, Stony Brook University School of Medicine, HSC T15-060, Stony Brook, NY 11794, USA; [b] Department of Medicine, Mount Sinai School of Medicine, 1 Gustave L Levy Place, New York, NY 10029, USA; [c] Endocrinology Division, Department of Medicine, Mount Sinai School of Medicine, 1 Gustave L Levy Place, New York, NY 10029, USA; [d] Department of Endocrinology, ProHealth Care Associates, Ohio Drive, Lake Success, NY 11042, USA
* Corresponding author. 26 Research Way, East Setauket, NY 11733.
E-mail address: Deirdre.cocks.eschler@gmail.com

Endocrinol Metab Clin N Am 44 (2015) 381–397
http://dx.doi.org/10.1016/j.ecl.2015.02.006
0889-8529/15/$ – see front matter © 2015 Elsevier Inc. All rights reserved.

endo.theclinics.com

PA, pheochromocytoma, and ACC contribute to significant maternal and fetal morbidity and mortality. This article reviews the normal changes to the HPA axis in pregnancy and describes the diagnosis and management of adrenal disease during pregnancy.

Changes to the Hypothalamus-Pituitary-Adrenal Axis in Pregnancy

Changes in the HPA axis and the RAAS in pregnancy result in an increase in activity of both systems. Although the size and weight of the adrenal gland remain similar to the nonpregnant state, the zona fasciculata, the mostly cortisol-producing zone of the adrenal gland, is reported to increase in pregnancy.[1,2]

Hypothalamic-pituitary-adrenal axis

In healthy women, total and free plasma cortisol, adrenocorticotropic hormone (ACTH), corticotropin-releasing hormone (CRH), cortisol binding globulin (CBG), and urinary free cortisol (UFC) all increase in pregnancy. Placental CRH is similar to hypothalamic CRH,[3] although it does not follow a circadian pattern.[4] Placental CRH stimulates the placenta to produce ACTH,[5] which in turn stimulates the maternal adrenal glands to produce cortisol. In addition, the maternal adrenal glands are more responsive to ACTH during pregnancy,[6] resulting in an increase in free serum cortisol levels and UFC.[3] Although much of placental ACTH production is autonomous[7] and fails to respond to the negative feedback of glucocorticoids,[8] maternal serum cortisol has a positive feedback on placental CRH, further increasing its levels.[9] Placental CRH may also stimulate the maternal pituitary to release ACTH.[10] Estrogen from the placenta also plays a role by stimulating the production of CBG from the liver, resulting in increased bound and total serum cortisol levels. Progesterone from the placenta may have an antiglucocorticoid effect that contributes to the increase in free cortisol as well, because it creates a state of relative glucocorticoid resistance.[11] In addition, there may be an altered set point for pituitary ACTH response to cortisol feedback, with tissues more refractory to cortisol (**Box 1**).[6,7]

Although the initial increase in CBG early in pregnancy produces a transient reduction in free cortisol level, maternal ACTH levels increase in response, resulting in a normal cortisol level early in pregnancy[3] and increasing cortisol levels at as early as 11 weeks gestation.[12] A progressive increase has been described in total and free plasma cortisol, CBG, and 24-hour UFC levels throughout each trimester with free cortisol levels increasing by 1.2-fold, 1.4-fold, and 1.6-fold, and with 24 hour UFC level increasing 1.7-fold, 2.4-fold, and 3.1-fold compared with a control group in the first, second, and third trimesters respectively.[13] Maternal serum CRH, derived mostly from the placenta, becomes detectable then steadily begins to increase starting in the middle of the second trimester, with a sharp upswing at the end of gestation.[14,15] ACTH values also increase throughout pregnancy beginning in the late first trimester and peaking during labor and delivery.[16,17] CRH and ACTH levels return to nonpregnant values within 24 hours of delivery.[18] At 2 to 3 months postpartum, plasma free cortisol and UFC levels return to baseline but CBG and total plasma cortisol levels remain increased.[13] Although cortisol levels increase throughout pregnancy, diurnal variations of cortisol remain in pregnancy, but with a higher evening nadir.[4,6,12]

Renin-angiotensin-aldosterone system

Maternal progesterone levels increase throughout gestation, mostly as a result of placental progesterone production.[19] Progesterone acts as an antagonist to the mineralocorticoid receptor, likely at the renal tubule level.[20] This process results in an increase in sodium secretion[20] and an increase in aldosterone production.[21] This

---

Box 1
HPA axis changes in a normal pregnancy

- Increase in zona fasciculata in adrenal gland[1,2]

- Increase in total and free cortisol and UFC

  o Starting about 11 weeks' gestation

  o Free cortisol levels by 1.2-fold, 1.4-fold, and 1.6-fold and 24-hour UFC by 1.7-fold, 2.4-fold, and 3.1-fold in the first, second, and third trimesters respectively[13]

- Increase in ACTH

  o Beginning in the late first trimester, peaking during labor and delivery[16,17]

- Increase in CRH

  o Mostly from placental production

  o Detectable then steadily increases in middle of the second trimester, with a sharp increase at the end of gestation[13,15]

- Increase in CBG[13]

- Increase in aldosterone

  o Levels increase steadily up to 3-fold to 8-fold then plateau in the third trimester[21–23]

- Increase in plasma renin activity

  o Approximately 4-fold by eighth week; 7-fold at term[23]

- Increase in deoxycorticosterone.[24,26,27]

CRH and ACTH levels return to nonpregnant values within 24 hours of delivery,[18] and, at 2 to 3 months postpartum, plasma free cortisol and UFC levels return to baseline but CBG and total plasma cortisol levels remain increased.[13]

---

increase in aldosterone parallels that of progesterone and increases steadily throughout pregnancy, plateauing in the third trimester.[21–23] Mean plasma aldosterone increases 3-fold to 8-fold during pregnancy[22,23] and urinary aldosterone also increases throughout pregnancy,[23] whereas mean urinary sodium and potassium secretion remains constant.[23] Plasma renin activity (PRA) also increases throughout pregnancy up to almost 4-fold by the eighth week of pregnancy and 7-fold at term compared with the nonpregnant state[23]; largely because of an increase in renin substrate (angiotensinogen), which increases steadily until the 20th week of gestation.[23]

There have been different proposed mechanisms for such an upregulation in RAAS. The increase in prostaglandin synthesis and arterial venous shunt of the placental unit cause a decrease in systemic vascular resistance which are thought to initiate an activation of RAAS.[23] Extrarenal production of renin by the ovaries and maternal decidua as well as stimulation of renal renin release directly by estrogen[24,25] likely contribute to the early increase in renin. The direct effect of estrogen and the estrogen-stimulated increase in CBG from the liver contribute to the increase in PRA, promoting increased angiotensin II levels and ultimately, increased aldosterone production from the adrenal glands.[2,23–25] Deoxycorticosterone (DOC), also a potent mineralocorticoid, has an extra-adrenal origin during pregnancy; it is produced from progesterone, with levels increasing significantly in pregnancy.[24,26,27]

Despite the normal physiologic increase in renin and aldosterone levels in pregnancy, healthy pregnant women remain normotensive and normokalemic, likely because of the antimineralocorticoid effect of progesterone and the decrease in systemic vascular resistance in pregnancy.[24]

Adrenal Adenomas in Pregnancy

Cushing syndrome in pregnancy

Incidence and epidemiology CS is 3 times more common in women than in men.[28,29] Abnormal menses and difficulty conceiving are often present in women with CS, and therefore it is rare for a woman with CS to become pregnant.[30] Egg quality may be affected in CS, in part because of hypogonadotropic hypogonadism and possibly because of direct effects of cortisol itself, because glucocorticoid receptors have been found on granulosa cells.[31] In one study, the ovaries of women with CS tended to be smaller, with a decrease in the number of primordial follicles, a reduction in all phases of follicular activity, and the presence of patchy fibrosis that was similar to the ovaries of postmenopausal women.[32]

The cause of CS varies in the pregnant and nonpregnant populations. During pregnancy, adrenal adenomas account for 40% to 60% of cases (as opposed to 15% in the nonpregnant state), pituitary adenomas account for 15% to 40% (vs >60% in the nonpregnant state),[33,34] and ACC accounts for less than 10% of cases of CS in pregnancy.[33] This discrepancy is speculated to be caused by improved ovulation, and subsequently fertility, in adrenal versus pituitary CS because of the lack of increased adrenal androgen levels in adrenal CS.[3,33,34] In addition, some adrenal cells that become cortisol-secreting tumors have been shown to express luteinizing hormone (LH)/human chorionic gonadotropin (hCG) receptor, which is stimulated during pregnancy.[3] There have been many case reports of pregnancy-induced CS that resolved postpartum,[35] postulated to be caused by increased expression of LH/hCG receptors on adrenal tumors that become activated during pregnancy.[35–37]

Diagnosis A high degree of clinical suspicion must be present to detect CS in pregnancy because many symptoms overlap with a normal pregnancy, including weight gain, striae, hirsutism, acne, fatigue, central obesity, emotional liability, hypertension (HTN), and glucose intolerance. Signs and symptoms that makes CS more likely include muscle weakness; thick, dark, purple abdominal striae (**Fig. 1**); pathologic fractures; and hypokalemia (**Table 1**).[3,38,39]

In pregnant women without CS, only 40% had a suppression of plasma cortisol after a 1-mg dexamethasone suppression test (DST), a blunting effect that increased with advancing gestational age.[17,40] In one study, up to 82% of healthy pregnant women had an abnormal 1 mg DST in the peripartum period[41]; this effect persisted up to 5 weeks postpartum.[42] This finding may be caused by an altered HPA set point in pregnancy, such that higher cortisol levels are needed to suppress ACTH secretion, also compounded by the increase in total serum cortisol level that occurs in

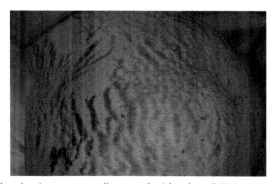

Fig. 1. Dark, thick striae in a woman diagnosed with adrenal CS in pregnancy.

Table 1
Cushing's evaluation: pregnant versus non-pregnant women

	Non-pregnancy	Pregnancy
1 mg DST	• Highly sensitivity in CD and adrenal CS • Test of choice to diagnose an adrenal incidentaloma[43] • False positives can occur with use of OCPs; altered dexamethasone metabolism (eg, certain antiepileptics)	• >80% normal pregnant women have false plus DST[41] • Recommend against its use[43]
24 hr UFC	• May be useful to diagnose cyclic CS[43] • Less reliable in renal failure, alcoholism, depression, morbid obesity	• Test of choice in pregnancy • At least >3 times upper limit normal in 2nd or 3rd trimester (mean 8-fold increase)[34,43]
Midnight salivary cortisol	• More sensitive for CD	• Not validated • Loss of diurnal cortisol variation (which is preserved but with higher nadir normal pregnancy)[4,6,12]
Imaging	• Typically pituitary MRI vs adrenal computed tomography depending on suspected etiology	• Pituitary MRI can be obtained without contrast safely in the 3rd trimester and likely safely in the 2nd trimester • Adrenal ultrasonography[34,44]
Etiology	• >60% due to pituitary adenoma	• 40–60% caused by adrenal adenoma (50% of primary adrenal CS failed to have suppressed ACTH)[33,34]

pregnancy.[34] The largest review of CS in pregnancy, by Lindsay and colleagues,[34] summarizes data from 136 pregnancies in 122 women who were diagnosed at an average gestation age of 18 weeks; there was a mean 8-fold increase in UFC level and a loss of diurnal serum cortisol variation in these women.

Accordingly, the Endocrine Society guidelines recommend a UFC level of more than 3 times the upper limit of normal in the second or third trimesters to be used in the diagnosis of CS in pregnancy, and recommend against the use of DST (given the high number of false-positives) as the initial evaluation for CS in pregnant women.[43] The role of salivary cortisol in establishing the diagnosis of CS in pregnancy has not been validated.

Once CS is suspected in pregnancy, establishing the cause may be more challenging than in the nonpregnant state. Although ACTH can be used in the nonpregnant state to identify ACTH-dependent versus ACTH-independent disease, half of pregnant patients with primary adrenal CS fail to have a suppressed serum ACTH level.[34] This finding may be caused by placental CRH stimulation of maternal ACTH release giving rise to detectable placental ACTH levels in maternal serum[3] as well as by a paradoxic dexamethasone stimulation of placental CRH and ACTH,[44] thus potentially creating increased ACTH levels in all pregnant women, but a false-positive increase of ACTH levels in those with adrenal tumors.

In the small number of patients tested, high-dose DSTs were able to identify all patients with ACTH-independent CS (whose cortisol levels failed to suppress); however, not all patients with pituitary-dependent CS had cortisol levels suppressed to less than 80% as expected in nonpregnant patients.[34] When high-dose dexamethasone suppression test fails to suppress or if ACTH level is low or borderline, an adrenal ultrasonography scan should be obtained. Adrenal ultrasonography identified 73% of adrenal adenomas in pregnancy so, if negative, an abdominal MRI scan without contrast should be obtained.[34,44]

Management Laparoscopic surgical resection is the treatment of choice for a cortisol-secreting adenoma discovered during pregnancy and can be done safely in the second trimester.[45,46] There is a trend toward an increase in live birth rate with treatment of CS in pregnancy, with no effect seen on premature birth or intrauterine growth restriction (IUGR) rates. However, these data may be limited by the small number of cases of CS syndrome in pregnancy, with many diagnosed later in pregnancy.[34]

There are fewer than 2 dozen reports of primary medical therapy used in the treatment of CS in pregnancy,[34,44] with metyrapone being the most commonly used drug. Metyrapone works rapidly to reduce cortisol levels by inhibiting the conversion of 11-deoxycortisol to cortisol. It can cause an increase in the accumulation of mineralocorticoid precursors and therefore can lead to HTN and, although controversial, likely increases the risk of preeclampsia.[44,47] Ketoconazole, also a steroidogenesis inhibitor, has been used successfully in 4 reported cases of CS in pregnancy, and without feminizing a male fetus in one case.[44,48] Although a population-based study of its use showed no negative outcomes,[49] hepatic dysfunction is possible and there have been reports of teratogenic effect in rats.[50] Both metyrapone and ketoconazole are pregnancy risk category C, indicating that a risk to the fetus cannot be ruled out. Mitotane, an adrenolytic, is a US Food and Drug Administration (FDA) category D pregnancy risk. Because of its teratogenic potential, it should not be used in pregnancy.[51] In the setting of pituitary-dependent CS, cabergoline, a dopamine agonist targeting the pituitary, has been found to be useful in treating some individuals with CS when used at high doses.[52] Studies of cabergoline used in lower doses in pregnancies complicated by prolactinomas show that it is safe and thus an FDA category B risk.[53–55] To date, there have been 2 published cases of cabergoline used for pituitary-dependent CS in pregnancy.[48,56]

Outcomes CS in pregnancy poses significant risks to the mother and the fetus. Maternal rates of HTN in pregnancy in patients with CS were almost 70%, with 14% having severe eclampsia,[34] some complicated by HELLP (hemolysis elevated liver enzymes low platelets) syndrome,[57] and a quarter with diabetes or impaired glucose tolerance.[34] Women were also at an increased risk of osteoporosis and fractures, cardiac failure, psychiatric illness, infection, and death.[34] In almost half of the cases, fetuses were born prematurely and almost one-quarter had IUGR. There was an increased risk of spontaneous abortions and stillbirths.[3,34,58]

Although the fetus is partially protected from hypercortisolism by placental 11-beta-HSD2 converting most of the cortisol to inactive cortisone, adverse fetal effects are probably related to placental and maternal changes from CS[34] as well as the high levels overwhelming this enzyme. In studies of neonates exposed to higher maternal cortisol (in the second trimester) and placental CRH (in the third trimester), there was a reduction in physical and neuromuscular development.[59,60]

Primary aldosteronism in pregnancy

Incidence and epidemiology PA, initially called Conn syndrome after the discovery of aldosterone-secreting adenomas, is a state of continued aldosterone synthesis and release, marked by high aldosterone and low renin values and is the most common endocrine cause of HTN. In the nonpregnant population, about two-thirds of PA cases are caused by bilateral adrenal hyperplasia and one-third are caused by an aldosterone-producing adenoma[61]; in more than 50% of these cases, serum potassium values are normal.[62] Adrenal cortical carcinoma, ectopic production of aldosterone, unilateral adrenal hyperplasia, and familial hyperaldosteronism are much rarer causes of PA.

PA is more common in women than in men and is often diagnosed when patients are 30 to 50 years old.[63] Recent studies indicate that PA may be responsible for up to 10% of all cases of HTN in nonpregnant patients, with an incidence higher in those with HTN with diabetes or obstructive sleep apnea and resistant HTN (HTN uncontrolled on 3 antihypertensive agents or controlled on $\geq$4 agents[61,62,64]).

PA is uncommon in pregnancy, with fewer than 3 dozen cases reported in the literature.[2] As seen in CS in pregnancy, PA in pregnancy is most commonly caused by an adrenal adenoma,[8] with very few reported cases caused by familial hyperaldosteronism type 1, glucocorticoid-remediable hyperaldosteronism,[65,66] or idiopathic hyperaldosteronism.[67]

Several recent studies have found evidence for a role of LH or hCG receptors in aldosterone-producing adenomas (APAs).[68–70] Morris and colleagues[71] observed increased expression of LH/hCG receptors in tissue resected from an ACC that caused increased aldosterone levels in a pregnant woman. In a different case of PA in pregnancy caused by an APA, Albiger and colleagues[72] reported an increase of aldosterone secretion following in vivo hCG stimulation. Therefore, in some cases of PA in pregnancy, it is possible that the increased hCG levels that occur during pregnancy could stimulate aldosterone secretion and/or tumorigenesis via the LH/hCG receptor.

Diagnosis Although values vary by institution, in nonpregnant women, an aldosterone/renin ratio of greater than 20 ng/dL per ng/mL/h and plasma aldosterone concentration (PAC) greater than 10 ng/dL with a concomitantly suppressed renin level are typically accepted values for a positive screening test.[61]

Given the normal physiologic increases in renin and aldosterone in pregnancy and the lack of pregnancy-specific references ranges, the diagnosis of PA in pregnancy can be difficult to establish and a high index of suspicion must exist. Features indicating a possibility of PA in pregnancy include moderate to severe HTN, proteinuria, and hypokalemia, although all symptoms need not be present.[8,73] Some women with PA in pregnancy remain normotensive or even have an improvement in their HTN, possibly because of the antimineralocorticoid effects of progesterone.[67] In one report, in 23 women with PA in pregnancy who did not undergo surgery, blood pressure (BP) improved spontaneously in 14%.[73] Furthermore, PRA and PAC were measured during pregnancy in only 11 of 27 cases of PA in pregnancy reported and reviewed in the literature. All patients in this series had increased PAC; PRA was more variable and not suppressed in all patients.[73] Because of the antikaliuretic effects of progesterone, potassium values may be normal in pregnant women with PA.[74]

A proposed diagnostic algorithm includes screening with a PRA and PAC. Although pregnancy-specific reference ranges do not yet exist, the mean plasma aldosterone level increases up to 8-fold during pregnancy and PRA increases up to 4-fold by the eighth week of gestation and 7-fold at term.[20,21] Although high aldosterone and a nonsuppressed plasma renin level do not rule out PA, in patients who have an increased PAC and suppressed PRA, confirmatory testing is not necessary in pregnancy given the potential risks associated with volume expansion and angiotensin-converting enzyme inhibitor use in pregnancy. Abdominal ultrasonography or MRI scan can be performed if there is high clinical suspicion for an adrenal mass.[2,8]

Management Conservative management with BP control and potassium supplementation is the main goal of medical management of PA in pregnancy with confirmatory testing and subtype differentiation after delivery. Although mineralocorticoid receptor antagonists are the first line of treatment in patients who are not pregnant, they are not proved to be safe in pregnancy. Spironolactone crosses the placenta and is pregnancy FDA category C drug with use contraindicated in pregnancy because of the feminization of male rats.[75] However, in a case report, high doses of spironolactone used to treat a woman with Bartter syndrome in pregnancy resulted in 2 male fetuses born without signs of feminization, the oldest of whom had entered normal puberty.[76] Eplerenone is a more selective aldosterone receptor antagonist with 0.1% less binding affinity for the androgen receptor than spironolactone.[77] Eplerenone, pregnancy risk factor B, has been successfully used in controlling HTN and hypokalemia in a case of PA in pregnancy[78] as well as for Gitelman syndrome in pregnancy.[79]

If a unilateral mass is found on abdominal MRI and BP is not controlled with medications, a unilateral adrenalectomy should be considered to treat PA in pregnancy.[2,8]

Outcomes Maternal morbidity and mortality were increased in a review of 29 cases of PA in pregnancy. Eighty-five percent of these woman had an increased BP greater than 140/90 mm Hg and more than half had proteinuria. Complications included preterm delivery in more than 50% of the cases (61% in subset managed without surgery) and intrauterine fetal demise and placental abruption (with intrauterine fetal demise and placental abruption, all women had proteinuria).[73] In the 6 patients with PA who did not have hyporeninemia (<1.0 ng/mL/h), pregnancies were complicated by placental abruption or preterm delivery and intrauterine fetal growth restriction, leading the investigators to recommend that women with PA without suppressed renin level and/or with proteinuria should be aggressively managed and monitored closely for such complications.[73] In another review, rates of preeclampsia, placental abruption, fetal growth restriction, and cesarean delivery seen in PA were reported to be similar to those seen in the obstetric population with essential HTN.[2]

In the few reports of familial, glucocorticoid-remediable aldosteronism (FH1), the women with chronic HTN who become pregnant, although not at increased risk of preeclampsia compared with the general obstetric population, did experience a worsening of their HTN, with an increased risk of primary cesarean section delivery and a trend toward lower birth rates.[66] Given that ACTH enables gene expression in FH1, this worsening of HTN is speculated to be caused by the physiologic increase in ACTH level in pregnancy.[66]

Pheochromocytoma in pregnancy

Incidence and epidemiology Pheochromocytomas are rare, with an even rarer occurrence during pregnancy, estimated at an incidence of approximately 0.007%.[8,80] Similar to the nonpregnant state, pheochromocytomas are typically unilateral and sporadic, with 10% occurring as bilateral, malignant, or familial (eg, multiple endocrine neoplasia II, von Hippel-Lindau syndrome, and type 1 neurofibromatosis).[8,80] The diagnosis is particularly important because undiagnosed and/or untreated pheochromocytoma has high maternal and fetal mortality, ranging from 15% to 25%[81] in some studies to up to 40% to 50% in other studies.[81] Maternal and fetal morbidity and mortality decline significantly once the disorder is properly diagnosed and treated.

Clinical features The presenting symptoms of a pheochromocytoma can overlap with the normal symptoms of pregnancy, resulting in a delay in diagnosis. Uncontrolled HTN, either sustained or paroxysmal, is the most common presenting feature during pregnancy. Evaluation for pheochromocytoma should be strongly considered in the setting of labile or sustained HTN, particularly if accompanied by heat intolerance, palpitations, and impaired glucose tolerance.[82] Other symptoms may be present, and in one study of a cohort of 15 pregnant women with pheochromocytoma, 12 of 15 women presented with headaches in addition to HTN.[83]

HTN is often mistakenly attributed to preeclampsia, particularly if proteinuria is present as well. Pheochromocytoma can manifest at any time during pregnancy, whereas preeclampsia typically presents later in pregnancy, frequently at greater than 20 weeks' gestation. In addition, the HTN associated with pheochromocytoma persists postpartum, whereas the HTN associated with preeclampsia typically resolves.[84]

As pregnancy progresses, symptoms often become more apparent, with symptoms more evident with the pregnant woman lying supine, which causes the gravid uterus to compress the tumor and results in paradoxic supine HTN despite a normal BP measurement in the sitting or erect position.[80] Rat pheochromocytoma (PC 12) cells express estrogen receptors alpha and beta, and G-protein–coupled receptor 30. Treatment with estradiol greatly increases sex hormone binding globulin production and increases the number of estrogen receptor beta–positive cells in differentiated rat pheochromocytoma cells.[85] More studies are needed to assess whether there is an increase in estrogen receptors in pheochromocytoma tissue in human models. Rarer presenting symptoms have been reported, including dyspnea, chest pain, seizures, and postpartum pulmonary edema.[86]

Neuroblastomas can also present similarly during pregnancy and may be misdiagnosed as pheochromocytoma. A rare malignant tumor derived from the primitive neural crest cells of the adrenal medulla, neuroblastomas can present with HTN and increased 24-hour urine catecholamine levels and vanillylmandelic acid.[87]

Establishing the diagnosis of pheochromocytoma in pregnancy Similar to the diagnosis in the nonpregnant state, pheochromocytoma is diagnosed in the setting of quantification of 24-hour urinary fractionated metanephrines and catecholamines and plasma fractionated metanephrines, at least twice the upper limit of the normal range. Under normal circumstances, pregnancy and preeclampsia should not influence catecholamine levels.[84]

In a multicenter cohort study of 214 nonpregnant patients with pheochromocytoma compared with 644 patients without pheochromocytoma, plasma free metanephrines and urinary fractionated metanephrines had a higher sensitivity for diagnosing pheochromocytoma (99% and 97%, respectively) compared with plasma catecholamines (84%), urinary total metanephrines (77%), and urinary vanillylmandelic acid (64%); however, these tests need further analysis, specifically in pregnant women.[88]

Imaging used to localize pheochromocytoma If a pheochromocytoma is suspected during pregnancy, the imaging modality recommended is MRI without gadolinium, and/or ultrasonography; however, the ultrasonography is often limited by the gravid uterus and has limited utility in diagnosing extra-adrenal tumors. Other tests, such as stimulation tests and 123-I-metaiodobenzylguanidine scintigraphy, are not considered safe for use during pregnancy.

Medical management of pheochromocytoma in pregnancy There is no clear consensus on the treatment of pheochromocytomas diagnosed during pregnancy and most data are limited to small case studies. Medical therapy, regardless of whether surgical intervention occurs during pregnancy, is a vital aspect of treatment and typically involves alpha-adrenergic blockade with subsequent beta-adrenergic blockade 10 to 14 days later. Alpha-receptor blockade functions to decrease BP and control for expansion of blood volume in pregnant women with pheochromocytoma. Phenoxybenzamine is the drug of choice during pregnancy (pregnancy class C), although it does cross the placenta and can potentially cause transient hypotension in the neonate.[89] Beta-blockade can be initiated after alpha-blockade to control for tachycardia. Antihypertensive drugs during pregnancy can cause fetal issues, including hypoxia and intrauterine growth retardation, as well as placental ischemia and placental abruption. These risks need to be balanced with the potential complications from uncontrolled HTN, such as hypertensive crisis, pulmonary edema, and cardiac and cerebral complications.[84]

Surgical management of pheochromocytoma in pregnancy Surgery is the definitive treatment of pheochromocytoma; however, the timing must be coordinated with respect to trimester of pregnancy and fetal status. If diagnosed early in pregnancy, appropriate medical treatment should be initiated until surgery can occur, with the optimal time for surgical resection being during the second trimester. If diagnosed later in pregnancy, medical treatment should be initiated and surgery deferred until after delivery. Preoperatively, alpha-receptor blockade with subsequent beta-blockade should be initiated. Laparoscopic adrenalectomy is recommended if the tumor mass is less than 7 cm; however, if diagnosed after 24 weeks of gestation, open surgical removal is preferred, timed with elective cesarean section closer to delivery. Cesarean section can be performed simultaneously with resection of the mass with a reduction in maternal and fetal mortality compared with vaginal delivery (31% vs 19%) because of the release of catecholamines during vaginal delivery.[89]

Patients require postoperative assessment as well as close monitoring because of the possibility of incomplete resection of tumor and recurrence or development of a malignant adrenal mass. In addition, genetic screening is recommended to assess for hereditary causes of pheochromocytoma, including multiple endocrine neoplasia 2A and von Hippel-Lindau syndromes.[89]

Adrenocortical Carcinoma in Pregnancy

Incidence and epidemiology

ACC is a rare cancer with an estimated incidence of slightly less than 1 case per million in the general population.[90,91] The prognosis for ACC is poor, with a 5-year survival rate of around 30%.[92–94] More than half of all ACCs are hormone secreting, with cortisol and androgen secretion being the most common.[95,96] ACC is more common in women than in men. There is a bimodal age distribution with the first peak occurring in childhood and a second during the fourth to fifth decades.[92,97] Data regarding ACC during pregnancy are limited to case reports, likely as a result of the rarity of the disease as well as the decreased fertility in those women with hypercortisolism and hyperandrogenism. When diagnosed during pregnancy, reported adverse fetal outcomes include premature birth, intrauterine growth retardation, stillbirth, and intrauterine death.[98] Frequently, there is a delay in diagnosis occurring after delivery.[96]

Clinical presentation

The presentation of an ACC during pregnancy often relates to the aberrant excess hormone production, frequently cortisol alone or in combination with androgens, from the tumor. In one study of 12 pregnant women with ACC, 75% of patients presented with HTN, diabetes, muscle wasting, morphologic changes, virilization, depression, and/or local or regional manifestations or tumor enlargement. One patient had symptomatic hypoglycemia, possibly caused by insulinlike growth factor 2 (IGF-2) hypersecretion; however, this relationship was not firmly established. Two-thirds of patients showed local or metastatic extension and all except 1 patient had surgical resection during pregnancy or postpartum.[96] In another case of a pregnancy complicated by ACC, LH/HCG receptor overexpression on the tumor resulted in excess maternal cortisol and androgen secretion causing partial virilization and ambiguous genitalia in the 46XX female infant.[71]

Genetic factors

The 2 most commonly observed genetic mutations in ACC are IGF-2 overexpression and constitutive activation of the Wnt/beta-catenin pathway.[99] In addition, the sonic hedgehog (SHH) pathway proteins seem to be upregulated in adult ACCs and down-regulated in pediatric ACCs.[100]

Imaging

The risk for malignancy with adrenal tumors increases with tumor size. At clinical presentation, ACCs are often large tumors, measuring more than 6 cm in diameter, and are sometimes found to be invading the adrenal vein and inferior vena cava.[101] Imaging modalities are limited during pregnancy; however, with high clinical suspicion for an adrenal mass, MRI should be considered. In addition to ACC, the differential diagnoses of an adrenal tumor greater than 4 cm should include a large adenoma, myelolipoma, adrenal metastasis from a different primary cancer, pheochromocytoma, adrenal cyst, ganglioneuroma, or other rare tumors of the adrenal gland (eg, sarcomas or lymphomas).[102] Computed tomography scan characteristics suggestive of a low risk for malignancy include a homogeneous mass with less than or equal to 10 Hounsfield units and smooth margins.[102] On MRI scans, ACC appears heterogeneous on both T1-weighted and T2-weighted images because of the presence of internal hemorrhage and necrosis. High signal intensity within the tumor may be noted on T1-weighted images because of hemorrhagic byproducts, whereas high signal intensity on T2-weighted images may be caused by areas of necrosis. A heterogeneous decrease in signal intensity should further raise suspicion for ACC.[101]

Treatment

A paucity of data exists on treatment options for ACC diagnosed during pregnancy. Given the poor prognosis of this tumor, some investigators have suggested complete surgical resection of the adrenal tumor at the time of diagnosis, regardless of pregnancy trimester.[96]

Mitotane has been used in the treatment of endogenous hypercortisolism and adrenal carcinoma, with data suggesting that treatment may prolong recurrence-free survival in nonpregnant patients with ACC after radical resection.[103] There is concern regarding the teratogenic effects of mitotane use during pregnancy and risk of fetal transfer. A few case reports revealed successful conception on mitotane and use of mitotane during pregnancy without evidence of adrenal dysfunction in the infant[104]; however, the potential for fetal risks limits this as a treatment option.[105]

SUMMARY

Adrenal diseases, including CS, PA, pheochromocytoma, and ACC, are uncommon in pregnancy; a high degree of clinical suspicion must exist. Physiologic changes to the HPA axis in a normal pregnancy result in increased cortisol, renin, and aldosterone levels, thus making the diagnosis of CS and PA in pregnancy challenging. However, catecholamine levels are not altered in pregnancy and allow a laboratory diagnosis of pheochromocytoma that is similar to that of the nonpregnant state. In the case of PA, if BP is controlled with medical therapy, confirmatory testing, subtype differentiation, and surgery should occur after delivery. Surgical resection is the treatment of choice for a cortisol-secreting adenoma discovered during pregnancy and can be done safely in the second trimester. In the case of a pheochromocytoma, medical treatment should begin immediately and surgery optimized according to gestational age of the baby, with elective cesarean section and concomitant open removal of the pheochromocytoma recommended if diagnosed after 24 weeks' gestation. Regardless of gestational age, surgery is the treatment of choice for ACC in pregnancy. Although adrenal tumors in pregnancy result in significant maternal and fetal morbidity and sometimes mortality, early diagnosis and appropriate treatment often improve outcomes.

REFERENCES

1. Gibson M, Tulchinsky D. The maternal adrenal. In: Tulchinsky D, Ryan KJ, editors. Maternal-fetal endocrinology. Philadelphia: Saunders; 1980. p. 129–43.
2. Monticone S, Auchus RJ, Rainey WE. Adrenal disorders in pregnancy. Nat Rev Endocrinol 2012;8(11):668–78.
3. Karaca Z, Tanriverdi F, Unluhizarci K, et al. Pregnancy and pituitary disorders. Eur J Endocrinol 2010;162(3):453–75.
4. Magiakou MA, Mastorakos G, Rabin D, et al. The maternal hypothalamic-pituitary-adrenal axis in the third trimester of human pregnancy. Clin Endocrinol (Oxf) 1996;44(4):419–28.
5. Petraglia F, Sawchenko PE, Rivier J, et al. Evidence for local stimulation of ACTH secretion by corticotropin-releasing factor in human placenta. Nature 1987; 328(6132):717–9.
6. Nolten WE, Rueckert PA. Elevated free cortisol index in pregnancy: possible regulatory mechanisms. Am J Obstet Gynecol 1981;139(4):492–8.
7. Cousins L, Rigg L, Hollingsworth D, et al. Qualitative and quantitative assessment of the circadian rhythm of cortisol in pregnancy. Am J Obstet Gynecol 1983;145(4):411–6.
8. Kamoun M, Mnif MF, Charfi N, et al. Adrenal diseases during pregnancy: pathophysiology, diagnosis and management strategies. Am J Med Sci 2014;347(1): 64–73.
9. Robinson BG, Emanuel RL, Frim DM, et al. Glucocorticoid stimulates expression of corticotropin-releasing hormone gene in human placenta. Proc Natl Acad Sci U S A 1988;85(14):5244–8.
10. Sasaki A, Shinkawa O, Yoshinaga K. Placental corticotropin-releasing hormone may be a stimulator of maternal pituitary adrenocorticotropic hormone secretion in humans. J Clin Invest 1989;84(6):1997–2001.
11. Allolio B, Hoffmann J, Linton EA, et al. Diurnal salivary cortisol patterns during pregnancy and after delivery: relationship to plasma corticotrophin-releasing-hormone. Clin Endocrinol (Oxf) 1990;33(2):279–89.
12. Demey-Ponsart E, Foidart JM, Sulon J, et al. Serum CBG, free and total cortisol and circadian patterns of adrenal function in normal pregnancy. J Steroid Biochem 1982;16(2):165–9.
13. Jung C, Ho JT, Torpy DJ, et al. A longitudinal study of plasma and urinary cortisol in pregnancy and postpartum. J Clin Endocrinol Metab 2011;96(5):1533–40.
14. Goland RS, Wardlaw SL, Blum M, et al. Biologically active corticotropin-releasing hormone in maternal and fetal plasma during pregnancy. Am J Obstet Gynecol 1988;159(4):884–90.
15. McLean M, Bisits A, Davies J, et al. A placental clock controlling the length of human pregnancy. Nat Med 1995;1(5):460–3.
16. Carr BR, Parker CR Jr, Madden JD, et al. Maternal plasma adrenocorticotropin and cortisol relationships throughout human pregnancy. Am J Obstet Gynecol 1981;139(4):416–22.
17. Lindsay JR, Nieman LK. The hypothalamic-pituitary-adrenal axis in pregnancy: challenges in disease detection and treatment. Endocr Rev 2005;26(6):775–99.
18. Okamoto E, Takagi T, Makino T, et al. Immunoreactive corticotropin-releasing hormone, adrenocorticotropin and cortisol in human plasma during pregnancy and delivery and postpartum. Horm Metab Res 1989;21(10):566–72.
19. Ryan KJ. Placental synthesis of steroid hormones. In: Tulchinsky D, Gibson M, editors. Maternal-fetal endocrinology. Philadelphia: Saunders; 1980. p. 129–43.

20. Landau RL, Lugibihl K. Inhibition of the sodium-retaining influence of aldosterone by progesterone. J Clin Endocrinol Metab 1958;18(11):1237–45.
21. Ledoux F, Genest J, Nowaczynski W, et al. Plasma progesterone and aldosterone in pregnancy. Can Med Assoc J 1975;112(8):943–7.
22. Dorr HG, Heller A, Versmold HT, et al. Longitudinal study of progestins, mineralocorticoids, and glucocorticoids throughout human pregnancy. J Clin Endocrinol Metab 1989;68(5):863–8.
23. Wilson M, Morganti AA, Zervoudakis I, et al. Blood pressure, the renin-aldosterone system and sex steroids throughout normal pregnancy. Am J Med 1980;68(1):97–104.
24. Abdelmannan D, Aron DC. Adrenal disorders in pregnancy. Endocrinol Metab Clin North Am 2011;40(4):779–94.
25. Langer B, Grima M, Coquard C, et al. Plasma active renin, angiotensin I, and angiotensin II during pregnancy and in preeclampsia. Obstet Gynecol 1998; 91(2):196–202.
26. Casey ML, MacDonald PC. Extraadrenal formation of a mineralocorticosteroid: deoxycorticosterone and deoxycorticosterone sulfate biosynthesis and metabolism. Endocr Rev 1982;3(4):396–403.
27. Parker CR Jr, Cutrer S, Casey ML, et al. Concentrations of deoxycorticosterone, deoxycorticosterone sulfate, and progesterone in maternal venous serum and umbilical arterial and venous sera. Am J Obstet Gynecol 1983;145(4): 427–32.
28. Lindholm J, Juul S, Jorgensen JO, et al. Incidence and late prognosis of Cushing's syndrome: a population-based study. J Clin Endocrinol Metab 2001;86(1): 117–23.
29. Steffensen C, Bak AM, Rubeck KZ, et al. Epidemiology of Cushing's syndrome. Neuroendocrinology 2010;92(Suppl 1):1–5.
30. Lado-Abeal J, Rodriguez-Arnao J, Newell-Price JD, et al. Menstrual abnormalities in women with Cushing's disease are correlated with hypercortisolemia rather than raised circulating androgen levels. J Clin Endocrinol Metab 1998; 83(9):3083–8.
31. Myers M, Lamont MC, van den Driesche S, et al. Role of luteal glucocorticoid metabolism during maternal recognition of pregnancy in women. Endocrinology 2007;148(12):5769–79.
32. Iannaccone A, Gabrilove JL, Sohval AR, et al. The ovaries in Cushing's syndrome. N Engl J Med 1959;261:775–80.
33. Buescher MA, McClamrock HD, Adashi EY. Cushing syndrome in pregnancy. Obstet Gynecol 1992;79(1):130–7.
34. Lindsay JR, Jonklaas J, Oldfield EH, et al. Cushing's syndrome during pregnancy: personal experience and review of the literature. J Clin Endocrinol Metab 2005;90(5):3077–83.
35. Achong N, D'Emden M, Fagermo N, et al. Pregnancy-induced Cushing's syndrome in recurrent pregnancies: case report and literature review. Aust N Z J Obstet Gynaecol 2012;52(1):96–100.
36. Lacroix A, Hamet P, Boutin JM. Leuprolide acetate therapy in luteinizing hormone–dependent Cushing's syndrome. N Engl J Med 1999;341(21):1577–81.
37. Chui MH, Ozbey NC, Ezzat S, et al. Case report: Adrenal LH/hCG receptor overexpression and gene amplification causing pregnancy-induced Cushing's syndrome. Endocr Pathol 2009;20(4):256–61.
38. Prebtani AP, Donat D, Ezzat S. Worrisome striae in pregnancy. Lancet 2000; 355(9216):1692.

39. Tajika T, Shinozaki T, Watanabe H, et al. Case report of a Cushing's syndrome patient with multiple pathologic fractures during pregnancy. J Orthop Sci 2002;7(4):498–500.

40. Odagiri E, Ishiwatari N, Abe Y, et al. Hypercortisolism and the resistance to dexamethasone suppression during gestation. Endocrinol Jpn 1988;35(5):685–90.

41. Greenwood J, Parker G. The dexamethasone suppression test in the puerperium. Aust N Z J Psychiatry 1984;18(3):282–4.

42. Owens PC, Smith R, Brinsmead MW, et al. Postnatal disappearance of the pregnancy-associated reduced sensitivity of plasma cortisol to feedback inhibition. Life Sci 1987;41(14):1745–50.

43. Nieman LK, Biller BM, Findling JW, et al. The diagnosis of Cushing's syndrome: an Endocrine Society Clinical Practice Guideline. J Clin Endocrinol Metab 2008;93(5):1526–40.

44. Lim WH, Torpy DJ, Jeffries WS. The medical management of Cushing's syndrome during pregnancy. Eur J Obstet Gynecol Reprod Biol 2013;168(1):1–6.

45. Angelico R, Ciangola IC, Mascagni P, et al. Laparoscopic adrenalectomy for hemorrhagic adrenal pseudocyst discovered during pregnancy: report of a case. Surg Laparosc Endosc Percutan Tech 2013;23(5):e200–4.

46. Toutounchi S, Makowska A, Krajewska E, et al. Laparoscopic treatment of Cushing's syndrome in a woman in late pregnancy - a case presentation. Wideochir Inne Tech Malo Inwazyjne 2011;6(4):261–3.

47. Connell JM, Cordiner J, Davies DL, et al. Pregnancy complicated by Cushing's syndrome: potential hazard of metyrapone therapy. Case report. Br J Obstet Gynaecol 1985;92(11):1192–5.

48. Berwaerts J, Verhelst J, Mahler C, et al. Cushing's syndrome in pregnancy treated by ketoconazole: case report and review of the literature. Gynecol Endocrinol 1999;13(3):175–82.

49. Kazy Z, Puho E, Czeizel AE. Population-based case-control study of oral ketoconazole treatment for birth outcomes. Congenit Anom (Kyoto) 2005;45(1):5–8.

50. Amaral VC, Nunes GP Jr. Prednisone reduces ketoconazole-induced skeletal defects in rat fetuses. Arch Toxicol 2009;83(9):863–71.

51. Leiba S, Weinstein R, Shindel B, et al. The protracted effect of o,p'-DDD in Cushing's disease and its impact on adrenal morphogenesis of young human embryo. Ann Endocrinol (Paris) 1989;50(1):49–53.

52. Pivonello R, De Martino MC, Cappabianca P, et al. The medical treatment of Cushing's disease: effectiveness of chronic treatment with the dopamine agonist cabergoline in patients unsuccessfully treated by surgery. J Clin Endocrinol Metab 2009;94(1):223–30.

53. Lebbe M, Hubinont C, Bernard P, et al. Outcome of 100 pregnancies initiated under treatment with cabergoline in hyperprolactinaemic women. Clin Endocrinol (Oxf) 2010;73(2):236–42.

54. Ono M, Miki N, Amano K, et al. Individualized high-dose cabergoline therapy for hyperprolactinemic infertility in women with micro- and macroprolactinomas. J Clin Endocrinol Metab 2010;95(6):2672–9.

55. Stalldecker G, Mallea-Gil MS, Guitelman M, et al. Effects of cabergoline on pregnancy and embryo-fetal development: retrospective study on 103 pregnancies and a review of the literature. Pituitary 2010;13(4):345–50.

56. Woo I, Ehsanipoor RM. Cabergoline therapy for Cushing disease throughout pregnancy. Obstet Gynecol 2013;122(2 Pt 2):485–7.

57. Castro RF, Maia FF, Ferreira AR, et al. HELLP syndrome associated to Cushing's syndrome–report of two cases. Arq Bras Endocrinol Metabol 2004;48(3):419–22 [in Portuguese].
58. Chico A, Manzanares JM, Halperin I, et al. Cushing's disease and pregnancy: report of six cases. Eur J Obstet Gynecol Reprod Biol 1996;64(1):143–6.
59. Ellman LM, Schetter CD, Hobel CJ, et al. Timing of fetal exposure to stress hormones: effects on newborn physical and neuromuscular maturation. Dev Psychobiol 2008;50(3):232–41.
60. Gillman MW, Rich-Edwards JW, Huh S, et al. Maternal corticotropin-releasing hormone levels during pregnancy and offspring adiposity. Obesity (Silver Spring) 2006;14(9):1647–53.
61. Galati SJ, Hopkins SM, Cheesman KC, et al. Primary aldosteronism: emerging trends. Trends Endocrinol Metab 2013;24(9):421–30.
62. Rossi GP, Bernini G, Caliumi C, et al. A prospective study of the prevalence of primary aldosteronism in 1,125 hypertensive patients. J Am Coll Cardiol 2006; 48(11):2293–300.
63. Fujiyama S, Mori Y, Matsubara H, et al. Primary aldosteronism with aldosterone-producing adrenal adenoma in a pregnant woman. Intern Med 1999;38(1): 36–9.
64. Persell SD. Prevalence of resistant hypertension in the United States, 2003-2008. Hypertension 2011;57(6):1076–80.
65. Hamilton E, O'Callaghan C, O'Brien RM, et al. Familial hyperaldosteronism type 1 in pregnancy. Intern Med J 2009;39(2):135–6.
66. Wyckoff JA, Seely EW, Hurwitz S, et al. Glucocorticoid-remediable aldosteronism and pregnancy. Hypertension 2000;35(2):668–72.
67. Ronconi V, Turchi F, Zennaro MC, et al. Progesterone increase counteracts aldosterone action in a pregnant woman with primary aldosteronism. Clin Endocrinol (Oxf) 2011;74(2):278–9.
68. Nicolini G, Balzan S, Morelli L, et al. LH, progesterone, and TSH can stimulate aldosterone in vitro: a study on normal adrenal cortex and aldosterone producing adenoma. Horm Metab Res 2014;46(5):318–21.
69. Rao CV. Human adrenal LH/hCG receptors and what they could mean for adrenal physiology and pathology. Mol Cell Endocrinol 2010;329(1–2):33–6.
70. Saner-Amigh K, Mayhew BA, Mantero F, et al. Elevated expression of luteinizing hormone receptor in aldosterone-producing adenomas. J Clin Endocrinol Metab 2006;91(3):1136–42.
71. Morris LF, Park S, Daskivich T, et al. Virilization of a female infant by a maternal adrenocortical carcinoma. Endocr Pract 2011;17(2):e26–31.
72. Albiger NM, Sartorato P, Mariniello B, et al. A case of primary aldosteronism in pregnancy: do LH and GNRH receptors have a potential role in regulating aldosterone secretion? Eur J Endocrinol 2011;164(3):405–12.
73. Okawa T, Asano K, Hashimoto T, et al. Diagnosis and management of primary aldosteronism in pregnancy: case report and review of the literature. Am J Perinatol 2002;19(1):31–6.
74. Ehrlich EN, Lindheimer MD. Effect of administered mineralocorticoids or ACTH in pregnant women. Attenuation of kaliuretic influence of mineralocorticoids during pregnancy. J Clin Invest 1972;51(6):1301–9.
75. Messina M, Biffignandi P, Ghigo E, et al. Possible contraindication of spironolactone during pregnancy. J Endocrinol Invest 1979;2(2):222.
76. Groves TD, Corenblum B. Spironolactone therapy during human pregnancy. Am J Obstet Gynecol 1995;172(5):1655–6.

77. Young WF Jr. Adrenal causes of hypertension: pheochromocytoma and primary aldosteronism. Rev Endocr Metab Disord 2007;8(4):309–20.
78. Cabassi A, Rocco R, Berretta R, et al. Eplerenone use in primary aldosteronism during pregnancy. Hypertension 2012;59(2):e18–9.
79. Morton A, Panitz B, Bush A. Eplerenone for Gitelman syndrome in pregnancy. Nephrology (Carlton) 2011;16(3):349.
80. Girling J, Martineau M. Thyroid and other endocrine disorders in pregnancy. Obstet Gynaecol Reprod Med 2010;20(9):265–71.
81. Lenders JW. Pheochromocytoma and pregnancy: a deceptive connection. Eur J Endocrinol 2012;166(2):143–50.
82. Keely E. Endocrine causes of hypertension in pregnancy–when to start looking for zebras. Semin Perinatol 1998;22(6):471–84.
83. Salazar-Vega JL, Levin G, Sanso G, et al. Pheochromocytoma associated with pregnancy: unexpected favourable outcome in patients diagnosed after delivery. J Hypertens 2014;32(7):1458–63 [discussion: 1463].
84. Dong D, Li H. Diagnosis and treatment of pheochromocytoma during pregnancy. J Matern Fetal Neonatal Med 2014;27(18):1930–4.
85. Gebhart VM, Jirikowski GF. Estrogen dependent expression of sex hormone binding globulin in PC 12 cells. Steroids 2014;81:26–30.
86. Kamari Y, Sharabi Y, Leiba A, et al. Peripartum hypertension from pheochromocytoma: a rare and challenging entity. Am J Hypertens 2005;18(10):1306–12.
87. Refaat MM, Idriss SZ, Blaszkowsky LS. Case report: an unusual case of adrenal neuroblastoma in pregnancy. Oncologist 2008;13(2):152–6.
88. Lenders JW, Pacak K, Walther MM, et al. Biochemical diagnosis of pheochromocytoma: which test is best? JAMA 2002;287(11):1427–34.
89. Oliva R, Angelos P, Kaplan E, et al. Pheochromocytoma in pregnancy: a case series and review. Hypertension 2010;55(3):600–6.
90. Golden SH, Robinson KA, Saldanha I, et al. Clinical review: Prevalence and incidence of endocrine and metabolic disorders in the United States: a comprehensive review. J Clin Endocrinol Metab 2009;94(6):1853–78.
91. Kebebew E, Reiff E, Duh QY, et al. Extent of disease at presentation and outcome for adrenocortical carcinoma: have we made progress? World J Surg 2006;30(5):872–8.
92. Allolio B, Fassnacht M. Clinical review: Adrenocortical carcinoma: clinical update. J Clin Endocrinol Metab 2006;91(6):2027–37.
93. Crucitti F, Bellantone R, Ferrante A, et al. The Italian Registry for Adrenal Cortical Carcinoma: analysis of a multiinstitutional series of 129 patients. The ACC Italian Registry Study Group. Surgery 1996;119(2):161–70.
94. Luton JP, Cerdas S, Billaud L, et al. Clinical features of adrenocortical carcinoma, prognostic factors, and the effect of mitotane therapy. N Engl J Med 1990;322(17):1195–201.
95. Fassnacht M, Libe R, Kroiss M, et al. Adrenocortical carcinoma: a clinician's update. Nat Rev Endocrinol 2011;7(6):323–35.
96. Abiven-Lepage G, Coste J, Tissier F, et al. Adrenocortical carcinoma and pregnancy: clinical and biological features and prognosis. Eur J Endocrinol 2010;163(5):793–800.
97. Wajchenberg BL, Albergaria Pereira MA, Medonca BB, et al. Adrenocortical carcinoma: clinical and laboratory observations. Cancer 2000;88(4):711–36.
98. Murakami S, Saitoh M, Kubo T, et al. A case of mid-trimester intrauterine fetal death with Cushing's syndrome. J Obstet Gynaecol Res 1998;24(2):153–6.

99. Fassnacht M, Kroiss M, Allolio B. Update in adrenocortical carcinoma. J Clin Endocrinol Metab 2013;98(12):4551–64.
100. Gomes DC, Leal LF, Mermejo LM, et al. Sonic hedgehog signaling is active in human adrenal cortex development and deregulated in adrenocortical tumors. J Clin Endocrinol Metab 2014;99(7):E1209–16.
101. Elsayes KM, Mukundan G, Narra VR, et al. Adrenal masses: MR imaging features with pathologic correlation. Radiographics 2004;24(Suppl 1):S73–86.
102. Else T, Kim AC, Sabolch A, et al. Adrenocortical carcinoma. Endocr Rev 2014; 35(2):282–326.
103. Terzolo M, Angeli A, Fassnacht M, et al. Adjuvant mitotane treatment for adrenocortical carcinoma. N Engl J Med 2007;356(23):2372–80.
104. Kojori F, Cronin CM, Salamon E, et al. Normal adrenal function in an infant following a pregnancy complicated by maternal adrenal cortical carcinoma and mitotane exposure. J Pediatr Endocrinol 2011;24(3-4):203–4.
105. Tripto-Shkolnik L, Blumenfeld Z, Bronshtein M, et al. Pregnancy in a patient with adrenal carcinoma treated with mitotane: a case report and review of literature. J Clin Endocrinol Metab 2013;98(2):443–7.

Adrenocortical Carcinoma

Review of the Pathologic Features, Production of Adrenal Steroids, and Molecular Pathogenesis

Yasuhiro Nakamura, MD, PhD[a], Yuto Yamazaki, MD[a],
Saulo J. Felizola, MD, PhD[a], Kazue Ise[a], Ryo Morimoto, MD, PhD[b],
Fumitoshi Satoh, MD, PhD[b], Yoichi Arai, MD, PhD[c],
Hironobu Sasano, MD, PhD[a],*

KEYWORDS

- Adrenocortical carcinoma • Weiss criteria • Molecular pathology • Steroidogenesis
- Immunohistochemistry

KEY POINTS

- Adrenocortical carcinoma (ACC) is a rare malignant neoplasm with an aggressive biological behavior.
- The Weiss criteria of adrenocortical malignancy are known as the most reliable tool for histopathological scoring system.
- Genomic features of adrenocortical carcinoma have been recently reported and may be used for the diagnosis of ACC.
- ACC cases may be hormonally functional, and immunohistochemical analysis of steroidogenic enzymes is utilized for the analysis of intratumoral production of corticosteroids.

INTRODUCTION

Adrenocortical carcinoma (ACC) is a rare malignant neoplasm arising from adrenocortical parenchymal cells. ACC is also known to have unique features compared with other tumors. In particular, ACC often secretes several types of steroid hormones with a pattern of disorganized steroidogenesis. This article summarizes the clinical,

The authors have nothing to disclose.
[a] Department of Pathology, Tohoku University Graduate School of Medicine, 2-1 Seiryo-machi, Aoba-ku, Sendai 980-8575, Japan; [b] Division of Nephrology, Endocrinology, and Vascular Medicine, Department of Medicine, Tohoku University Graduate School of Medicine, 2-1 Seiryo-machi, Aoba-ku, Sendai 980-8575, Japan; [c] Department of Urology, Tohoku University Graduate School of Medicine, 2-1 Seiryo-machi, Aoba-ku, Sendai 980-8575, Japan
* Corresponding author. Department of Pathology, Tohoku University School of Medicine, 2-1 Seiryo-machi, Aoba-ku, Sendai 980- 8575 Japan.
E-mail address: hsasano@patholo2.med.tohoku.ac.jp

Endocrinol Metab Clin N Am 44 (2015) 399–410
http://dx.doi.org/10.1016/j.ecl.2015.02.007
0889-8529/15/$ – see front matter © 2015 Elsevier Inc. All rights reserved.

histopathological, and biological features of ACC that are relevant to its pathogenesis, diagnosis and prognosis.

CLINICAL AND HISTOPATHOLOGICAL FEATURES OF ADRENOCORTICAL CARCINOMA

The incidence of ACC is estimated to be approximately 0.7 to 2 cases per 1 million population, accounting for 0.05% to 2% of all malignant tumors.[1] The age distribution of ACC is bimodal; the first peak is in early infancy under the age of 5 years, mainly derived from hereditary syndromes such as the Li-Fraumeni and Beckwith-Wiedemann syndromes.[2] The second peak is the fourth to fifth decades of life. The frequency in both genders is similar, but some reports indicate a slightly higher incidence in women.[2] The average overall survival in ACC cases was reported to be 14.5 months, with a 5-year mortality rate of approximately 75% to 90%.[3,4] Presently, only 30% of all ACCs are potentially curable at early stages after diagnosis. Metastases of ACC have been detected in the liver (48%–85%), lung (30%–60%), lymph nodes (7%–20%), and bones (7%–13%).[5,6] Clinical staging of ACC is usually based on the presence or absence of invasion or distant metastases.[7] Tumor size and weight are also reliable clinical parameters of staging ACC. Appropriate cut-off value of tumor weight (50 g) and tumor size (6.5 cm) indicates the high sensitivity (91%) and specificity (100%) in distinguishing ACC from adrenocortical adenoma (ACA).[8]

The histological diagnosis of ACC is pivotal in order to establish the final diagnosis. The Weiss criteria of adrenocortical malignancy comprise the most reliable histopathological scoring system differentiating ACC from ACA (**Table 1**).[9–11] ACC can be diagnosed by the presence of at least 3 of the 9 Weiss criteria. Three relate to cytological features (nuclear grade, mitoses and atypical mitoses); three refer to tumor structure (clear cells, diffuse architecture, and confluent necrosis), and three relate to invasion (venous invasion, sinusoidal invasion, and capsular infiltration). Most ACC cases are associated with relatively high scores in the Weiss criteria and do not pose major diagnostic challenges or problems for surgical pathologists involved in the diagnosis of resected adrenal neoplasms. However, occasionally some cases such as pediatric tumors or adrenocortical oncocytomas do pose diagnostic challenges if the final diagnosis is based solely on the Weiss criteria. In addition, as in any of the histopathological scoring

Table 1
Summary of Weiss criteria

Criteria	Scoring Points	
	0	1
Nuclear grade (Fuhrmann nuclear grade system)	I/II	III/IV
Mitoses	<6/10 HPF	≥6/10 HPF
Atypical mitoses	−	+
Clear cell component	<25%	≥25%
Diffuse architecture	<1/3	≥1/3
Confluent necrosis	−	+
Venous invasion	−	+
Sinusoidal invasion	−	+
Capsular infiltration	−	+

Three or more of the following 3 criteria indicate malignancy. Nuclear grade assessed by Fuhrmann nuclear grade, and grade III and/or IV indicates malignancy in adrenal tumors.
Abbreviation: HPF, high power fields.
Data from Refs.[9–11]

systems, interobserver differences among surgical pathologists are also by no means negligible factors, particularly when the tumors are possibly low grade carcinomas. Therefore, diagnostic markers other than histopathological factors augmenting this scoring system as an auxiliary diagnostic modality have been explored.

IMMUNOHISTOCHEMICAL MARKERS IN ADRENOCORTICAL CARCINOMA

Several immunohistochemical markers have been reported to be of diagnostic value in the differential diagnosis of resected adrenocortical neoplasms. These include the Ki67 proliferative index, p53, insulin-like growth factor (IGF)-II, cyclin E, β-catenin, and steroidogenic factor-1 (SF1).[11]

The Ki67 proliferative index is one of the most widely employed diagnostic immuno-histochemical markers in differentiating ACC from ACA. A Ki67 labeling index of more than 5% confirms the diagnosis of ACC.[12] However, a cut-off value in the range of 2.5% to 5% between carcinoma and adenoma has been proposed.[13] In addition, the Ki67 labeling index has also been reported to serve as a reliable prognostic factor in patients with ACC. For instance, Morimoto and colleagues[14] reported that a Ki67 labeling index over 7% was associated with significantly worse clinical outcomes in patients with ACC. However, because of the enormous intratumoral heterogeneity of ACC, determining the sites in which Ki67 labeling index is obtained markedly influenced the results. In particular, the question of whether the Ki67 labeling index should be calculated as the average of the entire tumor specimen or rather the summation of hot spots in the specimens has not been resolved. This flaw or limitation should be kept in mind when applying the Ki67 labeling index.

Overexpression of IGF-II has been reported in approximately 60% to 90% of ACC cases, and only rarely in ACA.[15,16] Epidermal growth factor receptor (EGFR) and p21 were also reported to be overexpressed in ACC.[17,18] Stojadinovic and colleagues[19] compared immunohistochemical markers between ACA and ACC: p21 (36.4% vs 69.4%), p53 (0% vs 5.4%), mdm-2 (36.4% vs 20.4%), and p27 (68.8% vs 94.4%). SF1 immunohistochemistry has been generally considered the most reliable method of identifying the primary lesion as being of adrenocortical origin.[20]

GENETIC OR MOLECULAR ASPECTS IN ADRENOCORTICAL CARCINOMA

It has been recently elucidated that several genes are related to the pathogenesis of ACC. Most ACC cases are sporadic, but several hereditary syndromes have been reported to be associated with the development of ACC, such as the Li-Fraumeni syndrome (TP53 gene mutation), the Beckwith-Wiedemann syndrome (11p15.5 chromosomal lesion alteration), multiple endocrine neoplasia type 1 (11q13 chromosomal lesion loss),[21–23] and Gardner syndrome (inactivating mutation of APC genes located in 5q21 chromosomal lesion).[24] The Li-Fraumeni syndrome occurs as a result of a germ line mutation of the TP53 gene, and the loss of heterozygosity at 17p13.1 results in the development of several malignant neoplasms such as breast cancer, hematological neoplasia, brain tumor, and ACC.[25,26] In particular, R175H and R337H are common mutations detected in southern Brazil, which are associated with a 10- to 15-fold increase in the occurrence of ACC.[27,28] Somatic mutations of TP53 genes have also been identified in sporadic ACC demonstrating overexpression of p53 protein in carcinoma cells.[29–31] The Beckwith-Wiedemann syndrome occurs as a result of an 11p15.5 chromosomal alteration, and presents with various developmental abnormalities, and some pediatric malignancies. This chromosomal lesion is linked to overexpression of factors of ACC tumorigenesis, IGF-II, CDKN1C, and H19.[32] Among those previously mentioned, the best recognized is IGF-II, which is overexpressed 100-fold in 60% to 90% of ACCs.[15,16]

MICRORNA PROFILES IN ADRENOCORTICAL CARCINOMA

Aberrant expression of microRNAs (miRs) may also play a role in the pathogenesis of ACC. MiRs are short (18 to 25 nucleotides) noncoding RNAs that regulate specific gene expression in the level of transcription in adhesion to mRNA by complementary sequence. In ACC, several miRs have been reported to be correlated with clinical and pathologic features of the tumors. In 2014, Duregon and colleagues[33] reported that miR-483-3p, miR-483-5p, and miR-210 expression levels were elevated, while miR-195 expression levels were lower in ACC, compared with ACA. In addition, these miRs were also reported to be associated with clinicopathological features of ACC.[33] These three miRs are all known to target IGF-II. High expression levels of miR-210 were positively associated with hypoxic conditions, and were also reported to be associated with aggressive clinical characteristics and a poor prognosis, Furthermore, high miR-210 expression levels significantly correlated with a high Ki67 labeling index and the presence of necrosis.[33] Interestingly, they reported that miR-483-3p, miR-483-5p, and miR-210, which are upregulated in ACC in general, were all significantly downregulated in oncocytic variant tumors, compared with other histological variants (classical and myxoid variants) of ACC.[33] Oncocytic variants of ACC are noted to express rich mitochondria in their cytoplasm, and are associated with an even poorer prognosis, compared with other ACC histological variants. Oncocytic ACC is difficult to diagnose by Weiss criteria, unless it clearly identifies the malignant potential findings, including coagulation necrosis, distant metastasis, invasion to adjacent organs and venous invasion. This reason is that several component of Weiss criteria, including nuclear atypism, diffuse architecture, and eosinophilic (oxyphilic) cytoplasm are commonly observed in both benign and malignant oncocytic adrenal neoplasms.[34,35] These miRs might be valuable in diagnosis of oncocytic ACC, distinguishing it from other histological variants of ACC. However, the distinction between adrenal oncocytic adenoma and carcinoma is still controversial.

MiRs can be detected not only in the tumor tissues, but also circulation of the patients, and if these miRs can be of clinical value, the analysis of miRs in the sera from patients with ACC can provide important information as to the clinical postoperative follow-up in terms of early detection of recurrence or metastasis.

ENDOCRINE FEATURES OF ADRENOCORTICAL CARCINOMA

Functional tumors account for approximately 60% of all ACC cases.[8,36] However, symptoms caused by hormone oversecretion are only present in about 40% of all cases of ACC. The most common hormone that is secreted by ACC is cortisol, and patients may present with signs/symptoms of Cushing syndrome such as hypertension, glucose intolerance or frank diabetes, osteoporosis, central obesity, acne, and/or hirsuitism. Functional tumors produce cortisol in 30% to 40% of cases, androgens in 20% to 30% of cases, estrogen in 6% to 10% of cases, and aldosterone in 2% to 2.5% of cases (**Fig. 1**).[2] Among such symptoms, virilization was reported in 24% of all ACCs, reported as a characteristic feature of presentation, because adrenal androgen precursors could not necessarily be efficiently converted into glucocorticoids.[2] In general, ACCs rarely produce and secrete a single steroid hormone in excess and usually are associated with overproduction and hypersecretion of multiple hormones and precursors. Most cases (24%–35%) produce different types of steroid hormones.[2,37,38] Therefore, excessive production or secretion of a single

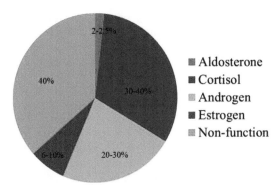

- Aldosterone
- Cortisol
- Androgen
- Estrogen
- Non-function

Fig. 1. The types of hormones produced and secreted in functional ACC cases based on previous reports. Functional cases account for approximately 60% of all ACCs, and 24% to 35% are associated with overproduction and hypersecretion of biologically active adrenocortical steroid hormones. (*Data from* Ng L, Libertino J. Adrenocortical carcinoma: diagnosis, evaluation and treatment. J Urol 2003;169:5–11.)

adrenocortical steroid usually indicates benign nature of adrenocortical neoplasm, but there are several exceptions. Aldosterone- or estrogen-producing ACCs, although rare, have been reported. The remaining cases, which are nonfunctional, are incidentally detected by computed tomography (CT) or MRI or nonspecific symptoms because of the relatively large nature of the retroperitoneal mass, such as back pain, abdominal mass, weakness, fever, and myalgias.[1] The clinical features of functional ACC are summarized in **Table 2**.[1,2]

ALDOSTERONE-PRODUCING ADRENOCORTICAL CARCINOMA

The incidence of pure aldosterone-producing ACC (APAC) is extremely low, accounting for only 2% of all cases.[2] The clinical presentation of this type of tumor is identical to that seen in primary aldosteronism from benign tumors and hyperplasia, namely hypertension and hypokalemia. The most common cause of primary aldosteronism

Table 2 Characteristics of functional adrenocortical carcinoma			
Hormones	**Frequency**	**Dominancy**	**Clinical Presentation**
Aldosterone	2%–2.5%	Women	Hypokalemia and hypertension
Cortisol	30%–40%	—	Cushing syndrome
Androgen	20%–30%	Women, children	Virilization, hirsuitism, and acne
Estrogen	6%–10%	Middle-aged men	Female: precocious puberty and post-menopausal bleeding Male: gynecomastia
Nonfunctional	40%	—	Tumor growth, abdominal mass, and weakness

Data from Allolio B, Fassnacht M. Clinical review: adrenocortical carcinoma: clinical update. J Clin Endocrinol Metab 2009;91(6):2027–37; and Ng L, Libertino J. Adrenocortical carcinoma: diagnosis, evaluation and treatment. J Urol 2003;169:5–11.

is aldosterone-producing adenoma (35%), bilateral idiopathic hyperaldosteronism (60%), although APAC cases are extremely rare, with less than 1% with Conn syndrome.[39,40] Four published cases were reported as APAC without hypertension.[41–45] These cases all presented with either hypokalemia or an abdominal mass, associated with a systolic blood pressure of 120 to 130 mm Hg. However, the mechanisms underlying the lack of hypertension in these rare cases have not been elucidated. Approximately 60 APAC cases have been previously reported. Seccia and colleagues[44] summarized these cases that report a peak incidence was in the fourth decade of life, with a female predominance (57%). Metastases were detected in 10% of the cases examined; median overall survival was 546 days, and median recurrence-free survival was 212 days. Plasma aldosterone concentration was increased on average by 14-fold, and plasma renin activity was suppressed in 55% in all cases.

CORTISOL-PRODUCING ADRENOCORTICAL CARCINOMA

Cortisol-producing ACC is the most common type, occurring in 30% to 40% of all ACCs. Combined hypersecretion of both cortisol and androgens is the most common hormonal pattern seen and suggests the presence of malignancy. Clinical presentations include features of Cushing syndrome such as hypertension, obesity, acne, and glucose intolerance or frank diabetes.[2,46] Abvien and colleagues reported that 63% of 202 ACC cases had evidence of cortisol hypersecretion. Sasano and colleagues reported 9 ACC cases (6 cases with Cushing syndrome, 1 case with primary aldosteronism, 2 cases without clinically symptoms associated with steroidogenic abnormalities). Six of these 9 cases expressed all the steroidogenic enzymes required for synthesis of cortisol or aldosterone only in small compact or clear cells; however, many carcinoma cells did not express steroidogenic enzymes required for synthesis of biologically active steroids. In these cases, 21-hydroxylase activity was markedly low, and 11-beta hydroxylase activity was moderately low, whereas, 17-alpha hydroxylase was positive in tumor cells. This disorganized steroidogenic enzyme expression indicates overproduction of precursor products of aldosterone or cortisol.[47]

ANDROGEN-PRODUCING ADRENOCORTICAL CARCINOMA

The frequency of androgen-producing ACC is approximately 20% to 30% of all ACCs. However, pure androgen-producing ACC is rare. Androgen and cortisol cosecreting ACCs are hormonally predominant. These cosecreting tumors occur more frequently in female and pediatric patients. Androgen-producing ACC is female dominant, males accounting for 10%–35%, because the presentation is clinically more apparent in females.[48–50] In pediatric cases, almost all adrenal tumors are functional, and virilization is the most frequent presentation. Pure androgen-secreting adrenal tumors (PASATs) comprise 40% to 60% of all pediatric adrenal tumors.[50] Most pediatric adrenocortical tumors are associated with a relatively good clinical course following the resection, with 90% overall long-term survival.[51]

Two recent studies concerning adult cases of PASAT were published.[52,53] Cordera and colleagues[52] and Moreno and colleagues[53] reported that approximately 50% of all female PASATs are malignant utilizing the Weiss criteria. Hirsuitism, acne, and clitoral enlargement are the common presening signs. Moreno and colleagues[53] found that malignant PASATs demonstrated 2.6-fold higher testosterone levels than benign PASATs. Tumor sizes and weights are also significantly higher in malignant PASATs.[52,53]

ESTROGEN-PRODUCING ADRENOCORTICAL CARCINOMA

Estrogen-producing ACC is a very rare type of functional ACC, accounting for approximately 6% to 10% of all ACCs. Common findings in female cases are precocious puberty or postmenopausal bleeding, while gynecomastia, testicular atrophy, and diminished libido may occur in men. Most cases occur between 24 and 45 years in men.[54,55] The criteria for confirmation of pure estrogen-producing ACC remains controversial elevation of serum estrogen levels indicates extraglandular aromatization of adrenal steroid precursors. Secretion of estrogen in ACC requires the local expression of aromatase and 17 β-hydroxysteroid dehydrogenase. It is also postulated that part of estrone is derived directly from ACC, and the rest is derived from the peripheral conversion of androstenedione into estrone.[56,57]

IMMUNOHISTOCHEMICAL EVALUATION OF FUNCTIONAL ADRENOCORTICAL CARCINOMA

ACC secretes various types of steroid hormones. In addition to the clinical presentation caused by overproduction of these steroid hormones, immunohistochemical analysis is pivotal in identifying the potential capacity of steroid production. Immunohistochemistry of steroidogenic enzymes expression including 3β-hydroxysteroid dehydrogenase (3βHSD), 17α-hydroxylase (P450c17), 21-hydroxylase (P450c21), 11β-hydroxylase (P450c11), DHEA-sulfotransferase (DHEA-ST), 17β-hydroxysteroid dehydrogenase type 5 (17β-HSD5), and aromatase should be performed on tumor specimens **(Fig. 2)**.[47,58] However, immunohistochemical analysis of these enzymes is quite difficult, and their expression pattern is different from that of ACA. Sasano[58] previously named these patterns of intratumoral steroidogenesis of ACC as "disorganized steroidogenesis", resulting in intratumoral heterogeneity of steroidogenesis and

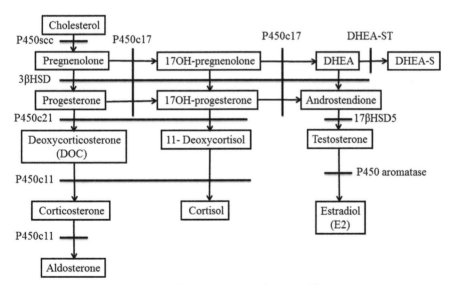

Fig. 2. The summary of pathway of steroidogenesis. (*Adapted from* Sasano H. Localization of steroidogenic enzymes in adrenal cortex and its disorders. Endocr J 1994;41:471–82; and Sasano H, Suzuki T, Nagura H, et al. Steroidogenesis in human adrenocortical carcinoma: biochemical activities, immunohistochemistry, and in situ hybridization of steroidogenic enzymes and histopathologic study in nine cases. Hum Pathol 1993;24:397–404.)

subsequently overproduction and oversecretion of precursor steroids. In addition, the discrepancy between the expression levels of mRNA and protein has been reported in several steroidogenic enzymes, such as P450c17, which has not been reported in any of the cases of ACA.[58] Here is shown representative illustrations of this pivotal immunohistochemical analysis of steroidogenic enzymes in ACC associated with Cushing syndrome and amenorrhea before surgery (**Fig. 3**). Clinically, serum levels of cortisol (32.88 μg/dL), testosterone (189 ng/dL), and DHEA-S (4000 ng/mL) are remarkably elevated. It is indeed appreciated that 3β-HSD and 17β-HSD5 staining are diffusely positive, but P450c17 and DHEA-ST are only partially immunopositive in carcinoma cells (see **Fig. 3**), indicative of disorganized steroidogenesis or intratumoral heterogeneity of adrenocortical steroidogenesis. Aromatase is negative, indicating the absence of estrogen production in this case (see **Fig. 3**).

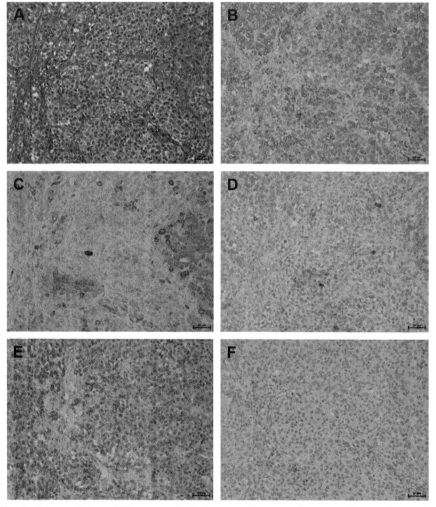

Fig. 3. Representative ACC case with Cushing syndrome and amenorrhea evaluated by immunohistochemical analysis, showing H&E staining (A), the expressions of 3β-HSD (B), P450c17 (C), DHEA-ST (D), 17β-HSD5 (E), and aromatase (F) (original magnification ×200).

SUMMARY AND FUTURE PROSPECTIVE

In this article, the current status of clinical, histopathological, and biological character-istics of ACC was briefly summarized. The Weiss criteria of adrenocortical malignancy is generally considered of diagnostic value, but it is also clear that histopathological or morphologic diagnosis alone may not be sufficient to provide the definitive final diag-nosis of ACC. Molecular/cell biological aspects and functional status could provide significant information to augment the Weiss criteria. Hormonally, most ACCs are functional, and the production of several adrenal cortical steroid hormones and precursors is considered characteristic of adrenocortical malignancy.

REFERENCES

1. Allolio B, Fassnacht M. Clinical review: adrenocortical carcinoma: clinical update. J Clin Endocrinol Metab 2006;91(6):2027–37.
2. Ng L, Libertino J. Adrenocortical carcinoma: diagnosis, evaluation and treatment. J Urol 2003;169:5–11.
3. Veytsman I, Nieman L, Fojo T. Management of endocrine manifestations and the use of mitotane as a chemotherapeutic agent for adrenocortical carcinoma. J Clin Oncol 2009;27:4619–29.
4. Balasubramaniam S, Fojo T. Practical considerations in the evaluation and man-agement of adrenocortical cancer. Semin Oncol 2010;37(6):619–26.
5. Schulick RD, Brennan MF. Long-term survival after complete resection and repeat resection in patients with adrenocortical carcinoma. Ann Surg Oncol 1999;6: 719–26.
6. Wajchenberg BL, Albergaria Pereira MA, Medonca BB. Adrenocortical carci-noma: clinical and laboratory observations. Cancer 2000;88:711–36.
7. Xichun S, Alberto A, Castro CY. Adrenal cortical carcinoma with concomitant myelolipoma in a patient with hyperaldosteronism. Arch Pathol Lab Med 2005; 129(6):144–7.
8. Aubert S, Wacrenier A, Leroy X, et al. Weiss system revisited: a clinicopathologic and immunohistochemical study of 49 adrenocortical tumors. Am J Surg Pathol 2002;26(12):1612–9.
9. Weiss LM. Comparative histologic study of 43 metastasizing and nonmetastasiz-ing adrenocortical tumors. Am J Surg Pathol 1984;8:163–9.
10. Weiss LM, Medeiros LJ, Vickery AL Jr. Pathologic features of prognostic signifi-cance in adrenocortical carcinoma. Am J Surg Pathol 1989;13:202–6.
11. Papotti M, Libè R, Duregon E, et al. The Weiss score and beyond—histopathol-ogy for adrenocortical carcinoma. Horm Cancer 2011;2:333–40.
12. McNicol AM. Lesions of the adrenal cortex. Arch Pathol Lab Med 2008;132(8): 1263–71.
13. Schmitt A, Saremaslani P, Schmid S, et al. IGFII and MIB1 immunohistochemistry is helpful for the differentiation of benign from malignant adrenocortical tumours. Histopathology 2006;49:298–307.
14. Morimoto R, Satoh F, Murakami O, et al. Immunohistochemistry of a proliferation marker Ki67/MIB1 in adrenocortical carcinomas: Ki67/MIB1 labeling index is a predictor for recurrence of adrenocortical carcinomas. Endocr J 2008;55(1): 49–55.
15. Gicquel C, Raffin-Sanson ML, Gaston V, et al. Structural and functional abnormal-ities at 11p15 are associated with the malignant phenotype in sporadic adreno-cortical tumors: study on a series of 82 tumors. J Clin Endocrinol Metab 1997; 82:2559–65.

16. Wilkin F, Gagne N, Paquette J, et al. Pediatric adrenocortical tumors: molecular events leading to insulin-like growth factor II gene overexpression. J Clin Endocrinol Metab 2000;85(5):2048–56.

17. Kamio T, Shigematsu K, Sou H, et al. Immunohistochemical expression of epidermal growth factor receptors in human adrenocortical carcinoma. Hum Pathol 1990;21:277–82.

18. Edgren M, Eriksson B, Wilander E, et al. Biological characteristics of adrenocortical carcinoma: a study of p53, IGF, EGF-r, Ki-67 and PCNA in 17 adrenocortical carcinomas. Anticancer Res 1997;17:1303–9.

19. Stojadinovic A, Brennan MF, Hoos A, et al. Adrenocortical adenoma and carcinoma: histopathological and molecular comparative analysis. Mod Pathol 2003;16(8):742–51.

20. Sasano H, Shizawa S, Suzuki T, et al. Transcription factor adrenal 4 binding protein as a marker of adrenocortical malignancy. Hum Pathol 1995;26(10):1154–6.

21. Görtz B, Roth J, Speel EJ, et al. MEN1 gene mutation analysis of sporadic adrenocortical lesions. Int J Cancer 1999;80:373–9.

22. Heppner C, Reincke M, Agarwal SK, et al. MEN1 gene analysis in sporadic adrenocortical neoplasms. J Clin Endocrinol Metab 1999;84:216–9.

23. Kjellman M, Roshani L, Teh BT, et al. Genotyping of adrenocortical tumors: very frequent deletions of the MEN1 locus in 11q13 and of a 1-centimorgan region in 2p16. J Clin Endocrinol Metab 1999;84:730–5.

24. Tissier F, Cavard C, Groussin L, et al. Mutations of beta-catenin in adrenocortical tumors: activation of the Wnt signaling pathway is a frequent event in both benign and malignant adrenocortical tumors. Cancer Res 2005;65:7622–7.

25. Sutter JA, Grimberg A. Adrenocortical tumors and hyperplasias in childhood—etiology, genetics, clinical presentation and therapy. Pediatr Endocrinol Rev 2006;4:32–9.

26. Ljungman M. Dial 9-1-1 for p53: mechanisms of p53 activation by cellular stress. Neoplasia 2000;2:208–25.

27. Ribeiro RC, Sandrini F, Figueiredo B, et al. An inherited p53 mutation that contributes in a tissue-specific manner to pediatric adrenal cortical carcinoma. Proc Natl Acad Sci U S A 2001;98:9330–5.

28. DiGiammarino EL, Lee AS, Cadwell C, et al. A novel mechanism of tumorigenesis involving pH-dependent destabilization of a mutant p53 tetramer. Nat Struct Biol 2002;9:12–6.

29. Miyamoto H, Kubota Y, Shuin T, et al. Bilateral adrenocortical carcinoma showing loss of heterozygosity at the p53 and RB gene loci. Cancer Genet Cytogenet 1996;88:181–3.

30. Gupta D, Shidham V, Holden J, et al. Value of topoisomerase II alpha, MIB-1, p53, E-cadherin, retinoblastoma gene protein product, and HER-2/neu immunohistochemical expression for the prediction of biologic behavior in adrenocortical neoplasms. Appl Immunohistochem Mol Morphol 2001;9:215–21.

31. Pinto EM, Billerbeck AE, Fragoso MC, et al. Deletion mapping of chromosome 17 in benign and malignant adrenocortical tumors associated with the Arg337His mutation of the p53 tumor suppressor protein. J Clin Endocrinol Metab 2005;90:2976–81.

32. Sparago A, Cerrato F, Vernucci M, et al. Microdeletions in the human H19 DMR result in loss of IGF2 imprinting and Beckwith-Wiedemann syndrome. Nat Genet 2004;36:958–60.

33. Duregon E, Rapa I, Votta A, et al. MicroRNA expression patterns in adrenocortical carcinoma variants and clinical pathologic correlations. Hum Pathol 2014;45(8): 1555–62.

34. Mearini L, Del Sordo R, Costantini E, et al. Adrenal oncocytic neoplasm:a systematic review. Urol Int 2013;91:125–33.
35. Ohtake H, Kawamura H, Matsuzaki M, et al. Oncocytic adrenocortical carcinoma. Ann Diagn Pathol 2010;14:204–8.
36. Hough AJ, Hollifield JW, Page DL, et al. Prognostic factors in adrenal cortical tumors. A mathematical analysis of clinical and morphologic data. Am J Clin Pathol 1979;72:390–9.
37. Wooten MD, King DK. Adrenal cortical carcinoma. Epidemiology and treatment with mitotane and a review of the literature. Cancer 1993;72:3145–55.
38. Icard P, Chapuis Y, Andreassian B, et al. Adrenocortical carcinoma in surgically treated patients: a retrospective study on 156 cases by the French Association of Endocrine Surgery. Surgery 1992;112:972–9.
39. Ganguly A. Primary aldosteronism. N Engl J Med 1998;339:1828–34.
40. Vallotton MB. Primary aldosteronism. Part I. Diagnosis of primary hyperaldosteronism. Clin Endocrinol (Oxf) 1996;45:47–52.
41. Muthusethupathi MA, Vimala A, Jayakumar M, et al. Normotensive primary aldosteronism due to adrenocortical carcinoma. Nephron 1998;79:247–8.
42. Yamazaki H, Abe Y, Katoh Y, et al. Establishment of an adrenocortical carcinoma xenograft with normotensive hyperaldosteronism in vivo. APMIS 1998;106:1056–60.
43. Song MS, Seo SW, Bae SB, et al. Aldosterone-producing adrenocortical carcinoma without hypertension. Korean J Intern Med 2012;27:221–3.
44. Seccia TM, Fassina A, Nussdorfer GG, et al. Aldosterone-producing adrenocortical carcinoma: an unusual cause of Conn's syndrome with an ominous clinical course. Endocr Relat Cancer 2005;12:149–59.
45. Young WF. Primary aldosteronism: renaissance of a syndrome. Clin Endocrinol (Oxf) 2007;66:607–18.
46. Abiven G, Coste J, Groussin L, et al. Clinical and biological features in the prognosis of adrenocortical cancer: poor outcome of cortisol-secreting tumors in a series of 202 consecutive patients. J Clin Endocrinol Metab 2006;91:2650–5.
47. Sasano H, Suzuki T, Nagura H, et al. Steroidogenesis in human adrenocortical carcinoma: biochemical activities, immunohistochemistry, and in situ hybridization of steroidogenic enzymes and histopathologic study in nine cases. Hum Pathol 1993;24:397–404.
48. Cavlan D, Bharwani N, Grossmanc A. Androgen and estrogen-secreting adrenal cancers. Semin Oncol 2010;37(6):638–48.
49. Mendonca BB, Lucon AM, Menezes CA, et al. Clinical, hormonal and pathological findings in a comparative study of adrenocortical neoplasms in childhood and adulthood. J Urol 1995;154:2004–9.
50. Fassnacht M, Allolio B. Clinical management of adrenocortical carcinoma. Best Pract Res Clin Endocrinol Metab 2009;23:273–89.
51. Sandrini R, Ribeiro RC, DeLacerda L. Childhood adrenocortical tumors. J Clin Endocrinol Metab 1997;82:2027–31.
52. Cordera F, Grant C, van Heerden J. Androgen-secreting adrenal tumors. Surgery 2003;134:874–80.
53. Moreno S, Montoya G, Armstrong J, et al. Profile and outcome of pure androgen-secreting adrenal tumors in women: experience of 21 cases. Surgery 2004;136:1192–8.
54. Barcelo B, Abascal J, Ardaiz J, et al. Feminizing adrenocortical carcinoma in a postmenopausal woman. Postgrad Med J 1979;55:406–8.

55. McKenna TJ, O'Connell Y, Cunningham S, et al. Steroidogenesis in an estrogen-producing adrenal tumor in a young woman: comparison with steroid profiles associated with cortisol and androgen-producing tumors. J Clin Endocrinol Metab 1990;70:28–34.

56. Zayed A, Stock JL, Liepman MK, et al. Feminization as a result of both peripheral conversion of androgens and direct estrogen production from an adrenocortical carcinoma. J Endocrinol Invest 1994;17:275–8.

57. Kimura M, Itoh N, Tsukamoto T, et al. Aromatase activity in an estrogen-producing adrenocortical carcinoma in a young man. J Urol 1995;153:1039–40.

58. Sasano H. Localization of steroidogenic enzymes in adrenal cortex and its disorders. Endocr J 1994;41:471–82.

Adrenocortical Carcinoma

Eric Baudin, MD, PhD, Endocrine Tumor Board of Gustave Roussy (Department of Endocrine Oncology and Nuclear Medicine)[a,b,c,*]

KEYWORDS

- Adrenocortical carcinoma • Prognosis • Predictors • Surrogate • Survival
- Metastasis • Mitotane • Chemotherapy

KEY POINTS

- Major breakthroughs have been achieved in the identification of relevant molecular alterations in adrenocortical carcinoma, but no simple actionable target has emerged.
- Progresses in the prognostic risk stratification constitute the basis of future stratified medical strategies and evaluations.
- Making therapeutic advances against adrenocortical carcinoma is a formidable challenge facing patients and clinicians with expert centers and networking as a basis of progress.
- R0 surgery of more than 90% of localized ACC patients is a unmet need.

Adrenocortical carcinoma (ACC) originates from the adrenal cortex and is typically defined by positive immunostaining for steroidogenic factor 1 (SF1), melanA (Mart1) markers but without staining for cytokeratins and chromogranin A.[1–4] As for all endocrine tumors, malignancy is ascertained by the presence of local or distant spread. No absolute criteria of malignancy exists for the diagnosis of ACC in those tumors confined to the adrenal gland, but a Weiss score of 3 or higher is generally considered to establish the diagnosis.[3,4] In addition, several studies have shown that a Ki67 index higher than or equal to 2.5% to 5% was associated with an abnormal Weiss score or a higher risk of recurrence.[5–9]

The incidence of ACC is less than 0.7 to 1.5 per 1 million people per year.[10–12] Because of the low incidence of ACC, a limited number of prospective studies have investigated potential therapies. In addition, the use of mitotane, a major drug

Dr E. Baudin has received honoraria and grants from HRA Pharma. All other authors have nothing to disclose.

[a] Département de Médecine, Gustave Roussy, 114, rue Édouard-Vaillant, Paris South University, Villejuif Cedex 94805, France; [b] Département de Nucléaire et de Cancérologie Endocrinienne, Gustave Roussy, 114, rue Édouard-Vaillant, Paris South University, Villejuif Cedex 94805, France; [c] Faculté de Médecine, INSERM UMR 1185, 63 rue Gabriel Péri, F-94276 Le Kremlin-Bicêtre, Université Paris Sud, Paris, France
* Gustave Roussy, 114, rue Édouard-Vaillant, Paris South University, Villejuif Cedex 94805, France.
E-mail address: eric.baudin@gustaveroussy.fr

metabolism inducer but also a drug with delayed antitumor activity, in most patients with ACC makes the conclusions from previous trials uncertain. Thus, advances in the understanding and management of ACC largely depend on the history of mitotane prescription, findings in retrospective studies, expert consensus, and clinicians' experience from expert centers. The implementation of networks for ACC, such as the European Network for the Study of Adrenal Tumors (ENSAT), the demonstration of the feasibility of phase 3 trials but also recent recommendations, constitute major steps forward.[3,4] This review focuses on the therapeutic management of adult patients with sporadic ACC.

CHARACTERIZATION BEFORE THERAPY

ACC must be precisely characterized according to standardized criteria as defined by ENSAT and the European Society for Medical Oncology recommendations.[4] Although the criteria are simple, lack of accurate characterization of patients with ACC in most retrospective studies, including absence of Weiss criteria, proliferative index, and resection status (R status), makes their final conclusions uncertain.

The minimum information that should be included in records of all patients with ACC is given in **Box 1**. Genetic disorders that affect less than 5% of adult patients with ACC are looked for in case of familial history or age younger than 40 years at diagnosis and have been extensively reviewed recently.[13] Approximately 80% of patients with ACC present with symptoms (tumor burden or hormone-related manifestations)[14–19] and two-thirds of patients with ACC produce steroids.[20] ACC hypersecretion can concern both active steroids (mainly glucocorticosteroids and

---

Box 1
Parameters to be characterized in patients with ACC at the time of therapeutic interventions

- Age and comorbidity, genetic background, performance status
- Weiss global score, including the precise count of mitosis/50 HPF
- Percentage of Ki 67 index in the most active regions (number of cells analyzed to be specified)
- Presence of tumor-related or hormone-related symptoms
- Secretory status: type and magnitude of secretions
- c/pTNM UICC and/or ENSAT staging including:
  - Modality of imaging
  - Disease-free interval
  - Number and location of abnormal lymph nodes at imaging or positive at pathology
  - Presence and type of venous invasion or adjacent organ invasion
  - Number and type of tumor organs
- Resection status of the primary, number of lymph nodes resected, tumor spillage/hemorrhage during surgery
- Mitotane history, highest plasma level reached in case of second-line therapy
- Signed informed consent for bioresource use when available

Abbreviations: c/p, clinical/pathological; HPF, high power field.

androgens but also estrogens or mineralocorticosteroids) and nonactive precursors with variable clinical impact. The presence of clinical symptoms should be recorded as well as the magnitude of hormone secretions.

At the time of diagnosis, based on thoracic and abdomen computed tomography (CT) and the analysis of multicentric studies, ACC patients typically present with a large primary tumor mass and are classified ENSAT stage I, II, III, or IV in 5% to 6%, 33% to 50%, 10% to 26% or 21% to 35% of cases, respectively.[12,21–23] Frequent upstaging to stage III of patients preoperatively misclassified as stage II justifies preoperative cautious radiologic analysis.[24] Within the stage III ACC subgroup, the usual sites of local involvement include adipose tissue surrounding the tumor, adjacent organs, renal vein or vena cava, and lymph nodes in 39 (85.3%), 14 (20.6%), 19 (27.9%), and 7 (10.3%), respectively, in a recent study.[22,25] The range of positive lymph nodes in patients with ACC varied between 20% and 50% in the absence or presence of routine lymph node dissection.[26] Half of distant metastases are present initially and half occur during follow-up.[27] The usual sites of metastatic involvement are mainly the liver and lungs, and less frequently, bone, peritoneum, and other sites.[16–18,27–29] At the time of the discovery of recurrences, local recurrences are present in to 57% to 63% of cases and distant metastases in 27% to 36% of cases.[30–32]

Routine use of [^{18}F]fluorodeoxyglucose (FDG) positron emission tomography (PET) still needs validation.[4,33,34] However, in our center, FDG-PET/CT is routinely performed at initial staging or at the time of recurrence when surgical resection is planned.

After surgery, the resection status and the Weiss score as well as the proliferative index are determined, including Ki67 measurements. Based on recommendations and the emerging role of the proliferative index as major diagnostic and prognostic tools in recent studies, standardization and the precise count of mitoses and the Ki67 labeling index should be included in the pathology reports.

The biology of ACC has recently been studied extensively.[35] Although the clinical application of molecular alterations remains unknown, they constitute the cornerstone of future progress. The existence of several predisposition syndromes suggested the involvement of several driver genes in the pathogenesis of ACC: Li-Fraumeni syndrome (*TP53*), Beckwith-Wiedemann syndrome (mapped to the 11p15.5 region containing genes coding IGFII, H19, and p57^{KIP2}), familial adenomatous polyposis (Wnt/β-catenin signaling *APC*), and Lynch syndromes (MSH2, MSH6, MLH3, PRS2).[13] Numerous genetic and molecular studies, combining several techniques (comparative genomic hybridization, transcriptome, miRNAome, methylome, exome sequencing) have recently been performed on adrenocortical tumors, including carcinoma.[35–39] These studies have confirmed the involvement of several key pathways, including the p53, Wnt/β-catenin, and IGFII pathways but also found that other driver genes such as *CDKN2A*, *RB1*, *TERT*, and *MENIN* can be involved in the control of the cell cycle or chromatin remodeling. Alteration in microRNA (miRNA) profiling or hypermethylation of the CpG island methylator phenotype in up to 50% of cases of ACC has also been described.[37–39]

PROGNOSIS: TOWARD PROGNOSTIC RISK STRATIFICATION

Although previously described as dismal, the prognosis of ACC is more heterogeneous than previously believed and long-term survivors exist. Factors that have hampered a precise prognostic stratification of these tumors in the past include the scarcity of ACC, the absence of validated TNM classification, and the lack of strict criteria of malignancy, which makes stage I or II ACC tumor behavior uncertain. Historically, the presence of metastases and tumor resectability constituted the keystones of prognostic stratification.[10,40] More recently, the Union for International Cancer Control (UICC) and ENSAT established the first TNM stage classifications, and the resection status was implemented allowing for refined prognostication.[22,29,41,42] Within the TNM staging system, ENSAT classification has been found to more accurately predict the outcome of patients with ACC, but recent studies suggest that the N status or severe vena cava invasion may behave like stage IV ACC, suggesting that refinements in the stratification of TNM are still needed.[16,25,29,43,44] Also, the relevance of stage I or II ENSAT subcategories is debated.[15,17–19,22,23,42] **Table 1** summarizes the evolution of TNM classifications in patients with ACC and new proposals based on recent studies.

After adjustment for TNM classification, several studies claimed that age,[12,14,15,17–19,23,29,42] the presence of hormone-related symptoms or steroid biomarkers,[14,17–19] Weiss score and/or proliferative index and/or differentiation,[9,15,17–19,27,29,42,45–47] and the R status also play an important prognostic role.[29,42,48] Recent publications based on a large number of patients and patients who were more precisely characterized enable elaboration of a prognostic stratification of patients with ACC in the adjuvant and palliative setting (**Fig. 1**).[15,16]

In patients with localized ACC, one recent study from the ENSAT group investigated the risk of recurrence and overall survival (OS) in 319 patients with stage I to III R0 ACC and in a validation cohort of 250 patients.[15] This study identified younger age, stage III or less, and low Ki67 labeling as the most significant parameters to predict recurrence-free survival. Based on these results and previous studies,[12,15,17,18,25,46,49] risk stratification in the management of these patients in the adjuvant setting can be envisaged based on a grading system that includes Weiss criteria and/or mitotic count and/or Ki67 analyses as well as the R status, age, and stage, as shown in **Fig. 1A**. This stratification is critical to adapt the adjuvant strategy in these patients.

In patients with ACC with advanced stage III to IV, another recent study of the ENSAT network, which analyzed 444 patients with advanced stage III to IV ACC, found that the stage as redefined by a new modified ENSAT (mENSAT) classification in which the presence of N positive moves from stage III to IV and which takes into account the number of tumor organs (see **Table 1**), has a major prognostic role together with 4 other parameters grouped together under the label GRAS.[16] After adjustment for a new mENSAT TNM classifications, GRAS parameters, as defined by grade (Weiss score <6 or >6 or Ki67 <20% or >20%), resection status of the primary, age younger than or older than 50 years, and absence or presence of tumor-related or hormone-related symptoms at diagnosis, were also found prognostic of OS. Similar parameters were previously found to play a major role in predicting recurrence in patients with localized ACC. Based on these results, a risk stratification of the management of patients with stage III to IV ACC in the palliative setting can be envisioned based on mENSAT new TNM staging and GRAS parameters, as shown in **Fig. 1B**.

At the time of recurrence, the prognostic impact of disease-free interval as well as R0 status was reported in several studies.[32,40,50–52] In addition, another study[30] suggested that feasaibility of complete surgery at the time of partial response (PR) to mitotane therapy may constitute another way to stratify the patients in terms of best first-line options, as shown in **Fig. 2**.

Similarly, molecular markers from genomic and epigenomic analyses are emerging and need to be applied to the aforementioned criteria.[35–39]

Table 1
TNM classifications in patients with ACC and proposals for new classifications

Stage	UICC	ENSAT	mENSAT	mENSAT + GRAS[b]
I	T1 (≤5 cm) N0, M0	T1 (≤5 cm) N0, M0	—	T1-2, favorable GRAS
II	T2 (>5 cm) N0, M0	T2 (>5 cm) N0, M0	—	II-A: T1-2, unfavorable GRAS II-B: T1-2, pejorative GRAS
III	T3N0 or, N1	T3-T4 or, Any T-N1, M0	T3, or T4, N0, M0	III-A: mENSAT stage III and favorable GRAS III-B: mENSAT stage III and unfavorable GRAS III-C: mENSAT stage III and pejorative GRAS
IV	T3N1 or T4 or M1	M1	Any T-N1, M1 IV-A: 2 tumor organs[a] IV-B: 3 tumor organs IV-C: >3 tumor organs	IV-A: mENSAT stage IV-A or B and favorable GRAS IV-B: mENSAT stage IV-A or B and unfavorable GRAS IV-C: mENSAT IV-C or mENSAT-IV-A or B and pejorative GRAS

mENSAT classification is based on the results of Ref.[16] ENSAT-GRAS new proposal takes into account references listed in the section on prognosis.
M1; presence of distant metastasis; N1, positive lymph nodes; T1, ≤5 cm; T2, <5 cm; T3, infiltration of surrounding tissue; T4, invasion of adjacent organs or renal vein/vena cava.

[a] Tumor organ counts include the primary and lymph nodes if not resected.

[b] GRAS parameters are considered favorable if grading defined by Ki67 is <20%, primary R0 resection status performed, age <50 y and absence of symptoms at diagnosis. GRAS parameters are classified unfavorable in case of age >50 y, or presence of symptoms at diagnosis. GRAS parameters are classified as pejorative in case of: grading as defined by Ki67 >20% and/or primary R1-2 resection status.

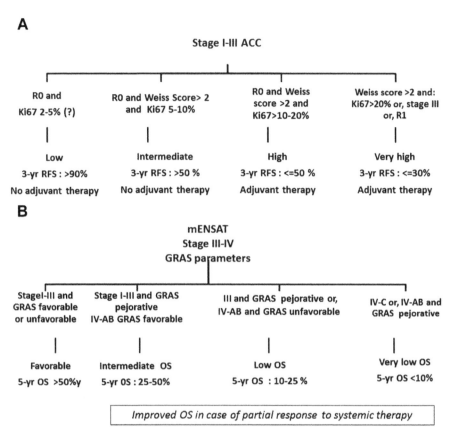

Fig. 1. (*A*) Proposals for stratification of the risk of recurrence in patients with stage I to III ACC. RFS, recurrence-free survival. (*B*) Proposals for 5-year OS risk stratification for patients with advanced stage III to IV ACC. Please refer to **Table 1** for GRAS definitions.

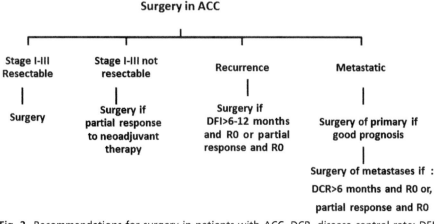

Fig. 2. Recommendations for surgery in patients with ACC. DCR, disease control rate; DFI, disease-free interval; R0, margin free resection expected.

Hypermethylation status, miRNA profile, or p53 mutations constitute valuable candidates that could integrate a future clinicomolecular prognostic classification of patients with ACC.[35,53]

TREATMENT

Tumor growth is the main cause of death in patients with ACC, and there has been no major breakthrough in recent decades. In addition, no shift toward lower stage at the discovery of the disease has been observed.[12,18,23] However, emerging standardization of ACC management throughout the world through recommendations, emergent targets, and the recent demonstration of the feasibility of phase 3 trials within networks constitute remarkable keystones for the future. During the last decade, the role of mitotane in the management of patients with ACC has been reinforced, the combination of mitotane with etoposide-doxorubicin-cisplatin (MEDP) has been selected as the standard treatment for patients with advanced ACC; preliminary targeted therapy approaches have failed and future targets for ACC management have emerged. The therapeutic options for patients with advanced ACC remain limited and mostly palliative. New protocols including phase 1 trials, even as first line, are urgently needed.

CONTROL OF HORMONE-RELATED SYMPTOMS

In many patients with ACC, steroid hypersecretion may be reduced by the administration of mitotane as monotherapy.[3,4] This compound, through its combined antitumor and antisecretory effects, reduces steroid production by tumor cells.[13,54–56] However, in some patients with ACC, major cortisol secretion may rapidly compromise short-term survival, and the use of metyrapone, ketoconazole, or etomidate, administered either alone or in combination, as a complement of mitotane is effective in rapidly blocking hypercortisolism.[57]

CONTROL OF TUMOR GROWTH

Current recommendations for the treatment of patients with ACC are based on retrospective studies but also 10 single-arm phase 2 and 2 phase 3 studies (**Tables 2–4**). Stratification of therapeutic management has recently been implemented.[4] Mitotane therapy and the combination of mitotane with locoregional therapies or cisplatinum-based cytotoxic chemotherapy remain the basis for the therapeutic management of these patients. Surgery remains the only curative treatment modality. There is no demonstration that median OS has improved in the past decades.[12,23]

SURGERY

ACC resection is the only curative treatment.[29,42] As stated in recommendations,[3,4,58,59] surgery should respect the rules of oncologic surgery and be performed within expert centers by expert surgeons and through laparotomy. In European guidelines, laparoscopy is accepted in cases of tumors smaller than 8 to 10 cm with no evidence of invasion. In all cases, not only expert surgeons but also expert multidisciplinary teams and active prospective registration of patients within dedicated databases are mandatory. Retrospective studies that compared the risk of recurrence in patients operated on by laparotomy or laparoscopy have shown comparable[60–63] or higher risk of recurrence after laparoscopy.[45,64,65] The absence of clear pathologic definitions of so-called stage I to II ACC in these studies as well as potential biases

Table 2
Tumor response rate to monotherapy in patients with ACC

Author, Year; Design (n)	Drug/Line	Dosage (g/d)	World Health Organization/ RECIST Criteria	Response (%)	Duration (mo)
Venkatesh et al,[81] 1989; retrospective (72)	M/1	NR	No	21 (29)	NA
Luton et al,[82] 1990; retrospective (37)	M/1	3–20	No	5 (13)	5–25
Decker et al,[83] 1991; prospective (36)	M/1	6	Yes	8 (22)	3–82
Pommier et al,[84] 1992; retrospective (29)	M/1	NA	No	7 (24)	NA
Haak et al,[85] 1994; retrospective (55)	M/1	4–8	Yes	15 (27)	2–190
Barzon et al,[86] 1997; retrospective (11)	M/1	4–8	Yes	2 (18)	12–21
Williamson et al,[87] 2000; prospective (16)	M/2	4–10	Yes	2 (13)	NA
Baudin et al,[88] 2001; prospective (13)	M/1	6–12	Yes	4 (33)	10–48
Gonzalez et al,[30] 2007; retrospective (52)	M/1	NA	No	13 (19)	NA
Decker et al,[83] 1991; phase 2 (16)	D/1	60 mg/m^2	No	3 (19)	3–51

Abbreviations: D, doxorubicin; M, mitotane.

in all series constitute significant limitations that preclude definitive conclusions. Pre-selection of R0 patients likely occurs in studies on laparoscopy as well as an increased number of patients referred at the time of recurrences for studies on laparotomy. To date, only half of all patients with ACC have been potentially resectable at diagnosis,[42] and the rate of R0 resection ranges between 53% and 58% in most modern series[18,29,31,60,66] but reached 76% to 89% in tertiary referral centers.[31,65] Thus, the increased rate of R0 resection at first surgery of adrenal tumors should be considered as the primary objective of all centers and networks worldwide. Tracks toward this objective encompass the restriction of adrenal surgery for suspected adrenal tumors to expert centers as well as better selection of resectable tumors. In addition, although the added value and definition of expert centers is still debated,[12,62,66,67] it is common sense to state that only such centers offer expert surgeons within a multidisciplinary team as well as adequate follow-up and registration.

Oncologic surgical resection standards (en bloc adrenal gland resection, margin-free resection, no tumor spillage, conversion to laparotomy in case of difficult dissection) must be strictly respected. For some patients with locally advanced tumor, the surgery requires en bloc resection of surrounding peritoneal tissue and adjacent organs. However, routine nephrectomy is not recommended in all patients. A lymphadenectomy may improve the prognosis or the staging, but its extent remains to be specified.[26] ACC with extension into the renal vein, vena cava, or right atrium may require thrombectomy, cardiopulmonary bypass, hepatectomy for local spread or exposure, and vena cava reconstruction.[43,44,68,69]

At the time of recurrence, surgery is recommended for patients with favorable prognostic factors, including a disease-free interval from previous surgery that is

Table 3
Tumor response rate to first-line cytotoxic chemotherapy in patients with ACC

Author, Year; Design (n)	Drugs	ACC Stage IV (%)	WHO/ RECIST Criteria	Response (%)	Disease Control Rate Duration (mo) (Range)
Williamson et al,[87] 2000; phase 2 (45)	E, P	94	SWOG	11	NA
Van Slooten et al,[96] 1983; retrospective (11)	(M)C, D, P	100	WHO	18	(6–9)
Bukoswski et al,[97] 1983; phase 2 (37)	M, P	100	No	30	Median 7.9 (1.4–36)
Khan et al,[98] 2000; phase 2 (22)	M, S	Not all	No	36	Median 7 (3–13)
Fassnacht et al,[28] 2012; phase 3 (153)	M, S	99	RECIST	9	Median 2.1
Schlumberger et al,[99] 1991; retrospective (14)	M, F, D, P	100	WHO	23	NA (4–42)
Bonacci et al,[100] 1998; retrospective (18)	M, E, P	88	WHO	33	NA (8–26)
Berruti et al,[70] 2005; phase 2 (72)	M, E, D, P	87	WHO	55	Median 9
Abraham et al,[101] 2002; phase 2 (36)	M, E, D, V	100	WHO	14	Median 12
Urup et al,[102] 2013; phase 2 (21)	M, Doc, P	100	RECIST	21	Median 3
Fassnacht et al,[28] 2012; phase 3 (151)	M, E, D, P	100	RECIST	23	Median 5
Lerario et al,[107] 2014; phase 1 (19)	M, Cixutumumab	100	RECIST	5	Median 1.5 (2.6–48)

Series are classified as a function of mitotane prescription, number, and type of drugs. Duration is expressed in median and ranges when available or percentage of control at a fixed date.

Abbreviations: C, cisplatin; D, doxorubicin; Doc, docetaxel; E, etoposide; F, 5-fluorouracil; M, mitotane; (M), signifies that mitotane was not given in all patients; NA, not available; P, paclitaxel; S, streptozotocin; SWOG, Southwest Oncology Group; V, vincristine; WHO, World Health Organization.

longer than 6 to 12 months, and achievable R0 resection.[31,32,40,50–52] If not possible, surgery may be reconsidered at the time of objective response.[30,70,71] In the palliative setting, surgery of the primary is also recommended in patients with favorable prognostic parameters if an R0 resection can be achieved.[16] Surgery of metastases is considered on a case-by-case basis and performed mainly in patients with favorable prognostic factors, sustained PR, and long-term survival with R0 resection expectations.[51,52] In all cases, postoperative mortality less than 5% is expected. **Fig. 2** recapitulates the use of ACC surgery in patients with ACC.

LOCOREGIONAL GUIDED THERAPY

Interventional radiology techniques may offer an alternative approach to surgery to control tumor growth and to improve secretory status in the palliative setting. They are recommended in combination with mitotane therapy in patients with advanced

Table 4
Tumor response rate to post-first-line cytotoxic chemotherapy in patients with ACC[a]

Author, Year; Design (n)	Drugs/Line	ACC Stage IV (%)	WHO/ RECIST Criteria	Response (%)	Disease Control Rate Duration (mo) (Range)
Baudin et al,[105] 2002; retrospective (12)	M, I	81	RECIST	0	NA (1.5–4)
Khan et al,[103] 2004; retrospective (9)	M, Cy, V, T, C	18	WHO	11	Median 6.7 (3–11)
Sperone et al,[104] 2010; retrospective (29)	M, F, G	87	RECIST	7	Median 5.3 (1–43)
Fassnacht et al,[28] 2012; phase 3 (86)	M, S	100	RECIST	NA	Median 2.2
Fassnacht et al,[28] 2012; phase 3 (101)	M, E, D, P	100	RECIST	NA	Median 5.5
Quinkler et al,[112] 2008; retrospective (10)	(M)G-Erlotinib	100	RECIST	0	NA (8)
Wortmann et al,[116] 2010; retrospective (10)	(M)Ca-Avastin	100	RECIST	0	Median 2.1
Kroiss et al,[90] 2012; phase 2 (35)	(M)Sunitinib	NA	RECIST	0	Median 2.9 (6–11)
Berruti et al,[4] 2012; phase 2 (9)	Paclitaxel-Sorafenib	20	RECIST	0	—
Sullivan et al,[115] 2014; phase 2 (13)	Axitinib	100	RECIST	0	Median 5.5 (1.8–10.9)
Haluska et al,[108] 2010; phase 1 (14)	(M)Figitumumab	NA	RECIST	0	43%–3 mo
Naing et al,[110] 2013; phase 1 (26)	(M)Cixutumumab-Temsirolimus	NA	RECIST	5	42%–6 mo
Fassnacht et al,[109] 2015; phase 3 (90)	Linsatinib	NA	RECIST	3	Median 1.5

Series are classified as a function of mitotane prescription, number, and type of drugs. Duration is expressed in median and ranges when available or percentage of control at a fixed date. (M) signifies that most patients, but not all, received concomitant mitotane therapy.

Abbreviations: C, cisplatin; Ca, capecitabin; Cy, cyclophosphamide; D, doxorubicin; E, etoposide; F, 5-fluorouracil; G, gemcitabine; I, irinotecan; M, mitotane; NA, not available; S, streptozotocin; T, teniposide; V, vincristine; WHO, World Health Organization.

[a] All patients received previous chemotherapy with at least mitotane and cisplatinum or streptozotocin except for Naing and Fassnacht, in which series only 50% of patients with ACC previously received cisplatinum therapy.

ACC with favorable prognostic factors.[4] The local rate of tumor control provided by these tools is superior to systemic options, justifying the increasing use of these modalities in patients with ACC.

Thermal ablation techniques, namely radiofrequency ablation and cryotherapy, are effective for curing small (<3 cm) metastatic lesions in the liver, lung, and bone. Minimal morbidity, short recovery time, and repeatability in the same organ are major advantages of these techniques.[72–74] Transarterial chemoembolization (TACE) consists of the injection of an emulsion of lipiodol (Guerbet, Aulnay sous Bois, France) and chemotherapy directly into the liver arterial supply. In one retrospective study using platinum-based TACE as second-line treatment,[75] an 83% rate of liver tumor control was reported at 3 months, and this was observed especially in patients with small metastases (≤ 3 cm).

RADIOTHERAPY

Radiotherapy (RT) is recommended in patients with ACC in the adjuvant setting in case of R1 resection in the European guidelines or in all stage III patients in the French guidelines.[4] In the palliative setting, RT is recommended to control bone or brain metastases. Proximity of the adrenals to critical organs, such as the kidney, stomach, intestine, and spinal cord, and radioresistance of ACC were supposed to argue against the use of RT in the setting of ACC. Recent technical improvements in RT techniques include stereotactic RT, intensity-modulated radiation therapy, and breathing motion monitoring techniques. Data from the German ACC registry also suggest a role for adjuvant RT after a macroscopically complete resection. Median dose was 50.4 Gy (range, 41.4–56 Gy), given in 1.8-Gy to 2.0-Gy daily fractions. Local recurrence appeared in 2 of 14 patients in the RT group and in 11 of 14 patients in the control group.[76] These recurrences developed in the adrenalectomy bed and the adjacent ipsilateral and contralateral interaortocaval lymph nodes. These results were confirmed in only 1 of 2 recently published studies, but none of these studies reported an improved OS rate.[77,78] Stereotactic RT was shown to provide a favorable effect when used for the management of metastasis to the adrenals with limited toxicity and in the palliative setting, showing a 27% response rate according to RECIST (Response Evaluation Criteria In Solid Tumors) in selected patients.[79] These results suggest an increasing role of RT in the future to control unresectable primary ACC, local recurrence, and the treatment of liver or lung metastases in patients with ACC.

MITOTANE THERAPY

Mitotane constitutes the most studied and specific systemic option for patients with ACC, but the mechanism of its antitumor action remains unknown.[80] Mitotane therapy is recommended in both the adjuvant setting in patients with ACC at high risk of recurrence and in the palliative setting in all patients, in combination with locoregional or other systemic options.[4] Mitotane is the only drug approved in Europe for the treatment of advanced ACC.

In the palliative setting, 6 retrospective and 3 prospective studies have analyzed the antitumor role of this drug as monochemotherapy in patients with unresectable ACC.[30,81–88] As described in **Table 2**, various dosages of the drug were used in a minimum of 11 to a maximum of 72 patients as first-line therapy in most cases. PRs were reported in 13% to 33% of cases, with response duration of 2 to 190 months. In the absence of placebo-controlled randomized trials, the real benefit of mitotane therapy on OS remains unknown. In addition, the delayed modality of action of this drug makes the feasibility of such a trial questionable in the future. Based on these results and progress in the prognostic stratification of patients with ACC with unresectable stage III to IV advanced disease, current recommendations suggest the use of mitotane in all patients in combination with either locoregional therapies or other systemic options in patients with favorable or poor prognostic parameters, respectively.[4]

The side effects of mitotane are diverse and target mainly the digestive (nausea, vomiting, diarrhea) and neurologic systems (vertigo, dizziness, somnolence, blurred vision, poor verbalization, and slow ideation). Awareness of these side effects is critical and requires dedicated education of patients and providers. Digestive secondary effects occur early and are believed to be related to a direct effect of the drug on the digestive mucosa. Because of its cytotoxic effect on the adrenals and the inhibitory effect on steroidogenesis, adrenal insufficiency is a logical consequence of mitotane therapy that requires both glucocorticoid and mineralocorticoid substitution. As a rule, the appearance of digestive cytotoxic effects requires an increase in cortisol supplementation both to control the stress and as a diagnostic test to diagnose insufficient replacement of cortisol. Mitotane is a strong inducer of liver enzyme activity, including CYP3A4, with major relevance regarding concomitant therapy such as cortisol replacement, vitamin K antagonist, oral contraception, and combined antitumor therapies.[13,54–56,89,90] As a practical consequence of this mitotane induction of CYP3A4 activity, the routine cortisol replacement dosage is folded by 2 or 3 compared with patients treated for primary adrenal insufficiency; in addition, heparin and mechanical contraception methods are favored. Blood monitoring of mitotane should include electrolyte measurements, liver tests, and blood cell measurements, because their respective alterations constitute rare but potentially severe cytotoxic targets of the drug. The relevance of monitoring gonadal steroids or thyroid function tests remains debatable in the absence of related symptoms.[91] Dyslipidemia should be treated with drugs that do not interfere with CYP3A4 liver enzyme activity.

Eight retrospective studies have explored the role of mitotane therapy in the adjuvant setting[14,15,17,21,88,92–95] but no single trial has been performed. Compared to historical controls, improved recurrence-free survival was reported in 4 and improved OS in 3, and was restricted to patients with cortisol secretion in 1. Based on these limited results and the progress on prognostic stratification, mitotane adjuvant therapy is recommended in patients with ACC at high risk of recurrence as defined by Ki67 higher than 10% or R1 resection.[4] Because of the high risk of recurrence of stage III ACC, adjuvant mitotane therapy is also recommended in these patients in the French guidelines. Patients with ACC with Ki67 less than 10% should be enrolled in the ongoing ADIUVO (Efficacy of Adjuvant Mitotane Treatment) trial, which is investigating the role of mitotane in patients with stage I to III ACC after R0 resection on recurrence-free survival in the prospective setting.

CYTOTOXIC CHEMOTHERAPY

Apart from mitotane, only doxorubicin has been tested as monochemotherapy in first-line or post-first-line patients with stage IV ACC (see **Table 2**). With doxorubicin used in first line, a 19% objective response rate was reported in 1 study.[83] No confirmatory study has been published.

Apart from the 2 studies mentioned earlier, mitotane therapy has been combined with a cytotoxic agent in all studies but two that analyzed the results of first-line cytotoxic chemotherapy (see **Table 3**). In addition, no randomized trial comparing the antitumor role of mitotane combined or not with other chemotherapy has been published. Therefore, in 2015, the benefit of combining mitotane with other cytotoxic drugs compared with mitotane alone remains unknown. The results of the combination of etoposide and cisplatinum or cyclophosphamide, doxorubicin, cisplatin without mitotane has been published in 2 studies[87,96]; PR rates were 11% to 18% (see **Table 3**). Two phase 2 studies have analyzed the antitumor effect of mitotane combined with 1 single drug chemotherapy: cisplatinum or streptozotocin in 35 and 22 patients, respectively[97,98]; a PR of 30% has been reported with a 7.9-month median duration[97] and a 36% PR rate with a 7-month median duration.[98]

Five other studies have analyzed the antitumor effect of mitotane combined with cytotoxic polychemotherapy. PR rates between 14% and 55% were reported.[70,96,99–102] Cisplatinum or doxorubicin was the most frequently used drug. Response rate higher than 20% was reported in all series that used at least mitotane and cisplatinum chemotherapy with a disease control rate for 3 to 9 months. In patients pretreated with streptozotocin- or cisplatinum-based chemotherapy (see **Table 4**), 2 PRs in 28 patients were reported with the combination of gemcitabine and 5-fluorouracil and a time to progression of 5.3 months, which constitutes the best result reported to date.[103–105]

Recently, the first international randomized in locally advanced and metastatic adrenocortical carcinoma phase 3 trial (FIRMACT) performed in patients with ACC, which compared the OS of patients with advanced ACC randomized for either an MEDP or mitotane and streptozotocin (MS) regimen was published.[28] A nonstatistically significant gain in OS of 2.8 months was reported with a statistically significant impact of the MEDP arm on secondary end points like PR rate or progression-free survival (PFS) compared with the MS regimen. These results established MEDP as the first standard of chemotherapy in patients with advanced ACC.[4] The gain in OS (17.1 vs 4.7 months) in the subgroup of 119 patients with ACC who did not receive second-line chemotherapy but were given MEDP as first line also supports the use of MEDP as a standard. The PR rate or median PFS was 30% and 5 months or 11% and 2.1 months in the MEDP or MS arms, respectively. Based on these results, the use of streptozotocin in patients with ACC seems ineffective. Although these trials did not meet the primary end point, this first randomized study on ACC provided robust results to rationalize future phase 2 hypotheses. In parallel, it is well known that combining mitotane with other cytotoxic agents increases the rate of side effects.[97] Therefore, there is an urgent need for novel therapies for ACC that are both more effective and better tolerated than the current MEDP standard. With a 10% OR in second or third lines and 5.3-month time to progression, the combination of gemcitabine and 5-fluorouracil is recommended after cisplatinum-based chemotherapy, but no validation has been provided.[104]

MOLECULAR TARGETED THERAPIES

Few studies have investigated the use of targeted molecular therapies for ACC mostly in the post-first-line setting and in combination with mitotane (see **Tables 2** and **4**). Based on insulin growth factor 2 hyperexpression, and cell signaling through insulin growth factor 1 receptor (IGF-1R) and insulin receptor (IR), preclinical and phase 1 studies have investigated the role of IGF-1R inhibitors with PRs in some phase 1 studies[106,107] but not in all.[108] Recently, the negative results of a placebo-controlled phase 3 study analyzing the antitumor effect of linsitinib, a dual IGF-1R and IR small molecule inhibitor, on OS and PFS analyses were reported.[109] However, 4 of 139 patients clearly benefited from the drug, as shown by prolonged tumor responses, with no escape after 23 months or more. These results suggest a benefit of IGF-1R inhibition, as a single agent, in 3% of patients with ACC in whom the molecular background remains to be identified. Using the same approach, IGF-1R antibody cixutumumab combined with mitotane as first-line therapy for 19 cases of ACC, with 1 PR and a PFS of 6 weeks, was considered insufficient to proceed to a phase 2 study.[107] By contrast, the combination of cixutumumab with temsirolimus-mammalian target of rapamycin pathway inhibitor yielded interesting results, as shown by a 42% rate of stabilization at 6 months in a series of heavily pretreated ACCs.[110] These results await further confirmation. Prognostic characteristics of patients with ACC and plasma level mitotane levels were lacking, precluding precise conclusions. In 2 different series, 19 and 10 patients were treated with epidermal growth factor receptor inhibitors in combination with gemcitabine in one[111,112]; no PR was observed. Four patients with ACC received imatinib or everolimus in 2 studies, with no response.[113,114]

Preliminary experiences from several other endocrine cancers show prolonged tumor control with antiangiogenic therapy, but the benefit of this strategy has not yet been confirmed in patients with ACC. Two phase 2 trials analyzed the antitumor response to sunitinib or axitinib and reported no PR and median PFS of 83 days or 5 months in 35 or 13 pretreated patients with ACC, respectively.[90,115] In 2 additional phase 2 trials, combination of antiangiogenic agents with chemotherapy was investigated. In 1 study, bevacizumab plus capecitabine in 10 pretreated patients with ACC produced no PR and median PFS was 59 days.[116] In a second study, tumor progression was observed in all 9 patients at 2 months treated with the combination of sorafenib and taxol.[117] One recent phase 1 trial with the combination of imatinib with dacarbazine and capecitabine in 7 pretreated patients with ACC produced 1 PR.[118] These results show no role of antiangiogenic agents in patients with ACC, but the absence of pharmacokinetic analysis of these agents at the time of investigation makes the potential interaction of mitotane a possible explanation.[90]

PREDICTORS AND SURROGATE MARKERS OF RESPONSE

The elucidation of predictors of response to mitotane therapy or the MEDP regimen is a key step to select patients with ACC who are the most likely to respond and to encourage likely nonresponders to undergo first-line protocols with alternative agents. Studies of predictors and surrogate markers of response in patients with ACC in the recently published FIRMACT trials are ongoing.

PREDICTORS OF RESPONSE

Mitotane plasma level monitoring is recommended in ACC management with the objective of reaching 14 to 20 mg/L,[3,4] but this level is achieved in only up to 50% of patients with ACC.[3,4,18,85,88] Higher PR rates[85,88,119] and improved OS or recurrence-free survival have been reported[71,85,95,119,120] in retrospective studies when plasma mitotane levels higher than 14 mg/L were reached. One recent retrospective study confirmed the 14-mg/L mitotane plasma level as the best compromise to predict tumor response but also found a better sensitivity of 89% or specificity of 90% when the 10-mg/L or 20-mg/L cutoffs were used.[119] These results suggest a revision of the 14-mg/L to 20-mg/L standard plasma mitotane window to a standard of 10 to 30 mg/L.[119] Recent studies have shown that a high-dose strategy may increase the chance of obtaining earlier therapeutic plasma mitotane levels, but no statistical difference was observed.[121,122] Based on these recent results, we now use a maximum tolerated dose approach, as described in **Fig. 3**, based on the search for the highest tolerated dose maintained during at least 2 RECIST evaluations 2 to 3 months apart and a range of plasma mitotane levels between 10 and 30 mg/L. Other predictors of response to mitotane therapy have been proposed, including DNA repair gene excision repair complementation group 1,[71,123] high ribonucleotide reductase large subunit,[124] CYP2W1[125] and cortisol secretion,[14] but these have not been confirmed. In addition, 1 recent study[119] failed to show any additional value of mitotane metabolite measurements, especially 1,1-(o,p'-dichlorodiphenyl) acetic acid.

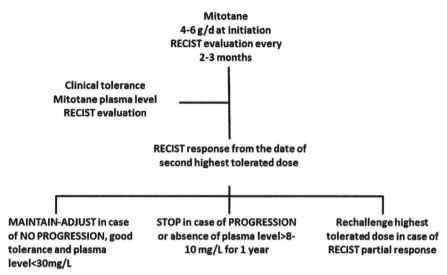

Fig. 3. Mitotane therapy management in the palliative setting at Gustave Roussy in 2015.

SURROGATES OF RESPONSE

Four retrospective studies have reported a relationship between complete response or PR and improved survival[19,70,71,101] but this was not confirmed in 1 study.[97] Prolonged median survival of responders more than 34 months was reported. These results suggest that responders should be reconsidered for proper personalized management, including locoregional options such as surgery. One preliminary study did not disclose any role for FDG-PET as an early surrogate of response.[34] Circulating tumor cells may also be a tool to consider in the future.[126]

FUTURE STRATEGIES FOR DEVELOPING TREATMENTS AGAINST ADRENOCORTICAL CARCINOMA

Looking for actionable targets in each patient with ACC is a major goal of personalized therapy. Major breakthroughs have been achieved in the identification of relevant molecular alterations in ACC but no simple actionable target has emerged. Among these molecular abnormalities, the overexpression of IGFII is the most frequent but its role as a target for therapy for ACC has been invalidated by a recent phase 3 clinical trial that failed to show any significant antitumor efficacy.[109,127,128] β-Catenin signaling and p53/Rb pathways as well as chromatin remodeling constitute the most frequent molecular alterations in ACC of various TNM stages.[35-39] CTNNB1 and TP53 mutations are present in 20% to 70% and 16% to 31% of patients with ACC, respectively,[35-39,53,128-130] but no simple targeting of such molecular abnormalities is available.

Next-generation sequencing allows for the analysis of a large set of genes in a time span compatible with clinical needs. In a recently published study, we screened new potentially targetable molecular abnormalities in a large cohort of advanced ACCs.[130] No simple actionable alteration of genes, including EGFR, BRAF, KIT, PIK3CA, RET, or PDGFR-A, that are targetable by available drugs was found. Based on the most common gene abnormalities detected (TP53

Box 2
Recommendations for future studies in ACC

- Patients with ACC who undergo any kind of therapeutic intervention should be subject to clear definition and to a thorough clinical and molecular standardized characterization of their disease

- Studies on prognostic stratification should still be implemented to achieve the most precise characterization of ACC outcomes within each TNM and GRAS subgroup

- Recommended therapeutic strategies used for patients with ACC should be prospectively recorded, once patient permission is granted, in dedicated registries to minimize missing data and to achieve progresses with historical therapies

- Mitotane plasma levels should be recorded at the time of new therapeutic evaluation as well as best response under mitotane therapy. Scenarios on the best modality of evaluation of new drug therapy in patients treated with mitotane should be clarified in near future

- Predictors of response to mitotane therapy and markers of resistance as well as surrogates of OS should be elucidated

- Researchers should develop parallel single-arm phase 2 clinical trials with similar primary end points in which PR or PFS is a major end point. In all cases, precise molecular characterization should be implemented at the time of enrollment and progression

- Efforts should be made to enroll patients with ACC within phase 1

- Phase 3 should remain the last step of drug validation, keeping in mind that a gain in 2 months of OS requires 300 patients per arm to provide statistically significant results. Stratification for mitotane therapy and prognostic parameters should be implemented

---

(15%), *ATM* (12.5%), and *CTNNB1* (10%) mutations, *CDK4* (cyclin-dependent kinase-4) amplification (17.9%) and *CDKN2A* (14.3%) and *CDKN2B* (10.7%) deletion genes, which are all directly or indirectly involved in controlling G1-S phase cell cycle progression, are the most commonly altered. We recently suggested that drugs targeting the cell cycle could be the most relevant new therapeutic approach.[130] Based on frequent gains of fibroblast growth factor receptors (FGFR) 1 to 4, we also suggested that the FGFR pathway could be a potential target for treatment in patients with ACC. Conversely, *HER2* (ERBB2) amplification was not present in ACC, in accordance with previous reports. Recently, a similar approach was conducted and similar conclusions were reached, with most frequent genomic abnormalities occurring on *TP53*, *CDKN21*, *CTNNB1*, and *ATM* and *NF1* and *MEN1* in more than 10% of cases.[131]

Making therapeutic advances against ACC, a rare cancer, is a formidable challenge facing patients and clinicians. The rarity of ACC makes phase 3 clinical trials as the basis of proof of concept a challengeable practice when urgent improvements are expected. However, recommendations such as those described in **Box 2** may help in the development of new treatments for ACC. These strategies are supported by multiple expert groups on different continents and international networking initiatives such as ENSAT.

ACKNOWLEDGMENTS

The members of the Endocrine Tumor Board of Gustave Roussy (Department of Endocrine Oncology and Nuclear Medicine), who served as co-authors for this article, are: Segolene Hescot, MD; Amandine Berdelou, MD; Isabelle Borget, PharmD; Caroline Caramella, MD; Frederic Dumont, MD; Desirée Deandreis, MD; Frederic Deschamps, MD; Eric Deutsch, MD, PhD; Abir Al Ghuzlan, MD; Marc Lombes, MD, PhD; Rossella Libe, MD; Angelo Paci, PharmD; Jean-Yves Scoazec, MD, PhD; Jacques Young, MD, PhD; Sophie Leboulleux, MD, PhD; Martin Schlumberger, MD, PhD.

REFERENCES

1. Weiss LM. Comparative histologic study of 43 metastasizing and nonmetastasizing adrenocortical tumors. Am J Surg Pathol 1984;8(3):163–9.
2. Sbiera S, Schmull S, Assie G, et al. High diagnostic and prognostic value of steroidogenic factor-1 expression in adrenal tumors. J Clin Endocrinol Metab 2010;95(10):E161–71.
3. Schteingart DE, Doherty GM, Gauger PG, et al. Management of patients with adrenal cancer: recommendations of an international consensus conference. Endocr Relat Cancer 2005;12(3):667–80.
4. Berruti A, Baudin E, Gelderblom H, et al. Adrenal cancer: ESMO clinical practice guidelines for diagnosis, treatment and follow-up. Ann Oncol 2012;23(Suppl 7): vii131–8.
5. Goldblum JR, Shannon R, Kaldjian EP, et al. Immunohistochemical assessment of proliferative activity in adrenocortical neoplasms. Mod Pathol 1993;6(6):663–8.
6. Terzolo M, Boccuzzi A, Bovio S, et al. Immunohistochemical assessment of Ki-67 in the differential diagnosis of adrenocortical tumors. Urology 2001; 57(1):176–82.
7. Gupta D, Shidham V, Holden J, et al. Value of topoisomerase II alpha, MIB-1, p53, E-cadherin, retinoblastoma gene protein product, and HER-2/neu immunohistochemical expression for the prediction of biologic behavior in adrenocortical neoplasms. Appl Immunohistochem Mol Morphol 2001;9(3):215–21.
8. Aubert S, Wacrenier A, Leroy X, et al. Weiss system revisited: a clinicopathologic and immunohistochemical study of 49 adrenocortical tumors. Am J Surg Pathol 2002;26(12):1612–9.
9. Stojadinovic A, Ghossein RA, Hoos A, et al. Adrenocortical carcinoma: clinical, morphologic, and molecular characterization. J Clin Oncol 2002;20(4):941–50.
10. Søreide JA, Brabrand K, Thoresen SO. Adrenal cortical carcinoma in Norway, 1970-1984. World J Surg 1992;16(4):663–7 [discussion: 668].
11. Kebebew E, Reiff E, Duh QY, et al. Extent of disease at presentation and outcome for adrenocortical carcinoma: have we made progress? World J Surg 2006;30(5):872–8.
12. Kerkhofs TM, Verhoeven RH, Van der Zwan JM, et al. Adrenocortical carcinoma: a population-based study on incidence and survival in the Netherlands since 1993. Eur J Cancer 2013;49(11):2579–86.
13. Else T, Kim AC, Sabolch A, et al. Adrenocortical carcinoma. Endocr Rev 2014; 35(2):282–326.
14. Abiven G, Coste J, Groussin L, et al. Clinical and biological features in the prognosis of adrenocortical cancer: poor outcome of cortisol-secreting tumors in a series of 202 consecutive patients. J Clin Endocrinol Metab 2006;91(7): 2650–5.
15. Beuschlein F, Weigel J, Saeger W, et al. Major prognostic role of Ki67 in localized adrenocortical carcinoma after complete resection. J Clin Endocrinol Metab 2015;100(3):841–9.

16. Libé R. Prognostic factors for synchronous stage III and IV adrenocortical carcinomas (ACC): an ENSAT study. 2015.

17. Else T, Williams AR, Sabolch A, et al. Adjuvant therapies and patient and tumor characteristics associated with survival of adult patients with adrenocortical carcinoma. J Clin Endocrinol Metab 2014;99(2):455–61.

18. Ayala-Ramirez M, Jasim S, Feng L, et al. Adrenocortical carcinoma: clinical outcomes and prognosis of 330 patients at a tertiary care center. Eur J Endocrinol 2013;169(6):891–9.

19. Berruti A, Fassnacht M, Haak H, et al. Prognostic role of overt hypercortisolism in completely operated patients with adrenocortical cancer. Eur Urol 2014;65(4): 832–8.

20. Arlt W, Biehl M, Taylor AE, et al. Urine steroid metabolomics as a biomarker tool for detecting malignancy in adrenal tumors. J Clin Endocrinol Metab 2011;96(12): 3775–84.

21. Icard P, Goudet P, Charpenay C, et al. Adrenocortical carcinomas: surgical trends and results of a 253-patient series from the French Association of Endocrine Surgeons study group. World J Surg 2001;25(7):891–7.

22. Fassnacht M, Johanssen S, Quinkler M, et al. Limited prognostic value of the 2004 International Union Against Cancer staging classification for adrenocortical carcinoma: proposal for a revised TNM classification. Cancer 2009;115(2):243–50.

23. Kutikov A, Mallin K, Canter D, et al. Effects of increased cross-sectional imaging on the diagnosis and prognosis of adrenocortical carcinoma: analysis of the National Cancer Database. J Urol 2011;186(3):805–10.

24. Miller BS, Gauger PG, Hammer GD, et al. Resection of adrenocortical carcinoma is less complete and local recurrence occurs sooner and more often after laparoscopic adrenalectomy than after open adrenalectomy. Surgery 2012; 152(6):1150–7.

25. Do Cao C, Leboulleux S, Borget I, et al. First prognostic analysis of stage iii adrenocortical carcinoma patients after complete resection: a retrospective French multicentric study from the INCA-COMETE network. European Congress of Endocrinology 2011 [abstract 414].

26. Reibetanz J, Jurowich C, Erdogan I, et al. Impact of lymphadenectomy on the oncologic outcome of patients with adrenocortical carcinoma. Ann Surg 2012; 255(2):363–9.

27. Assié G, Antoni G, Tissier F, et al. Prognostic parameters of metastatic adrenocortical carcinoma. J Clin Endocrinol Metab 2007;92(1):148–54.

28. Fassnacht M, Terzolo M, Allolio B, et al. Combination chemotherapy in advanced adrenocortical carcinoma. N Engl J Med 2012;366(23):2189–97.

29. Bilimoria KY, Shen WT, Elaraj D, et al. Adrenocortical carcinoma in the United States: treatment utilization and prognostic factors. Cancer 2008;113(11):3130–6.

30. Gonzalez RJ, Tamm EP, Ng C, et al. Response to mitotane predicts outcome in patients with recurrent adrenal cortical carcinoma. Surgery 2007;142(6):867–75 [discussion: 867–75].

31. Dy BM, Wise KB, Richards ML, et al. Operative intervention for recurrent adrenocortical cancer. Surgery 2013;154(6):1292–9 [discussion: 1299].

32. Erdogan I, Deutschbein T, Jurowich C, et al. The role of surgery in the management of recurrent adrenocortical carcinoma. J Clin Endocrinol Metab 2013; 98(1):181–91.

33. Deandreis D, Leboulleux S, Caramella C, et al. FDG PET in the management of patients with adrenal masses and adrenocortical carcinoma. Horm Cancer 2011;2(6):354–62.

34. Takeuchi S, Balachandran A, Habra MA, et al. Impact of 18F-FDG PET/CT on the management of adrenocortical carcinoma: analysis of 106 patients. Eur J Nucl Med Mol Imaging 2014;41(11):2066–73.

35. Assié G, Letouzé E, Fassnacht M, et al. Integrated genomic characterization of adrenocortical carcinoma. Nat Genet 2014;46(6):607–12.

36. Giordano TJ, Kuick R, Else T, et al. Molecular classification and prognostication of adrenocortical tumors by transcriptome profiling. Clin Cancer Res 2009;15(2): 668–76.

37. Barreau O, Assié G, Wilmot-Roussel H, et al. Identification of a CpG island methylator phenotype in adrenocortical carcinomas. J Clin Endocrinol Metab 2013; 98(1):E174–84.

38. Duregon E, Rapa I, Votta A, et al. MicroRNA expression patterns in adrenocortical carcinoma variants and clinical pathologic correlations. Hum Pathol 2014; 45(8):1555–62.

39. Juhlin CC, Goh G, Healy JM, et al. Whole-exome sequencing characterizes the landscape of somatic mutations and copy number alterations in adrenocortical carcinoma. J Clin Endocrinol Metab 2015;100(3):E493–502.

40. Schulick RD, Brennan MF. Long-term survival after complete resection and repeat resection in patients with adrenocortical carcinoma. Ann Surg Oncol 1999;6(8):719–26.

41. Lughezzani G, Sun M, Perrotte P, et al. The European Network for the Study of Adrenal Tumors staging system is prognostically superior to the International Union Against Cancer-staging system: a North American validation. Eur J Cancer 2010;46(4):713–9.

42. Asare EA, Wang TS, Winchester DP, et al. A novel staging system for adrenocortical carcinoma better predicts survival in patients with stage I/II disease. Surgery 2014;156(6):1378–85 [discussion: 1385–6].

43. Turbendian HK, Strong VE, Hsu M, et al. Adrenocortical carcinoma: the influence of large vessel extension. Surgery 2010;148(6):1057–64 [discussion: 1064].

44. Mihai R, Iacobone M, Makay O, et al. Outcome of operation in patients with adrenocortical cancer invading the inferior vena cava–a European Society of Endocrine Surgeons (ESES) survey. Langenbecks Arch Surg 2012;397(2):225–31.

45. Miller BS, Gauger PG, Hammer GD, et al. Proposal for modification of the ENSAT staging system for adrenocortical carcinoma using tumor grade. Langenbecks Arch Surg 2010;395(7):955–61.

46. Berruti A, Fassnacht M, Baudin E, et al. Adjuvant therapy in patients with adrenocortical carcinoma: a position of an international panel. J Clin Oncol 2010; 28(23):e401–2 [author reply: e403].

47. Volante M, Bollito E, Sperone P, et al. Clinicopathological study of a series of 92 adrenocortical carcinomas: from a proposal of simplified diagnostic algorithm to prognostic stratification. Histopathology 2009;55(5):535–43.

48. Johanssen S, Hahner S, Saeger W, et al. Deficits in the management of patients with adrenocortical carcinoma in Germany. Dtsch Arztebl Int 2010;107(50): 885–91.

49. De Reyniès A, Assié G, Rickman DS, et al. Gene expression profiling reveals a new classification of adrenocortical tumors and identifies molecular predictors of malignancy and survival. J Clin Oncol 2009;27(7):1108–15.

50. Bellantone R, Ferrante A, Boscherini M, et al. Role of reoperation in recurrence of adrenal cortical carcinoma: results from 188 cases collected in the Italian National Registry for Adrenal Cortical Carcinoma. Surgery 1997;122(6): 1212–8.

51. Gaujoux S, Al-Ahmadie H, Allen PJ, et al. Resection of adrenocortical carcinoma liver metastasis: is it justified? Ann Surg Oncol 2012;19(8):2643–51.
52. Datrice NM, Langan RC, Ripley RT, et al. Operative management for recurrent and metastatic adrenocortical carcinoma. J Surg Oncol 2012;105(7):709–13.
53. Ragazzon B, Libé R, Gaujoux S, et al. Transcriptome analysis reveals that p53 and {beta}-catenin alterations occur in a group of aggressive adrenocortical cancers. Cancer Res 2010;70(21):8276–81.
54. Veytsman I, Nieman L, Fojo T. Management of endocrine manifestations and the use of mitotane as a chemotherapeutic agent for adrenocortical carcinoma. J Clin Oncol 2009;27(27):4619–29.
55. Schteingart DE. Drugs in the medical treatment of Cushing's syndrome. Expert Opin Emerg Drugs 2009;14(4):661–71.
56. Van der Pas R, de Herder WW, Hofland LJ, et al. New developments in the medical treatment of Cushing's syndrome. Endocr Relat Cancer 2012;19(6): R205–23.
57. Kamenický P, Droumaguet C, Salenave S, et al. Mitotane, metyrapone, and ketoconazole combination therapy as an alternative to rescue adrenalectomy for severe ACTH-dependent Cushing's syndrome. J Clin Endocrinol Metab 2011; 96(9):2796–804.
58. Stefanidis D, Goldfarb M, Kercher KW, et al. SAGES guidelines for minimally invasive treatment of adrenal pathology. Surg Endosc 2013;27(11):3960–80.
59. Henry JF, Sebag F, Iacobone M, et al. Results of laparoscopic adrenalectomy for large and potentially malignant tumors. World J Surg 2002;26(8):1043–7.
60. Brix D, Allolio B, Fenske W, et al. Laparoscopic versus open adrenalectomy for adrenocortical carcinoma: surgical and oncologic outcome in 152 patients. Eur Urol 2010;58(4):609–15.
61. Porpiglia F, Fiori C, Daffara F, et al. Retrospective evaluation of the outcome of open versus laparoscopic adrenalectomy for stage I and II adrenocortical cancer. Eur Urol 2010;57(5):873–8.
62. Lombardi CP, Raffaelli M, De Crea C, et al. Endoscopic adrenalectomy: is there an optimal operative approach? Results of a single-center case-control study. Surgery 2008;144(6):1008–14 [discussion: 1014–5].
63. Donatini G, Caiazzo R, Do Cao C, et al. Long-term survival after adrenalectomy for stage I/II adrenocortical carcinoma (ACC): a retrospective comparative cohort study of laparoscopic versus open approach. Ann Surg Oncol 2014; 21(1):284–91.
64. Leboulleux S, Deandreis D, Al Ghuzlan A, et al. Adrenocortical carcinoma: is the surgical approach a risk factor of peritoneal carcinomatosis? Eur J Endocrinol 2010;162(6):1147–53.
65. Cooper AB, Habra MA, Grubbs EG, et al. Does laparoscopic adrenalectomy jeopardize oncologic outcomes for patients with adrenocortical carcinoma? Surg Endosc 2013;27(11):4026–32.
66. Hermsen IG, Kerkhofs TM, den Butter G, et al. Surgery in adrenocortical carcinoma: importance of national cooperation and centralized surgery. Surgery 2012;152(1):50–6.
67. Gratian L, Pura J, Dinan M, et al. Treatment patterns and outcomes for patients with adrenocortical carcinoma associated with hospital case volume in the United States. Ann Surg Oncol 2014;21(11):3509–14.
68. Chiche L, Dousset B, Kieffer E, et al. Adrenocortical carcinoma extending into the inferior vena cava: presentation of a 15-patient series and review of the literature. Surgery 2006;139(1):15–27.

69. Fabre D, Houballah R, Fadel E, et al. Surgical management of malignant tumours invading the inferior vena cava. Eur J Cardiothorac Surg 2014;45(3): 537–42 [discussion: 542–3].
70. Berruti A, Terzolo M, Sperone P, et al. Etoposide, doxorubicin and cisplatin plus mitotane in the treatment of advanced adrenocortical carcinoma: a large prospective phase II trial. Endocr Relat Cancer 2005;12(3):657–66.
71. Malandrino P, Al Ghuzlan A, Castaing M, et al. Prognostic markers of survival after combined mitotane- and platinum-based chemotherapy in metastatic adrenocortical carcinoma (ACC). Endocr Relat Cancer 2010;17(3):797–807.
72. Deschamps F, Farouil G, Ternes N, et al. Thermal ablation techniques: a curative treatment of bone metastases in selected patients? Eur Radiol 2014;24(8): 1971–80.
73. Ripley RT, Kemp CD, Davis JL, et al. Liver resection and ablation for metastatic adrenocortical carcinoma. Ann Surg Oncol 2011;18(7):1972–9.
74. Wood BJ, Abraham J, Hvizda JL, et al. Radiofrequency ablation of adrenal tumors and adrenocortical carcinoma metastases. Cancer 2003;97(3):554–60.
75. Cazejust J, De Baère T, Auperin A, et al. Transcatheter arterial chemoembolization for liver metastases in patients with adrenocortical carcinoma. J Vasc Interv Radiol 2010;21(10):1527–32.
76. Fassnacht M, Hahner S, Polat B, et al. Efficacy of adjuvant radiotherapy of the tumor bed on local recurrence of adrenocortical carcinoma. J Clin Endocrinol Metab 2006;91(11):4501–4.
77. Sabolch A, Feng M, Griffith K, et al. Adjuvant and definitive radiotherapy for adrenocortical carcinoma. Int J Radiat Oncol Biol Phys 2011;80(5):1477–84.
78. Habra MA, Ejaz S, Feng L, et al. A retrospective cohort analysis of the efficacy of adjuvant radiotherapy after primary surgical resection in patients with adrenocortical carcinoma. J Clin Endocrinol Metab 2013;98(1):192–7.
79. Ho J, Turkbey B, Edgerly M, et al. Role of radiotherapy in adrenocortical carcinoma. Cancer J 2013;19(4):288–94.
80. Hescot S, Slama A, Lombès A, et al. Mitotane alters mitochondrial respiratory chain activity by inducing cytochrome c oxidase defect in human adrenocortical cells. Endocr Relat Cancer 2013;20(3):371–81.
81. Venkatesh S, Hickey RC, Sellin RV, et al. Adrenal cortical carcinoma. Cancer 1989;64(3):765–9.
82. Luton JP, Cerdas S, Billaud L, et al. Clinical features of adrenocortical carcinoma, prognostic factors, and the effect of mitotane therapy. N Engl J Med 1990;322(17):1195–201.
83. Decker RA, Elson P, Hogan TF, et al. Eastern Cooperative Oncology Group study 1879: mitotane and adriamycin in patients with advanced adrenocortical carcinoma. Surgery 1991;110(6):1006–13.
84. Pommier RF, Brennan MF. An eleven-year experience with adrenocortical carcinoma. Surgery 1992;112(6):963–70 [discussion: 970–1].
85. Haak HR, Hermans J, van de Velde CJ, et al. Optimal treatment of adrenocortical carcinoma with mitotane: results in a consecutive series of 96 patients. Br J Cancer 1994;69(5):947–51.
86. Barzon L, Fallo F, Sonino N, et al. Adrenocortical carcinoma: experience in 45 patients. Oncology 1997;54(6):490–6.
87. Williamson SK, Lew D, Miller GJ, et al. Phase II evaluation of cisplatin and etoposide followed by mitotane at disease progression in patients with locally advanced or metastatic adrenocortical carcinoma: a Southwest Oncology Group Study. Cancer 2000;88(5):1159–65.

88. Baudin E, Pellegriti G, Bonnay M, et al. Impact of monitoring plasma 1,1-dichlorodiphenildichloroethane (o,p'DDD) levels on the treatment of patients with adrenocortical carcinoma. Cancer 2001;92(6):1385–92.

89. Van Erp NP, Guchelaar HJ, Ploeger BA, et al. Mitotane has a strong and a durable inducing effect on CYP3A4 activity. Eur J Endocrinol 2011;164(4): 621–6.

90. Kroiss M, Quinkler M, Johanssen S, et al. Sunitinib in refractory adrenocortical carcinoma: a phase II, single-arm, open-label trial. J Clin Endocrinol Metab 2012;97(10):3495–503.

91. Daffara F, De Francia S, Reimondo G, et al. Prospective evaluation of mitotane toxicity in adrenocortical cancer patients treated adjuvantly. Endocr Relat Cancer 2008;15(4):1043–53.

92. Bodie B, Novick AC, Pontes JE, et al. The Cleveland Clinic experience with adrenal cortical carcinoma. J Urol 1989;141(2):257–60.

93. Terzolo M, Angeli A, Fassnacht M, et al. Adjuvant mitotane treatment for adrenocortical carcinoma. N Engl J Med 2007;356(23):2372–80.

94. Grubbs EG, Callender GG, Xing Y, et al. Recurrence of adrenal cortical carcinoma following resection: surgery alone can achieve results equal to surgery plus mitotane. Ann Surg Oncol 2010;17(1):263–70.

95. Terzolo M, Baudin E, Ardito A, et al. Mitotane levels predict the outcome of patients with adrenocortical carcinoma treated adjuvantly following radical resection. Eur J Endocrinol 2013;169(3):263–70.

96. Van Slooten H, van Oosterom AT. CAP (cyclophosphamide, doxorubicin, and cisplatin) regimen in adrenal cortical carcinoma. Cancer Treat Rep 1983; 67(4):377–9.

97. Bukowski RM, Wolfe M, Levine HS, et al. Phase II trial of mitotane and cisplatin in patients with adrenal carcinoma: a Southwest Oncology Group study. J Clin Oncol 1993;11(1):161–5.

98. Khan TS, Imam H, Juhlin C, et al. Streptozocin and o,p'DDD in the treatment of adrenocortical cancer patients: long-term survival in its adjuvant use. Ann Oncol 2000;11(10):1281–7.

99. Schlumberger M, Brugieres L, Gicquel C, et al. 5-Fluorouracil, doxorubicin, and cisplatin as treatment for adrenal cortical carcinoma. Cancer 1991;67(12): 2997–3000.

100. Bonacci R, Gigliotti A, Baudin E, et al. Cytotoxic therapy with etoposide and cisplatin in advanced adrenocortical carcinoma. Br J Cancer 1998;78(4): 546–9.

101. Abraham J, Bakke S, Rutt A, et al. A phase II trial of combination chemotherapy and surgical resection for the treatment of metastatic adrenocortical carcinoma: continuous infusion doxorubicin, vincristine, and etoposide with daily mitotane as a P-glycoprotein antagonist. Cancer 2002;94(9):2333–43.

102. Urup T, Pawlak WZ, Petersen PM, et al. Treatment with docetaxel and cisplatin in advanced adrenocortical carcinoma, a phase II study. Br J Cancer 2013; 108(10):1994–7.

103. Khan TS, Sundin A, Juhlin C, et al. Vincristine, cisplatin, teniposide, and cyclophosphamide combination in the treatment of recurrent or metastatic adrenocortical cancer. Med Oncol 2004;21(2):167–77.

104. Sperone P, Ferrero A, Daffara F, et al. Gemcitabine plus metronomic 5-fluorouracil or capecitabine as a second-/third-line chemotherapy in advanced adrenocortical carcinoma: a multicenter phase II study. Endocr Relat Cancer 2010; 17(2):445–53.

105. Baudin E, Docao C, Gicquel C, et al. Use of a topoisomerase I inhibitor (irinotecan, CPT-11) in metastatic adrenocortical carcinoma. Ann Oncol 2002;13(11):1806–9.
106. Jones RL, Kim ES, Nava-Parada P, et al. Phase I study of intermittent oral dosing of the insulin-like growth factor-1 and insulin receptors inhibitor OSI-906 in patients with advanced solid tumors. Clin Cancer Res 2015;21(4):693–700.
107. Lerario AM, Worden FP, Ramm CA, et al. The combination of insulin-like growth factor receptor 1 (IGF1R) antibody cixutumumab and mitotane as a first-line therapy for patients with recurrent/metastatic adrenocortical carcinoma: a multi-institutional NCI-sponsored trial. Horm Cancer 2014;5(4):232–9.
108. Haluska P, Worden F, Olmos D, et al. Safety, tolerability, and pharmacokinetics of the anti-IGF-1R monoclonal antibody figitumumab in patients with refractory adrenocortical carcinoma. Cancer Chemother Pharmacol 2010;65(4):765–73.
109. Fassnacht M, Berruti A, Baudin E, et al. Linsitinib (OSI-906) versus placebo for patients with locally advanced or metastatic adrenocortical carcinoma: a double-blind, randomised, phase 3 study. Lancet Oncol 2015.
110. Naing A, Lorusso P, Fu S, et al. Insulin growth factor receptor (IGF-1R) antibody cixutumumab combined with the mTOR inhibitor temsirolimus in patients with metastatic adrenocortical carcinoma. Br J Cancer 2013;108(4):826–30.
111. Samnotra V, Vassilopoulou-Sellin R, Fojo T, et al. A phase II trial of gefinitinib monotherapy in patients with unresectable adrenocortical carcinoma. J Clin Oncol 2007 [abstract 15527].
112. Quinkler M, Hahner S, Wortmann S, et al. Treatment of advanced adrenocortical carcinoma with erlotinib plus gemcitabine. J Clin Endocrinol Metab 2008;93(6):2057–62.
113. Gross DJ, Munter G, Bitan M, et al. The role of imatinib mesylate (Glivec) for treatment of patients with malignant endocrine tumors positive for c-kit or PDGF-R. Endocr Relat Cancer 2006;13(2):535–40.
114. Fraenkel M, Gueorguiev M, Barak D, et al. Everolimus therapy for progressive adrenocortical cancer. Endocrine 2013;44(1):187–92.
115. O'Sullivan C, Edgerly M, Velarde M, et al. The VEGF inhibitor axitinib has limited effectiveness as a therapy for adrenocortical cancer. J Clin Endocrinol Metab 2014;99(4):1291–7.
116. Wortmann S, Quinkler M, Ritter C, et al. Bevacizumab plus capecitabine as a salvage therapy in advanced adrenocortical carcinoma. Eur J Endocrinol 2010;162(2):349–56.
117. Berruti A, Sperone P, Ferrero A, et al. Phase II study of weekly paclitaxel and sorafenib as second/third-line therapy in patients with adrenocortical carcinoma. Eur J Endocrinol 2012;166(3):451–8.
118. Halperin DM, Phan AT, Hoff AO, et al. A phase I study of imatinib, dacarbazine, and capecitabine in advanced endocrine cancers. BMC Cancer 2014;14:561.
119. Hermsen IG, Fassnacht M, Terzolo M, et al. Plasma concentrations of o,p'DDD, o,p'DDA, and o,p'DDE as predictors of tumor response to mitotane in adrenocortical carcinoma: results of a retrospective ENSAT multicenter study. J Clin Endocrinol Metab 2011;96(6):1844–51.
120. Wängberg B, Khorram-Manesh A, Jansson S, et al. The long-term survival in adrenocortical carcinoma with active surgical management and use of monitored mitotane. Endocr Relat Cancer 2010;17(1):265–72.
121. Mauclère-Denost S, Leboulleux S, Borget I, et al. High-dose mitotane strategy in adrenocortical carcinoma: prospective analysis of plasma mitotane measurement during the first 3 months of follow-up. Eur J Endocrinol 2012;166(2):261–8.

122. Kerkhofs TM, Baudin E, Terzolo M, et al. Comparison of two mitotane starting dose regimens in patients with advanced adrenocortical carcinoma. J Clin Endocrinol Metab 2013;98(12):4759–67.
123. Ronchi CL, Sbiera S, Kraus L, et al. Expression of excision repair cross complementing group 1 and prognosis in adrenocortical carcinoma patients treated with platinum-based chemotherapy. Endocr Relat Cancer 2009;16(3):907–18.
124. Volante M, Terzolo M, Fassnacht M, et al. Ribonucleotide reductase large subunit (RRM1) gene expression may predict efficacy of adjuvant mitotane in adrenocortical cancer. Clin Cancer Res 2012;18(12):3452–61.
125. Ronchi CL, Sbiera S, Volante M, et al. CYP2W1 is highly expressed in adrenal glands and is positively associated with the response to mitotane in adrenocortical carcinoma. PLoS ONE 2014;9(8):e105855.
126. Pinzani P, Scatena C, Salvianti F, et al. Detection of circulating tumor cells in patients with adrenocortical carcinoma: a monocentric preliminary study. J Clin Endocrinol Metab 2013;98(9):3731–8.
127. Drelon C, Berthon A, Val P. Adrenocortical cancer and IGF2: is the game over or our experimental models limited? J Clin Endocrinol Metab 2013;98(2):505–7.
128. El Wakil A, Lalli E. The Wnt/beta-catenin pathway in adrenocortical development and cancer. Mol Cell Endocrinol 2011;332(1-2):32–7.
129. Wasserman JD, Zambetti GP, Malkin D. Towards an understanding of the role of p53 in adrenocortical carcinogenesis. Mol Cell Endocrinol 2012;351(1):101–10.
130. De Martino MC, Al Ghuzlan A, Aubert S, et al. Molecular screening for a personalized treatment approach in advanced adrenocortical cancer. J Clin Endocrinol Metab 2013;98(10):4080–8.
131. Ross JS, Wang K, Rand JV, et al. Next-generation sequencing of adrenocortical carcinoma reveals new routes to targeted therapies. J Clin Pathol 2014;67(11): 968–73.

Surgical Management of Adrenocortical Carcinoma

Gustavo G. Fernandez Ranvier, MD[a], William B. Inabnet III, MD[b],*

KEYWORDS

- Adrenocortical tumor • Adrenocortical carcinoma
- Metastatic adrenocortical carcinoma • Open adrenalectomy • Mitotane treatment
- Chemotherapy for adrenocortical carcinoma

KEY POINTS

- Adrenocortical carcinoma (ACC) is one of the most aggressive malignant endocrine tumors.
- ACC has a bimodal age distribution, with the first peak occurring at the age of 5 years and the second in the fourth to sixth decade of life.
- A comprehensive biochemical evaluation is required before surgical resection.
- Complete surgical resection is the first-line treatment of ACC.
- The definite diagnosis of ACC is made by the presence of preoperative locoregional invasion or distant metastases on imaging studies or the presence of capsular or vascular invasion on postoperative pathology specimens.

INTRODUCTION

Adrenocortical carcinoma (ACC) is one of the most malignant endocrine tumors.[1,2] ACC occurs infrequently, with an incidence of 2 cases per million persons per year.[1,3–9] In the United States, ACC accounts for 0.2% of cancer-related deaths.[1,2] ACC is one of the most aggressive cancers, generally carrying a poor prognosis because most patients present with large tumors and advanced disease.[2] Adrenocortical carcinoma has a bimodal age distribution, with the first peak occurring at the age of 5 years and the second in the fourth to sixth decade of life.[2,8] Adrenocortical carcinoma is most common in women, with an female/male ratio ranging from 1.5:1 to

Disclosure: The authors have nothing to disclose.
[a] Division of Metabolic, Endocrine and Minimally Invasive Surgery, Department of Surgery, Mount Sinai Hospital, Icahn School of Medicine at Mount Sinai, 5 East 98th Street, Box 1259, New York, NY 10029, USA; [b] Department of Surgery, Mount Sinai Beth Israel, Icahn School of Medicine at Mount Sinai, First Ave at 16th St, Baird Hall, 16th Floor, Suite 20, New York, NY 10003, USA
* Corresponding author.
E-mail address: william.inabnet@mountsinai.org

2.5:1.[2,7,10–12] These tumors are most often sporadic, but may occur in patients with hereditary syndromes such as multiple endocrine neoplasia type 1 (MEN1), Li-Fraumeni syndrome, and Beckwith-Wiedemann syndrome.[13–15] The incidence is 10-fold to 15-fold higher in children in southern Brazil, where some environmental factors and genetic changes have been identified in the pathogenesis of adrenocortical carcinoma.[16–18] These tumors may be hormone-secreting tumors (functional), leading to Cushing syndrome or virilization, or may be nonfunctional.

Because ACC can lead to the rapid development of locoregional invasion or distant metastasis, the 5-year survival rate varies from 32% to 50% for patients with resectable tumors. The median survival rate is less than 1 year for patients who present with metastatic disease.[19,20] Detection of tumors at an early clinical stage is imperative for curative resection. Surgical resection of ACC remains the first-line treatment and accomplishing an initial complete resection (R0) of the tumor is the most important factor for treatment success.[1,2,21,22] It is important to understand that patients with ACC require a comprehensive assessment and plan for the treatment of their disease in the preoperative, operative, and postoperative periods that should be performed by a multidisciplinary group of specialists ideally with representation from radiology, nuclear medicine, endocrinology, endocrine surgery, medical oncology, pathology, and genetics.

Surgical techniques for the treatment of ACC have evolved in the last 2 decades. The classic open transabdominal or lumbar approaches have slowly been replaced by the laparoscopic approach for removal of benign adrenocortical tumors.[23,24] However, although there is an ongoing debate on the role of the laparoscopic approach for the treatment of ACC, open techniques remain the approach of choice for treating most malignant primary adrenal disorders.

The main focus of this article is to provide comprehensive insight into the surgical management of ACC with an up-to-date review of surgical decision making.

MOLECULAR PATHOGENESIS

The molecular events involved in the development of sporadic ACC remain poorly understood.[24] As in colorectal cancer, a multistep tumor progression model has also been proposed for ACC.[19] Mutations of the TP53 gene (chromosome 17p13) are the most frequent mutations reported in human cancers.[25] The common finding of loss of heterozygosity (LOH) at the 17p13 locus in sporadic ACC suggests an important role of the TP53 tumor suppressor gene in the pathogenesis of sporadic ACC.[26,27] Specific germline mutations have been identified in some high-risk populations, such as a subset of children from a southern Brazilian population with one of highest incidences of ACC, occurring 10 to 15 times more frequently than the general population.[16–18] In this population, a distinct TP53 germline mutation (R337H) has been identified in up to 97% of children with adrenocortical tumors.[28–30] However, only a fraction of patients with ACC harbor a mutation of TP53, indicating that there are likely to be other molecular events responsible for the pathogenesis of ACC that have not been yet identified.[28–36]

Other chromosomal syndromes have been strongly implicated in the pathogenesis of ACC. Alterations of the DNA methylation of 11p15, the area of abnormality in Beckwith-Wiedemann syndrome, have been implicated in the pathogenesis of ACC.[37] The chromosomal locus 11p15 harbors the coding region for insulinlike growth factor (IGF)-2. Both the LOH at 11p15 and the overexpression of IGF-2 have been associated with the development of sporadic ACC.[26,38,39]

In contrast with the more commonly seen sporadic ACC, a subset of adrenocortical tumors are associated with hereditary cancer syndromes.[15] The Li-Fraumeni syndrome (breast cancer, soft tissue and bone sarcoma, brain tumors, and ACC) is associated with inactivating germline mutations of the TP53 tumor suppressor gene on chromosome 17p.[40-42] The Beckwith-Wiedemann syndrome (Wilms tumor, neuroblastoma, hepatoblastoma, and ACC), is associated with abnormalities in 11p15. MEN1, parathyroid, pituitary, pancreatic neuroendocrine tumors, and adrenal adenomas, as well as carcinoma, are associated with inactivating mutations of the MEN1 gene on chromosome 11q. Unilateral or bilateral adrenal tumors can be found in 20% to 40% of patients with MEN1; most are benign tumors, usually nonfunctional, but they can present with excess production of aldosterone or cortisol. A small subset of patients with MEN1 develop ACC.[43]

PRESENTATION

A careful history and physical examination should be performed to exclude signs and symptoms of pheochromocytoma, primary aldosteronism, hyperandrogenism, and Cushing syndrome. About 40% to 60% of all ACC tumors are functional and present with clinical symptoms related to hormone excess.[6,8,11,20,44,45] Adults with hormone-secreting ACC usually present with features of Cushing syndrome (50%–80%) and in some cases with an associated virilization syndrome consequent to the overproduction of both glucocorticoids and androgens. In some cases of severe hypercortisolism, patients present with signs and symptoms of mineralocorticoid excess as a consequence of glucocorticoid-mediated mineralocorticoid receptor activation.[8,46] The clinical symptoms associated with glucocorticoid excess (weight gain, weakness, and insomnia) usually develop rapidly over a period of 3 to 6 months. Patients who have coexisting hypersecretion of adrenal androgens may not experience the typical catabolic effects of glucocorticoid excess (muscle and skin atrophy). A less common presentation is virilization alone, but the presence of virilization in a patient with an adrenal neoplasm should increase suspicion of ACC.[15] Feminization and primary aldosteronism occur in fewer than 10% of cases.[47] Among all ACC tumors, about 20% to 30% are nonfunctioning tumors or have increased levels of adrenal steroid precursors without clinical manifestations of hormone hypersecretion. In these cases, patients usually present with clinical manifestations related to local tumor growth, such as early satiety, abdominal pain, and/or flank pain.[15,48] The remaining 20% to 30% are found incidentally as an adrenal mass detected on radiographic imaging performed for unrelated clinical reasons.

In children, most patients with ACC present with virilization (84%), whereas glucocorticoid excess alone (Cushing syndrome) or in association with other hormonal excess is uncommon.[49,50]

DIAGNOSTIC TOOLS AND DIFFERENTIATION BETWEEN BENIGN AND MALIGNANT ADRENOCORTICAL TUMORS
Biochemical/Hormonal Evaluation

The first step on diagnosis of a patient with an adrenal tumor is to determine whether it is functional or not. In the presence of an adrenal mass suspicious for ACC, a comprehensive hormonal evaluation is a mandatory step before surgery (**Table 1**).[48,51] Hormonal evaluation may help in establishing the adrenal origin of the tumor and provide tumor markers that can be useful during surveillance and follow-up after a surgical resection to estimate the presence of residual tumor or tumor recurrence.[25,48]

Adrenal carcinomas are typically inefficient steroid producers, but they secrete excessive amounts of adrenal steroid precursors because of decreased expression of several steroidogenic enzymes that may also result in diminished cortisol

Table 1
Biochemical work-up of patients with suspected ACC (ENSAT recommendations)

Hormonal Work-up	
Glucocorticoid excess (minimum 3 of 4 tests)	Dexamethasone suppression test (1 mg, 23 h) Excretion of free urinary cortisol (24-h urine) Basal cortisol (serum) Basal ACTH (plasma)
Sexual steroid and steroid precursors	DHEA-S (serum) 17-OH progesterone (serum) Androstenedione (serum) Testosterone (serum) 17β-estradiol (serum, only in men and postmenopausal women)
Mineralocorticoid excess	Potassium (serum) Aldosterone/renin ratio (if hypertension and/or hypokalemia)
Exclusion of pheochromocytoma (minimum 1 of 3 tests)	Metanephrines (plasma)

Abbreviations: ACTH, adrenocorticotropic hormone; DHEA-S, dehydroepiandrosterone sulfate; ENSAT, European Network for the Study of Adrenal Tumors.

production. Even in patients with no evidence of excess steroid production, more sensitive methods, such as gas chromatography/mass spectrometry, identify increased urinary metabolites of several steroids and precursors of androgens (pregnanediol, pregnanetriol, androsterone, etiocholanolone) or glucocorticoids (17-hydroxyproesterone, tetrahydro-11-deoxycortisol, cortisol, 6-hydroxy-cortisol, tetrahydrocortisol, and alpha-cortol); this is different from cortisol-secreting adenomas, which produce cortisol but do not produce high levels of adrenal steroid precursors or adrenal androgens.[52] Low serum aldosterone concentrations, but normal or high serum or urinary concentrations of aldosterone precursors (ie, deoxycorticosterone, 18-hydroxydeoxycorticosterone, corticosterone, 18-hydroxycorticosterone, tetrahydro-11-deoxycorticosterone [THDOC], and 5 alpha-THDOC) are found in most adrenal carcinomas, but not in adrenal adenomas.[52]

It is also mandatory to rule out the presence of a pheochromocytoma by determination of metanephrines in plasma and/or urine before attempting resection of any adrenal mass, and also to obtain plasma aldosterone and renin levels in patients with hypertension and/or hypokalemia.

Imaging

On imaging studies, both the size and appearance are important in distinguishing benign from malignant adrenal disorders. Computed tomography (CT) and magnetic resonance imaging (MRI) both contribute to the characterization of adrenal masses (**Figs. 1** and **2**).[53–55] These studies are also important for determining resectability and the relationship to adjacent structures. Suspicious features to consider at the time of evaluation are tumor size, heterogeneity, the presence of tumor calcification or central necrosis, tumor infiltration into surrounding tissue or invasion into organs, and functionality of the tumor. Malignant adrenocortical tumors are usually large with a median size of 13 cm (range, 8–29 cm), as reported in a large national cancer registry study.[2] On unenhanced CT imaging, most ACC has a washout of less than 50% and an attenuation of greater than 30 Hounsfield units, indicating low lipid

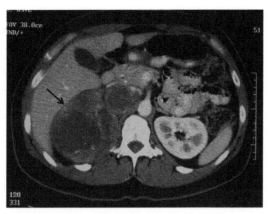

Fig. 1. CT imaging showing a large right adrenocortical carcinoma (*arrow*) with inferior vena cava compression.

content.[17] The most common sites of distant spread for ACC are the liver, lungs, lymph nodes, and bone (see **Fig. 2**).[8,56] For this reason, CT imaging of the chest and liver is typically included in the staging work-up if ACC is suspected based on the imaging evaluation or clinical presentation.

In a similar way, ACC most frequently presents as a large heterogeneous lesion with high intensity on T2-weighted images on MRI (see **Fig. 2**).[53] Similar features can also

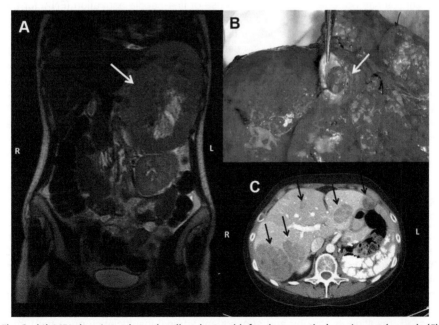

Fig. 2. (*A*) MRI showing a large locally advanced left adrenocortical carcinoma (*arrow*). (*B*) Specimen from the same patient after an en bloc resection showing tumor thrombus/invasion into the left renal artery (*arrow*). (*C*) CT imaging of the same patient with metastatic disease to the liver (*arrows*) 2 years after initial surgical resection.

be seen with pheochromocytoma, underscoring the need for biochemical assessment combined with radiologic evaluation. MRI/magnetic resonance angiography is the best method to determine invasion into adjacent organs and also the presence of tumor thrombosis (see **Fig. 2**).

PET scanning with fluorodeoxyglucose (FDG) is of value for identifying unilateral adrenal tumors with a high index of suspicion for malignancy as well as for determining the presence and extent of metastatic disease.[57–61] Although PET is more sensitive than CT or radiographic bone scans for distant metastases in a variety of clinical settings, false-negatives are possible and careful interpretation should be undertaken, especially when analyzing small lesions.[58] Furthermore, FDG-PET helps to differentiate benign from malignant lesions but it does not distinguish between adrenocortical or nonadrenocortical lesions (eg, metastases or adrenocortical carcinoma).[62]

The combination of PET-CT imaging improves the performance of PET and can also be useful for diagnosis of ACC, but it can be nonspecific in differentiating ACC from adenomas or pheochromocytoma.[55] With PET-CT, adrenal adenomas can be better differentiated from nonadenomas using a combination of CT attenuation measurements plus the intensity of FDG uptake.[63–65]

Other alternative PET scan tracers are under investigation.[62,66] Metomidate is the most widely used because it binds with high specificity and affinity to CYP11B (cytochrome P450, family 11, subfamily B) enzymes of the adrenal cortex. Because these enzymes are exclusively expressed in adrenocortical cells, uptake of labeled metomidate tracers has been shown to be highly specific for adrenocortical neoplasia versus pheochromocytomas or metastases.[62]

Role of Fine-Needle Aspiration Biopsy

Consensus has not been reached on the use of fine-needle aspiration (FNA) for the diagnosis of ACC.[53,54] FNA biopsies are of limited benefit in the evaluation of primary adrenocortical tumors because differentiation between benign and malignant tumors cannot be accurately established with needle biopsy alone. The only definitive diagnostic criterion for a malignant primary adrenocortical tumor is distant metastasis and/or the presence of local invasion. However, FNA can help distinguish a primary adrenal tumor from a metastatic lesion (usually in patients with known, advanced malignancies) or infectious/infiltrative causes.[53,67,68] However, if there is a high index of suspicion that an adrenal mass is ACC, FNA is generally discouraged because of the possibility of disrupting the tumor capsule or seeding the needle track.[69] If FNA is undertaken, it is essential that a diagnosis of pheochromocytoma be excluded with plasma metanephrines before the biopsy.

TREATMENT
Role of Preoperative Hormonal Therapy for Adrenocortical Carcinoma

According to the medical guidelines of the American Association of Endocrine Surgeons for the management of adrenal tumors, all patients suspected of having ACC should undergo biochemical testing to identify hormonal abnormalities and to determine whether the patient requires steroid replacement in cases of hypercortisolism.[51] Preoperative preparation is essential in patients with hypercortisolism. Depending on the functionality and hormonal characteristics, the contralateral gland may be suppressed, resulting in atrophy and subsequent adrenal insufficiency once the tumor has been removed. Current recommendations suggest that patients with clinical or subclinical Cushing syndrome be treated with 50 mg of intravenous hydrocortisone before the induction of anesthesia and 50 mg every 6 hours for 24 hours.[70] The dose of hydrocortisone should be then tapered by half per day until it is discontinued or a maintenance level has been reached. Assuming that only 1 adrenal gland has been surgically resected, the duration of the steroid therapy depends on the time to recovery of the hypothalamic-pituitary-adrenal axis, which can take up to 2 years in some cases.[71]

Surgical Treatment

Open adrenalectomy

Surgical resection remains the first-line treatment of ACC. Depending on tumor staging, there are different modalities and treatments. Most patients with a presumed localized ACC should undergo surgical resection because surgery is the only effective modality of treatment.[72] Because complete resection is the only curative option for localized disease, special care should be taken when dissecting the tumor margins to accomplish a complete R0 resection without violation of the tumor capsule. A complete surgical resection can be accomplished in those patients with potentially resectable disease stage classification (European Network for the Study of Adrenal Tumors [ENSAT] stage I–III; **Tables 2** and **3**). For potentially resectable tumors invading adjacent organs, surgery often needs to be extensive, with en bloc resection of involved organs such as the kidney, liver, spleen, pancreas, stomach, and colon.[1] Intracaval extension or tumor thrombus (see **Fig. 2**), which should be looked for on preoperative imaging, is not a contraindication to surgery; these findings may require cardiothoracic or subspecialty surgery collaboration and the use of cardiopulmonary bypass.[73]

ACC often spreads via lymphatic drainage. A benefit for routine lymphadenectomy during adrenalectomy was suggested in a report from the German ACC Study Group of 283 patients with completely resected ACC.[74] There was a significantly reduced risk for tumor recurrence and disease-related death in patients who underwent lymphadenectomy versus those who did not.

Although resection is technically possible for most patients with stage I to III disease, it is not curative for many, presumably because occult micrometastases are

Table 2	
TNM (tumor, node, metastasis) staging system for ACC	
Primary Tumor (T)	
TX	Primary tumor cannot be assessed
T0	No evidence of primary tumor
T1	Tumor ≤5cm in greatest dimension, no extra-adrenal invasion
T2	Tumor >5 cm in greatest dimension, no extra-adrenal invasion
T3	Tumor of any size with local invasion (periadrenal tissue), but not invading adjacent organs
T4	Tumor of any size with invasion of adjacent organs (kidney, diaphragm, great vessels, pancreas, spleen, liver)
Regional Lymph Nodes (N)	
NX	Regional lymph nodes cannot be assessed
N0	No regional lymph node metastasis
N1	Metastasis in regional lymph nodes
Distant Metastasis (M)	
M0	No distant metastasis
M1	Distant metastasis

Table 3 Comparison of UICC/WHO and ENSAT staging classification of ACC		
Stage	**UICC/WHO**	**ENSAT**
I	T1, N0, M0	T1, N0, M0
II	T2, N0, M0	T2, N0, M0
III	T3, N0, M0 T1–2, N1, M0	T3–4, N0, M0 T1–4, N1, M0
IV	T3, N1, M0 T4, N0–1, M0 Any M1	Any M1

Abbreviations: UICC, Union Internationale Contre le Cancer; WHO, World Health Organization.

present at the time of initial presentation, even with stage I disease.[1,6,75] As an example, in a single-center report of 202 consecutive cases of ACC, 40% of patients with stage I to III disease developed distant metastasis 2 years after diagnosis (27%, 46%, and 63% of patients with stage I, II, and III disease, respectively).[56]

Laparoscopic adrenalectomy

Laparoscopic adrenalectomy has largely replaced open techniques for the management of benign adrenal disorders, and laparoscopic removal of even large adrenal tumors can be performed safely by experienced surgeons.[76] However, debate still exists on the role of laparoscopic resection for ACC. Current guidelines on the surgical management of ACC clearly support open resection for known cases of ACC. Several retrospective studies have shown more frequent or earlier recurrences and a shorter disease-free survival when a laparoscopic approach is used for management of ACC.[77–79] In one study of 153 patients who underwent open adrenalectomy versus 6 laparoscopic resections, peritoneal carcinomatosis was observed in 8% of the patients with open resection in contrast with the development of carcinomatosis in 100% of patients undergoing laparoscopic resection.[77] In contrast, other studies have shown that the laparoscopic approach had comparable outcomes compared with open adrenalectomy in terms of oncologic outcomes, particularly for tumors up to 10 cm.[80–85] Nonetheless, current guidelines do not recommend a laparoscopic approach for known or highly suspected ACC.[51,77,78]

PATHOLOGY AND STAGING

The pathologic diagnosis of ACC is frequently challenging. The distinction between benign and malignant adrenocortical tumors should only be made by pathologists experienced in using the microscopic Weiss criteria (**Box 1**).[71,86] The only definitive diagnostic criterion for a malignant adrenocortical tumor is distant metastasis or the presence of local invasion. To date, the Weiss criteria are the most commonly used histopathologic system to determine adrenocortical malignancy.[71,86] In addition to the classic microscopic evaluation of ACC, other immunohistochemical markers have been proposed (Ki-67 proliferation index, TP53, IGF-2, cyclin E) but were not sufficiently discriminatory in distinguishing ACC from benign adrenal disorders.[70]

Although the best staging system for ACC is evolving, a variety of staging systems have been used for ACC.[20,37,45,87] The TNM (tumor, node, metastasis) staging system from the American Joint Commission on Cancer (AJCC)/International Union Against Cancer (UICC) (see **Tables 2** and **3**) is widely used but a new staging system proposed by ENSAT has gained popularity (see **Table 3**).[73] The ENSAT staging system has

> **Box 1**
> **Histopathologic features included in the Weiss criteria for evaluation of ACC**
>
> - Nuclear grade 3 to 4
> - Mitotic rate greater than 6/50 high-power fields
> - Less than 25% clear tumor cells in cytoplasm
> - Atypical mitoses
> - Diffuse architecture
> - Confluent necrosis
> - Venous invasion
> - Sinusoidal invasion
> - Capsular invasion
>
> On microscopic evaluation, the diagnosis of ACC is made with a score greater than or equal to 3, whereas a tumor with a score of 2 is of uncertain malignancy.

better prognostic stratification restricting stage IV tumors to patients with distant metastases. The superiority of the ENSAT staging system compared with the 2004 UICC/AJCC classification to determine prognosis of ACC was confirmed in an independent cohort study of 573 cases.[69]

POSTOPERATIVE MANAGEMENT
Therapeutic Agents for Hormonal Control

Adrenal hormonal function should be closely monitored in patients with ACC because patients may develop either adrenal insufficiency (caused by surgery or mitotane) or excess cortisol secretion (caused by persistent or recurrent tumor) in the perioperative period. In patients with hypercortisolism the administration of a specific adrenal enzyme inhibitor is often required. Controlling hypercortisolism is critical to avoid chemotherapy-induced or hypercortisolism-induced complications, such as immunosuppression-related infections or even death, from these endocrine complications rather than from tumor burden.

Metyrapone is a commonly used drug in patients with ACC and hypercortisolism. Ketoconazole is effective in benign adrenal disease, but is rarely effective to control the hypercortisolism in ACC. With the use of metyrapone, eucortisolemia can be achieved within a week. If eucortisolism is not achieved with metyrapone, a combination therapy with ketoconazole and mitotane can be used. A starting dosage of metyrapone 250 mg 4 times daily is recommended. This dosage can then be increased up to 6 g/d. If there is not appropriate response with metyrapone alone or it is not tolerated, ketoconazole is started at 200 mg 3 times per day, increasing daily as needed to 400 mg 3 times per day. Their effect can be assessed within a few days by measuring 24-hour urine cortisol levels. A combination of both drugs and mitotane may be necessary to achieve adequate control in some circumstances. In severe uncontrolled cases, addition of mifepristone, a glucocorticoid receptor antagonist, can be beneficial.[88] In patients who are unable to take drugs orally, intravenous etomidate (which blocks 11-beta-hydroxylase) can be used at a low dosage of 0.3 mg/kg/h. The use of etomidate requires a specialized team and appropriate hemodynamic monitoring.

Adrenal insufficiency is initially managed using replacement with intravenous hydrocortisone and then oral glucocorticoids for maintenance. Mitotane induces the metabolism of glucocorticoids, so higher-than-usual replacement doses are needed in patients receiving mitotane therapy. Aldosterone deficiency is replaced with the addition of fludrocortisone (0.1–0.3 mg daily) and adjusted to restore normal blood pressure and serum levels of potassium and renin. A small percentage of adult patients with ACC and a high percentage of pediatric patients with ACC present with virilization with/without hypercortisolism. Virilization is best treated with specific androgen blockage with androgen receptor inhibitors (bicalutamide at 50 mg/d) or 5-alpha reductase inhibition (finasteride at 5 mg/d).

Rare estrogen-producing ACC tumors can be treated with any of the antiestrogen therapies, including tamoxifen or aromatase inhibitors.

Mitotane Therapy

Mitotane is an adrenocorticolytic/adrenal enzyme inhibitor drug that has efficacy in patients with ACC.[89] It has been used in the adjuvant setting, for primary therapy for unresectable disease (stage IV), and for the treatment of disease recurrence, either alone or in combination with other cytotoxic agents.

Data showing the benefit of routine postoperative (adjuvant) administration of mitotane have been mixed, in large part because of the rarity of ACC and the lack of prospective randomized clinical trials. Although several uncontrolled reports suggest that adjuvant mitotane may delay or prevent recurrence in patients undergoing complete primary resection for nonmetastatic disease,[90–96] others have failed to show any benefit in terms of disease-free or overall survival.[11,20,44–46,97–99]

Despite the ongoing debate about who should be treated with mitotane, its use is generally recommended in those patients with metastatic disease or advanced localized disease in which a high recurrence rate is expected. The decision to use mitotane should be made on a case-by-case basis considering critical prognostic factors such as completeness of resection, proliferation rate, and accurate tumor staging to identify the high-risk patients with increased chances of tumor recurrence.[100–102]

Other Chemotherapy Protocols

It remains unknown whether chemotherapy alone or in combination with mitotane is more effective than adjuvant mitotane alone.

Adjuvant chemotherapy plus mitotane

A few prospective trials have explored combination regimens that contain mitotane. Although no chemotherapy regimen has been shown to improve overall survival in patients with advanced ACC, some of the more encouraging results have been with the combination of etoposide, doxorubicin, and cisplatin plus mitotane.[103,104]

Results with other chemotherapy drugs combined with mitotane are less promising.[105–107]

Chemotherapy without mitotane

Although they are frequently used, single agents such as cisplatin, cyclophosphamide, or doxorubicin are associated with poor response rates.[108,109] The overall result of chemotherapy protocols without the use of mitotane is discouraging.[108–111]

Radiation Therapy

It was thought that malignant adrenocortical tumors were radioresistant tumors; however, this is not likely to be true, at least in light of most recent studies.[112–114] Although there are no randomized trials testing the efficacy of adjuvant radiotherapy (RT) in patients with resected ACC, some support a benefit in certain patients who are at high risk for a local recurrence.[112,113] However, in a recent retrospective study of 16 patients with ACC who had undergone either surgery followed by adjuvant RT or surgery alone, the rate of local recurrence was not significantly reduced by adjuvant RT.[114] In addition, even in the studies that show an apparent benefit of adjuvant RT in decreasing local recurrences, neither disease-free nor overall survival was significantly better in irradiated patients.[112,113]

The currently available data in the literature support the palliative benefit of RT for unresectable local tumor that is causing local symptoms, or for distant symptomatic metastases, such as in bone, brain, and vena cava.[1,112,115,116]

Additional Surgery

Adrenocortical carcinoma with locally advanced, recurrent or metastatic disease

Locally advanced, recurrent, or metastatic ACC has a dismal prognosis. However, in those cases in which the tumor cannot be removed entirely, or in those cases with recurrent or distant metastatic disease, many studies have advocated that tumor debulking may have an impact on survival and at least some reports suggest that long-term survival rates are higher among patients who undergo resection of recurrent or metastatic disease,[1,11,21,44,87,117–119] although others disagree.[46]

In a study of 47 patients with ACC undergoing resection for locally recurrent or distant metastatic disease, the 5-year survival rates for patients with completely and incompletely resected locally recurrent disease were 57% and 0%, respectively.[119] Similar outcomes were reported in a study of 57 patients undergoing different surgical procedures for recurrent or metastatic ACC, with a 5-year survival of 41%, and median survival significantly longer for those with a disease-free interval greater than 12 months (6.6 vs 1.7 years). Another study of 28 patients undergoing resection for liver metastases from ACC (25 isolated, 3 with extrahepatic metastases), the 5-year survival rate was 39%.[118] The investigators concluded that, in selected patients with ACC liver metastases, resection is associated with an improvement in long-term survival, although it is not curative.

If complete resection is feasible, an aggressive surgical approach to locally recurrent disease, with the aim of achieving negative surgical margins, should be undertaken.[119–121] Resection may also be considered in the rare patients who present with limited, potentially resectable hepatic or pulmonary metastases. Resection of locally recurrent disease may also be indicated for patients in whom surgery is able to remove most, but not all, of the tumor burden or decrease severe hypercortisolism that is otherwise difficult to control.[4] This approach should be limited to selected patients with uncontrollable symptomatic hormone excess or those who are in imminent danger from organ invasion/compression.

Tumor debulking of nonresectable ACC should be considered on a case-by-case basis, taking into consideration the overall patient condition, tumor biology, rate of progression, and the histologic grade.[1] In those cases of invasive disease and tumors with high hormonal production, the patients may benefit from a palliative tumor reduction.[44,122] However, in some patients the presence of unresectable high-grade tumors may limit their treatment to palliation with medical management.[8]

Surveillance Strategy

For patients with a completely resected steroid-producing ACC, patients should be monitored every 3 months for 2 years with steroid tumor markers such as cortisol, dehydroepiandrosterone sulfate, androstenedione, testosterone, estradiol, or mineralocorticoid based on the steroid profile of the initial tumor. Careful interpretation of biochemical values should be undertaken in those patients receiving mitotane therapy because it alters steroid hormone levels and metabolism. The 24-hour urinary free cortisol excretion remains as the best index of cortisol production currently available.[123] Plasma adrenocorticotropic hormone (ACTH) levels may be used to measure reduction in cortisol (ACTH becomes detectable) and possible adrenal insufficiency (ACTH level increases beyond normal values).

PROGNOSIS

The overall survival for ACC is poor. It is estimated that the 5-year survival rate is approximately 32% to 50% for patients with resectable tumors and the median survival rate is less than 1 year for those with metastatic disease.[19,20] The most important clinical factors that determine prognosis of ACC are disease stage and completeness of resection.[8,11,20,29]

Tumor staging remains one of the best prognostic tools; however, survival may differ widely for any given tumor stage because many other factors, including genetic predisposition, could influence the outcomes.

SUMMARY

The molecular events involved in the pathogenesis of ACC remain unclear in most cases. Patients with ACC or with adrenal tumors suspicious for malignancy should be managed by a multidisciplinary team. A careful and comprehensive evaluation with biochemical and imaging studies is recommended for any adrenal mass concerning for malignancy. The gold-standard treatment of ACC is complete surgical resection with negative margins when possible. Mitotane therapy has been the mainstay of adjuvant therapy but controversy remains as to its utility in earlier stage disease. Although data are limited, there is some evidence that chemotherapy protocols can lead to extended survival in selected patients with advanced ACC.

REFERENCES

1. Schteingart DE, Doherty GM, Gauger PG, et al. Management of patients with adrenal cancer: recommendations of an international consensus conference. Endocr Relat Cancer 2005;12(3):667–80.
2. Bilimoria KY, Shen WT, Elaraj D, et al. Adrenocortical carcinoma in the United States: treatment utilization and prognostic factors. Cancer 2008;113(11): 3130–6.
3. Brennan MF. Adrenocortical carcinoma. CA Cancer J Clin 1987;37(6):348–65.
4. Dackiw AP, Lee JE, Gagel RF, et al. Adrenal cortical carcinoma. World J Surg 2001;25(7):914–26.
5. Fehaily MA, Duh QY. Adrenocortical carcinoma. In: Clark OH, Duh QY, Perrier N, et al, editors. Endocrine tumors: American Cancer Society, atlas of clinical oncology. Hamilton (ON): BC Decker; 2003. p. 123–30.
6. Allolio B, Fassnacht M. Clinical review: adrenocortical carcinoma: clinical update. J Clin Endocrinol Metab 2006;91(6):2027–37.
7. Hutter AM Jr, Kayhoe DE. Adrenal cortical carcinoma. Clinical features of 138 patients. Am J Med 1966;41(4):572–80.
8. Ng L, Libertino JM. Adrenocortical carcinoma: diagnosis, evaluation and treatment. J Urol 2003;169:5.
9. Hsing AW, Nam JM, Co Chien HT, et al. Risk factors for adrenal cancer: an exploratory study. Int J Cancer 1996;65:432.
10. Xiao XR, Ye LY, Shi LX, et al. Diagnosis and treatment of adrenal tumours: a review of 35 years' experience. Br J Urol 1998;82:199.

11. Luton JP, Cerdas S, Billaud L, et al. Clinical features of adrenocortical carcinoma, prognostic factors, and the effect of mitotane therapy. N Engl J Med 1990;322:1195.
12. Wooten MD, King DK. Adrenal cortical carcinoma. Epidemiology and treatment with mitotane and a review of the literature. Cancer 1993;72:3145.
13. Skogseid B, Larsson C, Lindgren PG, et al. Clinical and genetic features of adrenocortical lesions in multiple endocrine neoplasia type 1. J Clin Endocrinol Metab 1992;75(1):76–81.
14. Houdelette P, Chagnon A, Dumotier J, et al. Malignant adrenocortical tumor as a part of Wermer's syndrome. Apropos of a case. J Chir (Paris) 1989;126(6–7):385–7.
15. Else T, Kim AC, Sabolch A, et al. Adrenocortical carcinoma. Endocr Rev 2014; 35(2):282–326.
16. Sandrini R, Ribeiro RC, DeLacerda L. Childhood adrenocortical tumors. J Clin Endocrinol Metab 1997;82:2027.
17. Figueiredo BC, Stratakis CA, Sandrini R, et al. Comparative genomic hybridization analysis of adrenocortical tumors of childhood. J Clin Endocrinol Metab 1999;84:1116.
18. Figueiredo BC, Cavalli LR, Pianovski MA, et al. Amplification of the steroidogenic factor 1 gene in childhood adrenocortical tumors. J Clin Endocrinol Metab 2005;90(2):615.
19. Sidhu S, Sywak M, Robinson B, et al. Adrenocortical cancer: recent clinical and molecular advances. Curr Opin Oncol 2004;16(1):13–8.
20. Icard P, Goudet P, Charpenay C, et al. Adrenocortical carcinomas: surgical trends and results of a 253-patient series from the French Association of Endocrine Surgeons study group. World J Surg 2001;25(7):891–7.
21. Pommier RF, Brennan MF. An eleven-year experience with adrenocortical carcinoma. Surgery 1992;112(6):963–70 [discussion: 970–1].
22. Kendrick ML, Lloyd R, Erickson L, et al. Adrenocortical carcinoma: surgical progress or status quo? Arch Surg 2001;136(5):543–9.
23. Gagner M, Lacroix A, Prinz RA, et al. Early experience with laparoscopic approach for adrenalectomy. Surgery 1993;114(6):1120–4 [discussion: 1124–5].
24. Sidhu S, Marsh DJ, Theodosopoulos G, et al. Comparative genomic hybridization analysis of adrenocortical tumors. J Clin Endocrinol Metab 2002;87:3467.
25. Libè R, Fratticci A, Bertherat J. Adrenocortical cancer: pathophysiology and clinical management. Endocr Relat Cancer 2007;14(1):13–28.
26. Gicquel C, Bertagna X, Gaston V, et al. Molecular markers and long-term recurrences in a large cohort of patients with sporadic adrenocortical tumors. Cancer Res 2001;61:6762.
27. Bourcigaux N, Gaston V, Logié A, et al. High expression of cyclin E and G1 CDK and loss of function of p57KIP2 are involved in proliferation of malignant sporadic adrenocortical tumors. J Clin Endocrinol Metab 2000;85:322.
28. Ribeiro RC, Sandrini F, Figueiredo B, et al. An inherited p53 mutation that contributes in a tissue-specific manner to pediatric adrenal cortical carcinoma. Proc Natl Acad Sci U S A 2001;98:9330.
29. Latronico AC, Pinto EM, Domenice S, et al. An inherited mutation outside the highly conserved DNA-binding domain of the p53 tumor suppressor protein in children and adults with sporadic adrenocortical tumors. J Clin Endocrinol Metab 2001;86:4970.
30. Custódio G, Komechen H, Figueiredo FR, et al. Molecular epidemiology of adrenocortical tumors in southern Brazil. Mol Cell Endocrinol 2012;351(1):44–51.

31. Stojadinovic A, Ghossein RA, Hoos A, et al. Adrenocortical carcinoma: clinical, morphologic, and molecular characterization. J Clin Oncol 2002;20:941.
32. Ohgaki H, Kleihues P, Heitz PU. p53 mutations in sporadic adrenocortical tumors. Int J Cancer 1993;54:408.
33. Barzon L, Chilosi M, Fallo F, et al. Molecular analysis of CDKN1C and TP53 in sporadic adrenal tumors. Eur J Endocrinol 2001;145:207.
34. Libè R, Groussin L, Tissier F, et al. Somatic TP53 mutations are relatively rare among adrenocortical cancers with the frequent 17p13 loss of heterozygosity. Clin Cancer Res 2007;13:844.
35. Wagner J, Portwine C, Rabin K, et al. High frequency of germline p53 mutations in childhood adrenocortical cancer. J Natl Cancer Inst 1994;86:1707.
36. Reincke M, Karl M, Travis WH, et al. p53 mutations in human adrenocortical neoplasms: immunohistochemical and molecular studies. J Clin Endocrinol Metab 1994;78:790.
37. Sullivan M, Boileau M, Hodges CV. Adrenal cortical carcinoma. J Urol 1978; 120:660.
38. Gicquel C, Bertagna X, Schneid H, et al. Rearrangements at the 11p15 locus and overexpression of insulin-like growth factor-II gene in sporadic adrenocortical tumors. J Clin Endocrinol Metab 1994;78:1444.
39. Gicquel C, Raffin-Sanson ML, Gaston V, et al. Structural and functional abnormalities at 11p15 are associated with the malignant phenotype in sporadic adrenocortical tumors: study on a series of 82 tumors. J Clin Endocrinol Metab 1997;82:2559.
40. Li FP, Fraumeni JF Jr, Mulvihill JJ, et al. A cancer family syndrome in twenty-four kindreds. Cancer Res 1988;48:5358–62.
41. Bougeard G, Sesboüé R, Baert-Desurmont S, et al. Molecular basis of the Li-Fraumeni syndrome: an update from the French LFS families. J Med Genet 2008;45:535–8.
42. Chompret A, Abel A, Stoppa-Lyonnet D, et al. Sensitivity and predictive value of criteria for p53 germline mutation screening. J Med Genet 2001;38:43–7.
43. Schussheim DH, Skarulis MC, Agarwal SK, et al. Multiple endocrine neoplasia type 1: new clinical and basic findings. Trends Endocrinol Metab 2001;12:173–8.
44. Crucitti F, Bellantone R, Ferrante A, et al. The Italian Registry for Adrenal Cortical Carcinoma: analysis of a multiinstitutional series of 129 patients. The ACC Italian Registry Study Group. Surgery 1996;119:161.
45. Vassilopoulou-Sellin R, Schultz PN. Adrenocortical carcinoma. Clinical outcome at the end of the 20th century. Cancer 2001;92:1113.
46. Wajchenberg BL, Albergaria Pereira MA, Medonca BB, et al. Adrenocortical carcinoma: clinical and laboratory observations. Cancer 2000;88:711.
47. Griffin AC, Kelz R, LiVolsi VA. Aldosterone-secreting adrenal cortical carcinoma. A case report and review of the literature. Endocr Pathol 2014;25(3):344–9.
48. Fassnacht M, Allolio B. Clinical management of adrenocortical carcinoma. Best Pract Res Clin Endocrinol Metab 2009;23(2):273–89.
49. Michalkiewicz E, Sandrini R, Figueiredo B, et al. Clinical and outcome characteristics of children with adrenocortical tumors: a report from the International Pediatric Adrenocortical Tumor Registry. J Clin Oncol 2004;22:838.
50. Stewart JN, Flageole H, Kavan P. A surgical approach to adrenocortical tumors in children: the mainstay of treatment. J Pediatr Surg 2004;39:759.
51. Zeiger MA, Thompson GB, Duh QY, et al. American Association of Clinical Endocrinologists and American Association of Endocrine Surgeons Medical

Guidelines for the Management of Adrenal Incidentalomas: executive summary of recommendations. Endocr Pract 2009;15(5):450–3.

52. Arlt W, Biehl M, Taylor AE, et al. Urine steroid metabolomics as a biomarker tool for detecting malignancy in adrenal tumors. J Clin Endocrinol Metab 2011;96:3775.

53. Fassnacht M, Kenn W, Allolio B. Adrenal tumors: how to establish malignancy? J Endocrinol Invest 2004;27(4):387–99.

54. Ilias I, Sahdev A, Reznek RH, et al. The optimal imaging of adrenal tumours: a comparison of different methods. Endocr Relat Cancer 2007;14(3):587–99.

55. Heinz-Peer G, Memarsadeghi M, Niederle B. Imaging of adrenal masses. Curr Opin Urol 2007;17(1):32–8.

56. Abiven G, Coste J, Groussin L, et al. Clinical and biological features in the prognosis of adrenocortical cancer: poor outcome of cortisol-secreting tumors in a series of 202 consecutive patients. J Clin Endocrinol Metab 2006;91:2650.

57. Maurea S, Klain M, Mainolfi C, et al. The diagnostic role of radionuclide imaging in evaluation of patients with nonhypersecreting adrenal masses. J Nucl Med 2001;42:884.

58. Mackie GC, Shulkin BL, Ribeiro RC, et al. Use of [18F]fluorodeoxyglucose positron emission tomography in evaluating locally recurrent and metastatic adrenocortical carcinoma. J Clin Endocrinol Metab 2006;91:2665.

59. Becherer A, Vierhapper H, Pötzi C, et al. FDG-PET in adrenocortical carcinoma. Cancer Biother Radiopharm 2001;16:289.

60. Leboulleux S, Dromain C, Bonniaud G, et al. Diagnostic and prognostic value of 18-fluorodeoxyglucose positron emission tomography in adrenocortical carcinoma: a prospective comparison with computed tomography. J Clin Endocrinol Metab 2006;91:920.

61. Tenenbaum F, Groussin L, Foehrenbach H, et al. 18F-fluorodeoxyglucose positron emission tomography as a diagnostic tool for malignancy of adrenocortical tumours? Preliminary results in 13 consecutive patients. Eur J Endocrinol 2004; 150:789.

62. Hahner S, Sundin A. Metomidate-based imaging of adrenal masses. Horm Cancer 2011;2(6):348–53.

63. Metser U, Miller E, Lerman H, et al. 18F-FDG PET/CT in the evaluation of adrenal masses. J Nucl Med 2006;47:32.

64. Caoili EM, Korobkin M, Brown RK, et al. Differentiating adrenal adenomas from nonadenomas using (18)F-FDG PET/CT: quantitative and qualitative evaluation. Acad Radiol 2007;14:468.

65. Blake MA, Slattery JM, Kalra MK, et al. Adrenal lesions: characterization with fused PET/CT image in patients with proved or suspected malignancy–initial experience. Radiology 2006;238:970.

66. Hennings J, Lindhe O, Bergström M, et al. [11C]metomidate positron emission tomography of adrenocortical tumors in correlation with histopathological findings. J Clin Endocrinol Metab 2006;91:1410.

67. Jhala NC, Jhala D, Eloubeidi MA, et al. Endoscopic ultrasound-guided fine-needle aspiration biopsy of the adrenal glands: analysis of 24 patients. Cancer 2004;102:308.

68. Kocijancic K, Kocijancic I, Guna F. Role of sonographically guided fine-needle aspiration biopsy of adrenal masses in patients with lung cancer. J Clin Ultrasound 2004;32:12.

69. Mody MK, Kazerooni EA, Korobkin N. Percutaneous CT-guided biopsy of adrenal masses: immediate and delayed complications. J Comput Assist Tomogr 1995;19(3):434–9.

70. Shen WT, Lee J, Kebebew E, et al. Selective use of steroid replacement after adrenalectomy: lessons from 331 consecutive cases. Arch Surg 2006;141(8): 771–4 [discussion: 774–6].

71. Doherty GM, Nieman LK, Cutler GB Jr, et al. Time to recovery of the hypothalamic-pituitary-adrenal axis after curative resection of adrenal tumors in patients with Cushing's syndrome. Surgery 1990;108(6):1085–90.

72. Gaujoux S, Brennan MF. Recommendation for standardized surgical management of primary adrenocortical carcinoma. Surgery 2012;152(1):123–32.

73. Harrison LE, Gaudin PB, Brennan MF. Pathologic features of prognostic significance for adrenocortical carcinoma after curative resection. Arch Surg 1999; 134(2):181–5.

74. Reibetanz J, Jurowich C, Erdogan I, et al. Impact of lymphadenectomy on the oncologic outcome of patients with adrenocortical carcinoma. Ann Surg 2012; 255:363.

75. Hough AJ, Hollifield JW, Page DL, et al. Prognostic factors in adrenal cortical tumors. A mathematical analysis of clinical and morphologic data. Am J Clin Pathol 1979;72:390.

76. Kebebew E, Siperstein AE, Clark OH, et al. Results of laparoscopic adrenalectomy for suspected and unsuspected malignant adrenal neoplasms. Arch Surg 2002;137:948.

77. Gonzalez RJ, Shapiro S, Sarlis N, et al. Laparoscopic resection of adrenal cortical carcinoma: a cautionary note. Surgery 2005;138:1078.

78. Miller BS, Ammori JB, Gauger PG, et al. Laparoscopic resection is inappropriate in patients with known or suspected adrenocortical carcinoma. World J Surg 2010;34:1380.

79. Prager G, Heinz-Peer G, Passler C, et al. Applicability of laparoscopic adrenalectomy in a prospective study in 150 consecutive patients. Arch Surg 2004;139:46.

80. Lombardi CP, Raffaelli M, De Crea C, et al. Open versus endoscopic adrenalectomy in the treatment of localized (stage I/II) adrenocortical carcinoma: results of a multiinstitutional Italian survey. Surgery 2012;152(6):1158–64.

81. Zini L, Porpiglia F, Fassnacht M. Contemporary management of adrenocortical carcinoma. Eur Urol 2011;60:1055.

82. McCauley LR, Nguyen MM. Laparoscopic radical adrenalectomy for cancer: long-term outcomes. Curr Opin Urol 2008;18:134.

83. Porpiglia F, Fiori C, Daffara F, et al. Retrospective evaluation of the outcome of open versus laparoscopic adrenalectomy for stage I and II adrenocortical cancer. Eur Urol 2010;57:873.

84. Brix D, Allolio B, Fenske W, et al. Laparoscopic versus open adrenalectomy for adrenocortical carcinoma: surgical and oncologic outcome in 152 patients. Eur Urol 2010;58:609.

85. Available at: http://clinicaltrials.gov/ct2/show/NCT00777244?term=adrenocortical+carcinoma&rank=20. Accessed October 2, 2014.

86. Aubert S, Wacrenier A, Leroy X, et al. Weiss system revisited: a clinicopathologic and immunohistochemical study of 49 adrenocortical tumors. Am J Surg Pathol 2002;26:1612.

87. Macfarlane DA. Cancer of the adrenal cortex; the natural history, prognosis and treatment in a study of fifty-five cases. Ann R Coll Surg Engl 1958;23:155.

88. Castinetti F, Fassnacht M, Johanssen S, et al. Merits and pitfalls of mifepristone in Cushing's syndrome. Eur J Endocrinol 2009;160:1003.

89. Bertagna C, Orth DN. Clinical and laboratory findings and results of therapy in 58 patients with adrenocortical tumors admitted to a single medical center (1951 to 1978). Am J Med 1981;71:855.

90. Fassnacht M, Johanssen S, Fenske W, et al. Improved survival in patients with stage II adrenocortical carcinoma followed up prospectively by specialized centers. J Clin Endocrinol Metab 2010;95:4925.

91. Khorram-Manesh A, Ahlman H, Jansson S, et al. Adrenocortical carcinoma: surgery and mitotane for treatment and steroid profiles for follow-up. World J Surg 1998;22:605.

92. Terzolo M, Angeli A, Fassnacht M, et al. Adjuvant mitotane treatment for adrenocortical carcinoma. N Engl J Med 2007;356:2372.

93. Kasperlik-Załuska AA, Migdalska BM, Zgliczyński S, et al. Adrenocortical carcinoma. A clinical study and treatment results of 52 patients. Cancer 1995; 75:2587.

94. Dickstein G, Shechner C, Arad E, et al. Is there a role for low doses of mitotane (o,p'-DDD) as adjuvant therapy in adrenocortical carcinoma? J Clin Endocrinol Metab 1998;83:3100.

95. Kasperlik-Zaluska AA. Clinical results of the use of mitotane for adrenocortical carcinoma. Braz J Med Biol Res 2000;33:1191.

96. Schteingart DE. Adjuvant mitotane therapy of adrenal cancer - use and controversy. N Engl J Med 2007;356:2415.

97. Vassilopoulou-Sellin R, Guinee VF, Klein MJ, et al. Impact of adjuvant mitotane on the clinical course of patients with adrenocortical cancer. Cancer 1993;71:3119.

98. Haak HR, Hermans J, van de Velde CJ, et al. Optimal treatment of adrenocortical carcinoma with mitotane: results in a consecutive series of 96 patients. Br J Cancer 1994;69:947.

99. Barzon L, Fallo F, Sonino N, et al. Comment–Is there a role for low doses of mitotane (o,p'-DDD) as adjuvant therapy in adrenocortical carcinoma? J Clin Endocrinol Metab 1999;84:1488.

100. Terzolo M, Daffara F, Ardito A, et al. Management of adrenal cancer: a 2013 update. J Endocrinol Invest 2014;37(3):207–17.

101. Berruti A, Fassnacht M, Baudin E, et al. Adjuvant therapy in patients with adrenocortical carcinoma: a position of an international panel. J Clin Oncol 2010;28:e401.

102. Fassnacht M, Libé R, Kroiss M, et al. Adrenocortical carcinoma: a clinician's update. Nat Rev Endocrinol 2011;7:323.

103. Berruti A, Terzolo M, Sperone P, et al. Etoposide, doxorubicin and cisplatin plus mitotane in the treatment of advanced adrenocortical carcinoma: a large prospective phase II trial. Endocr Relat Cancer 2005;12:657.

104. Fassnacht M, Terzolo M, Allolio B, et al. Combination chemotherapy in advanced adrenocortical carcinoma. N Engl J Med 2012;366:2189.

105. Abraham J, Bakke S, Rutt A, et al. A phase II trial of combination chemotherapy and surgical resection for the treatment of metastatic adrenocortical carcinoma: continuous infusion doxorubicin, vincristine, and etoposide with daily mitotane as a P-glycoprotein antagonist. Cancer 2002;94:2333.

106. Bonacci R, Gigliotti A, Baudin E, et al. Cytotoxic therapy with etoposide and cisplatin in advanced adrenocortical carcinoma. Br J Cancer 1998; 78:546.

107. Sperone P, Ferrero A, Daffara F, et al. Gemcitabine plus metronomic 5-fluorouracil or capecitabine as a second-/third-line chemotherapy in advanced

adrenocortical carcinoma: a multicenter phase II study. Endocr Relat Cancer 2010;17:445.

108. Chun HG, Yagoda A, Kemeny N, et al. Cisplatin for adrenal cortical carcinoma. Cancer Treat Rep 1983;67:513.

109. Haq MM, Legha SS, Samaan NA, et al. Cytotoxic chemotherapy in adrenal cortical carcinoma. Cancer Treat Rep 1980;64:909.

110. Williamson SK, Lew D, Miller GJ, et al. Phase II evaluation of cisplatin and etoposide followed by mitotane at disease progression in patients with locally advanced or metastatic adrenocortical carcinoma: a Southwest Oncology Group Study. Cancer 2000;88:1159.

111. Khan TS, Sundin A, Juhlin C, et al. Vincristine, cisplatin, teniposide, and cyclophosphamide combination in the treatment of recurrent or metastatic adrenocortical cancer. Med Oncol 2004;21:167.

112. Polat B, Fassnacht M, Pfreundner L, et al. Radiotherapy in adrenocortical carcinoma. Cancer 2009;115:2816.

113. Fassnacht M, Hahner S, Polat B, et al. Efficacy of adjuvant radiotherapy of the tumor bed on local recurrence of adrenocortical carcinoma. J Clin Endocrinol Metab 2006;91:4501.

114. Habra MA, Ejaz S, Feng L, et al. A retrospective cohort analysis of the efficacy of adjuvant radiotherapy after primary surgical resection in patients with adrenocortical carcinoma. J Clin Endocrinol Metab 2013;98:192.

115. Sabolch A, Feng M, Griffith K, et al. Adjuvant and definitive radiotherapy for adrenocortical carcinoma. Int J Radiat Oncol Biol Phys 2011;80:1477.

116. Gröndal S, Cedermark B, Eriksson B, et al. Adrenocortical carcinoma. A retrospective study of a rare tumor with a poor prognosis. Eur J Surg Oncol 1990; 16:500.

117. Thompson NW, Cheung PS. Diagnosis and treatment of functioning and nonfunctioning adrenocortical neoplasms including incidentalomas. Surg Clin North Am 1987;67:423.

118. Gaujoux S, Al-Ahmadie H, Allen PJ, et al. Resection of adrenocortical carcinoma liver metastasis: is it justified? Ann Surg Oncol 2012;19:2643.

119. Schulick RD, Brennan MF. Long-term survival after complete resection and repeat resection in patients with adrenocortical carcinoma. Ann Surg Oncol 1999;6:719.

120. Datrice NM, Langan RC, Ripley RT, et al. Operative management for recurrent and metastatic adrenocortical carcinoma. J Surg Oncol 2012;105:709.

121. Bellantone R, Ferrante A, Boscherini M, et al. Role of reoperation in recurrence of adrenal cortical carcinoma: results from 188 cases collected in the Italian National Registry for Adrenal Cortical Carcinoma. Surgery 1997;122:1212.

122. Allolio B, Hahner S, Weismann D, et al. Management of adrenocortical carcinoma. Clin Endocrinol (Oxf) 2004;60:273.

123. van Seters AP, Moolenaar AJ. Mitotane increases the blood levels of hormone-binding proteins. Acta Endocrinol (Copenh) 1991;124:526.

Index

Note: Page numbers of article titles are in **boldface** type.

Endocrinol Metab Clin N Am 44 (2015) 453–484
http://dx.doi.org/10.1016/S0889-8529(15)00038-9
0889-8529/15/$ – see front matter © 2015 Elsevier Inc. All rights reserved.

Moving?

Make sure your subscription moves with you!

To notify us of your new address, find your **Clinics Account Number** (located on your mailing label above your name), and contact customer service at:

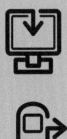

Email: journalscustomerservice-usa@elsevier.com

800-654-2452 (subscribers in the U.S. & Canada)
314-447-8871 (subscribers outside of the U.S. & Canada)

Fax number: 314-447-8029

Elsevier Health Sciences Division
Subscription Customer Service
3251 Riverport Lane
Maryland Heights, MO 63043

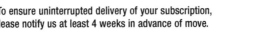

*To ensure uninterrupted delivery of your subscription,
please notify us at least 4 weeks in advance of move.

Printed and bound by CPI Group (UK) Ltd, Croydon, CR0 4YY

03/10/2024

01040494-0008